THE COMPLETE YOGA BOOK

THE
COMPLETE
YOGA BOOK

Yoga of Breathing,
Yoga of Posture,
and Yoga of Meditation

THREE VOLUMES IN ONE

JAMES HEWITT

SCHOCKEN BOOKS · NEW YORK

The line drawings of postures are by Ted Ripley. The Indian
illustrations are from the Richard von Garbe Collection published in Richard Schmidt's *Fakire und Fakirtum in alten und
modernen Indien* (Berlin, 1908).

Library of Congress Cataloging in Publication Data

Hewitt, James, 1928–
The complete yoga book.

Bibliography: p. 544
Includes indexes.
1. Yoga, Hatha.   2. Yoga.   I. Title.

RA781.7.H49 1978   613.7   77-15934

ISBN 0-8052-0969-7

Manufactured in the United States of America

First Schocken Books edition published in 1977

Contents

Preface

The philosophical, metaphysical, and religious bases of Yoga may be accepted or denied, in whole or in part; but there can be no gainsaying the rewards of greater health, vitality, and psychophysical poise that result from Yoga practice, as many thousands of men and women have discovered recently in the West. In the East yoga has been practised for thousands of years. Only in this century has it been introduced into Europe and America, but it is now firmly established. It has proved to be no passing fad, simply because it fulfils its promises, supplying the results expected of it at whichever level it is practised.

It is on the *practice* of Yoga, and also on the *practical* in Yoga, that I have concentrated in writing *Yoga of Breathing*, and in writing two complementary works, *Yoga of Posture* and *Yoga of Meditation*. The three volumes together comprise what is virtually an encyclopedia of Yoga practice and of practical Yoga. This practical approach is aimed at enriching the health and consciousness of people going about the complicated, stress-beset activity of present-day living. Yoga has always provided for the needs of 'householder Yogins' – men and women practising Yoga without withdrawing from family life and responsibilities.

In making a practical approach to Yoga we satisfy the demands of students who consider the rewards of psycho-physical health and poise worthy aims in themselves. We also provide the aspirant who wishes for 'higher consciousness' and mystical experience with the groundwork which equips him for the climb. The analogy with mountain climbing is apt, for the postures, breath controls, cleansing processes, and healthful eating habits and diet of physiological Yoga, called Hatha Yoga, prepare the aspirant for the subtle disciplines of psychical Yoga, called Raja Yoga. Raja Yoga refines consciousness and aims at the pinnacle of intuitive enlightenment (*samadhi*).

The three volumes are concerned mainly with these two Yogas, Hatha and Raja – the Yogas most widely practised in the West and most easily adaptable to occidental needs.

Yoga of Breathing is intended to establish the student securely in Yogic practice; to raise levels of health, energy, and psychophysical poise, through control of breathing, posture, hygiene, relaxation, and diet. Breath control (*pranayama*) is at the heart of the Yoga of breathing. It has been neglected in much of the literature of Yoga for Westerners, but in this book it is given the emphasis it deserves. An example of our direct and practical approach is that the *bandhas* and *mudras* of Hatha Yoga, which are special postures and muscle controls, are employed not for prolonged breath suspension and the arousal of mysterious energies, but for the enhancement of sexual health and fitness. *Yoga of Breathing* also includes a balanced programme of general postures.

Yoga of Posture presents by far the largest collection of postures (*asanas*) ever published – over 400. They include warm-up and limber-up exercises, which most Western students need before embarking on a programme of posturing; and modifications and simplifications of postures which can lead to full performance of the classic *asanas*. Thus there are programmes to suit any stage of suppleness.

Yoga of Meditation describes the most direct and practical techniques of meditation, including the traditional method of *Patanjali*, the transcendental meditation of Maharishi Mahesh Yogi, and recent Western experiments in auto-control of the involuntary nervous system using electrical biofeedback apparatus.

Each of the three volumes – *Yoga of Breathing*, *Yoga of Posture*, and *Yoga of Meditation* – stands on its own, but the three combine to make a clear and practical guide for practitioners of Yoga who wish to garner its many benefits for body and mind, and to improve the whole quality of everyday life. For Yoga is a life-science and a life-style.

Finally, a point concerning the printing of this book and of the two complementary volumes: I have followed the practice of many works written on Yoga for a mainly Western readership by omitting diacritical marks in the printing of words in Sanskrit, the classic language of Indian Yoga.

JAMES HEWITT

THE COMPLETE YOGA BOOK

Volume I

Yoga of Breathing

I Yoga and Yogas

WHAT IS YOGA?

Confusion will be avoided if we at once point out that there is Yoga as an end-goal and Yoga as a system of techniques and disciplines to reach the end-goal. Not only that: there are several systems, and therefore several Yogas. But the aim in each case is the same, though it is talked about in the language of a variety of religions and cultures. Strictly speaking, Yoga is Indian and Hindu; and for the Hindu mystic the supreme goal in living is absorption in *Brahman* – 'I am that.'

Who or what is *Brahman*? In the purest Yoga, which is that of the *upanishads*, *Brahman* is impersonal and imageless, and should not be confused with Brahma, a deity of the Hindu Trinity (the other members are Siva and Vishnu). *Brahman* as the One of world mysticism can be written about in a variety of ways, not all of them religious. Mysticism does not belong solely to the world religions, though it is linked closely with them. How does one classify Buddhism, which has no god, and looks on its founder, at a sophisticated level, as an enlightened man? Each age and culture finds its appropriate vocabulary for the One. In the West today, a psychological orientation makes Being, Self beyond empirical ego, and levels of consciousness the terms in which the loftiest aims of Yoga are most meaningfully discussed.

The Self to be realized beyond the ego in Indian Yoga is the *Atman*. Find the *Atman*, which is pure consciousness, through Yogic practice, and you find (the intuitive enlightenment called *samadhi*) that individual being and Cosmic Being have the same ground, and that *Atman* and *Brahman* are one. This realized union is called Yoga – the word comes from roots meaning 'union', and, the English 'yoke' is etymologically related.

A Yoga is also a system of physical and psychical controls whose aim is to make the practitioner aware of the identity of *Atman* and *Brahman*, or the ground of Being, or whatever concepts are found congenial. And even if you remain agnostic or sceptical towards the whole mystic concept, there remains such value in the bodily exercises and meditative techniques in terms of psycho-physical well-being that thousands of people practise Yoga with barely a thought for Yoga as a mystical goal. Their concern is with Yoga as practice.

THE SVETASVATARA UPANISHAD

The above points become clearer if we look at a concise description of Yoga practice and its powers found in the *Svetasvatara Upanishad*, 11, 8–15 (155)

If a wise man hold his body with its three erect parts (chest, neck, and head) even, and turn his senses with the mind towards the heart, he will then in the boat of *Brahman* cross all the torrents which cause fear.

Compressing his breathings let him who has subdued all motions, breathe forth through the nose with gentle breath. Let the wise man without fail restrain his mind, that chariot yoked with vicious horses.

Let him perform his exercises in a place level, pure, free from pebbles, fire, and dust, delightful by its sounds, its water, and bowers, not painful to the eye, and full of shelters and caves.

When Yoga is being performed, the forms which come first, producing apparitions in *Brahman*, are those of misty smoke, sun, fire, wind, fire-flies, lightnings, and a crystal moon.

When, as earth, water, light, heat, and ether arise, the fivefold quality of Yoga takes place, then there is no longer illness, old age, or pain for him who has obtained a body, produced by the fire of Yoga.

The first results of Yoga they call lightness, healthiness, steadiness, a good complexion, an easy pronunciation, a sweet odour, and slight excretions.

As a metal disk [mirror], tarnished by dust, shines bright again after it has been cleaned, so is the one incarnate person satisfied and free from grief, after he has seen the real nature of the self.

And when by means of the real nature of his self he sees, as by a lamp, the real nature of *Brahman*, then having known the unborn, eternal god, who is beyond all natures, he is freed from all fetters.

In the above quotation we see Yoga as goal (absorption in *Brahman*); Yoga as postures and breath controls; and Yoga as meditation and contemplation. The two most widely practised Yogas in the West are here indicated: the physiological Yoga, called Hatha Yoga, and the Yoga of mental mastery, called Raja Yoga. We will sometimes refer to them as the Yoga of Vitality and the Yoga of Meditation respectively. The Yoga of Posture is part of Hatha Yoga, or the Yoga of Vitality.

CLASSIFYING THE YOGAS

When it comes to classifying and grouping the systems of Yoga, one finds differences of opinion among the scholars. The reason for this is that the Yogas overlap and interpenetrate to such an extent that several classifications have validity. It is possible to use a system that incorporates several Yogas directly, and several others indirectly. And some people attempt nothing less than a synthesis of all the main Yogas. Swami Vivekananda and Sri Aurobindo have expounded this approach eloquently in their writings.

In *Yoga of Breathing* we will be describing methods taken from Hatha Yoga, which some people do not consider a Yoga at all, but a system of exercises that can serve other Yogas. But the main tradition sees it as purificatory preparation for Raja (Royal) Yoga. Hatha Yoga is the most widely practised Yoga in the West: it includes the well-known postures and breath controls.

The Yogas other than Hatha are mainly meditative and more directly aimed at Yoga as end-goal and union. Their practices will appear later in *Yoga of Meditation*. For the present it is sufficient to name them and indicate their nature briefly. However, even in performing the physical techniques of Hatha Yoga, to some extent one cannot avoid practising other Yogas.

At this stage the main Indian Yogas may be discerned as follows:

Jnana Yoga	Union by knowledge
Bhakti Yoga	Union by love and devotion
Karma Yoga	Union by action and service
Mantra Yoga	Union by voice and sound

Yantra Yoga	Union by vision and form
Laya and Kundalini Yoga	Union by arousal of latent psychic nerve-force
Tantric Yoga	A general term for the physio-logical disciplines. Also union by harnessing sexual energy
Hatha Yoga	Union by bodily mastery (principally of breath)
Raja Yoga	Union by mental mastery

Jnana Yoga

This is the path of spiritual knowledge and wisdom, suited to the intellectual temperament, in which the intellect penetrates the veils of ignorance that prevent man from seeing his True Self (*Atman*), which is other than the empirical ego. The disciplines of this path of the well-honed intellect are those of study and meditation.

Bhakti Yoga

This is the Yoga of strongly-focused love, devotion, and worship, at its finest in love of the One. The Hindu may concentrate his devotion upon a worshipped deity (Krishna is the most popular) or upon the divine principle as incarnated in a *guru*. Bhakti Yoga is accessible to Westerners with highly devotional temperaments; others are made to feel uncomfortable by some of the excesses. This could be said to be the favourite Yoga of the Indian masses. Its disciplines are those of rites and the singing of songs of praise. St Francis of Assisi is often mentioned as an example of a Christian *bhakti*.

Karma Yoga

This is the path of selfless action and service, without thought of the fruits of action. Its most eloquent exposition is the Lord Krishna's instruction of the young prince Arjuna in the *Bhagavad Gita*. Mahatma Gandhi, the father of modern India, could be looked on as a Karma Yogin.

Mantra Yoga

The practice of Mantra Yoga influences consciousness through repeating (aloud or inwardly) certain syllables, words, or phrases (*mantras*). A form of Mantra Yoga is being practised by many thousands of Westerners, in the form of the Transcendental Meditation taught by Maharishi Mahesh Yogi. Rhythmic repetition of *mantras* is called *japa*. The most highly-regarded *mantras* are 'OM' and 'OM MANE PADME HUM'.

Yantra Yoga
As Mantra Yoga influences consciousness through the vibrations of the voice and sound, so Yantra Yoga employs sight and form. The colourful *mandalas* of Northern India and Tibet are objects of contemplation to Yogins. The visualization may be with the inner eye, just as listening to a *mantra* may be with the inner ear. A *yantra* is a design with power to influence consciousness: it can be an objective picture, an inner visualization, or the design of a temple.

Laya and Kundalini Yoga
These combine many of the techniques of Hatha Yoga, especially prolonged breath suspension and a stable posture, with intense meditative concentration, so as to awaken the psychic nerve-force latent in the body, symbolized as serpent power (*kundalini*), which is coiled below the base of the spine. The force is taken up the spine, passing through several power centres (*chakras*), until it reaches a *chakra* in the crown of the head, when intuitive enlightenment (*samadhi*) is triggered. The physiological and concentrative disciplines are severe, and this is a Yoga best practised with personal supervision by a teacher.

Tantric Yoga
'Tantric' is applied as a general term to distinguish physiological systems from those that are non-physiological. Tantrism is also a form of Yoga, found mainly in Northern India and Tibet, in which control of the sexual energies has a prominent part, and the union of male and female (Yogi and Yogini), either actually or in an act of imaginative creation, has a ritualistic role. Tantric Yoga, of all the Yogas, guards its teachings and techniques most closely. This sexual Yoga may be looked upon with a measure of disapproval by adherents of some of the other schools.

Hatha Yoga
The word Hatha derives from two roots: *ha* means 'sun' and *tha* means 'moon'. The flow of breath in the right nostril is called the

'sun breath' and the flow of breath in the left nostril is the 'moon breath'. Central to all Hatha Yoga disciplines is the regulation of breath, the harmonizing of its positive (sun) and negative (moon), or male and female currents. Another meaning of the word Hatha is 'forced', but the term Forced Yoga would not do justice to the poised and gentle nature of most Yogic controls.

This is the Yoga best known and most widely practised in the West, and the subject of the majority of popular manuals on Yoga. Its best-known feature is posturing – in particular sitting with the legs crossed and the feet upturned on the thighs (Lotus Posture or *Padmasana*) and standing on the head (Headstand Posture or *Sirsasana*). *Asana*, which now means a Yogic posture, originally meant 'seat' or 'sitting method', an indication that the wide range of postures developed from a few basic positions for sitting in meditation.

Hatha Yoga exercises are practised extensively in the West for their practical benefits to the health of the nervous system, glands, and vital organs. When it is practised similarly in India it is sometimes called Ghatastha Yoga; but there physiological Yoga is less often separated from its over-all mystical setting and purpose.

Hatha Yoga may be viewed as a hygiene which takes into account the purification of the total organism. It may sound quotidian to some people to call this Yoga a hygiene, but there is a mainstream tradition that sees Hatha Yoga as a purificatory preparation for Raja Yoga, which is work upon consciousness itself. Such mental disciplining can best be effected in a healthy, relaxed body in which the energies have been equalized.

The French writer C. Kerneiz, writing under the pseudonym 'Felix Guyot', opened his book *Yoga : the Science of Health* (37) with these words:

> Keep well, remain young a long time, and live to a good old age, such is the threefold wish that the men of every race and country have, at all times, formulated at the bottom of their hearts. This threefold wish is a very natural one, for it is simply the expression of the most powerful and the most tenacious of instincts: self-preservation. Live! We want to live with the greatest amplitude possible.
>
> To fight against disease, when it comes, and to avert, as far as is possible, the threat of death which is in its train; to defer old age, and, by doing so, put off death itself, we have hygiene, which is only, it is

true, an autonomous but not independent province of the medical kingdom.

But there exists a science, practised in India and Tibet, and more or less throughout the whole of China, which is somewhat mysterious, for it is not taught to all comers. This science is traditional and its origin is lost in the night of time. It has precisely the same object as hygiene in Western countries: to keep its adepts in health and strength and to ward off old age and death for the longest time possible. This science of Life, which is only a branch of the secret of the Yogis, is called the Hatha Yoga.

Raja Yoga

Hatha Yoga is the most practical of Yogas, with its emphasis on promoting vibrant health and tapping the organism's latent energies. It has, too, an integrating and calming influence on the mind. But the direct work of mastering consciousness and stilling thought so as to become aware of the Ground of Being belongs to Raja or Royal Yoga. Raja Yoga is considered royal because the Yogin who practises this Yoga thereby becomes ruler over his mind.

Raja Yoga is closely associated with the systematization of Yoga techniques by Patanjali (who lived about the third or second century BC) in his *Yoga Sutras*. He lists *asanas* (postures) and *pranayama* (breath controls) among his 'eight limbs' of Yoga, and such classic texts as the *Hatha Yoga Pradipika*, the *Gheranda Samhita*, and the *Siva Samhita* follow Patanjali in seeing Hatha Yoga practices as providing a physiological hygiene that prepares the body for effective mental control. According to this view, Raja Yoga includes Hatha Yoga within its system.

Hatha Yoga works upon the body, purifying and perfecting it, and through the body upon the mind. Raja Yoga works upon the mind, refining and perfecting it, and through the mind upon the body. But just as some people practise the physiological Yogas with little or no thought for mental disciplines, so there are exponents of the mental Yogas who consider that the body will respond beneficially to control of consciousness without having to resort to anything more 'physical' than a stable posture in sitting for meditation. But a great number of Yogins combine the physiological Yoga of Breathing with the psychical Yoga of Meditation.

OVERLAPPING OF PATHS

From examination of the brief summary of the main Yoga systems just given, you will perceive that it would be difficult to practise any one of them without to some extent incorporating elements from others. Concentration, a central feature of Raja Yoga, operates in all the other paths in varying degrees. The devotion of Bhakti Yoga provides some motive power and affective feeling tone in performing the actions of Karma Yoga, the exercises of Hatha Yoga, the incantations of Mantra Yoga, the visualizations of Yantra Yoga, and so on – even the intellectual work of Jnana Yoga is not without this affective colouring. One could trace at some length this criss-crossing of Yoga paths.

THE CLASSIC TEXTS OF HATHA YOGA

The three main classic treatises on Hatha Yoga are the *Hatha Yoga Pradipika* ('Light on the Hatha Yoga'), the *Gheranda Samhita* ('Gheranda's Compendium'), and the *Siva Samhita* ('Siva's Compendium'). The first-named is considered to be the standard work.

These texts – like Patanjali's guide to Raja Yoga – were written tersely and in such a way that expansion and elucidation by teachers was required. Until recent times a teacher was essential, but now books (such as this one) can act as instructors in practical Yoga suited to the needs of the majority of men and women who have no desire to withdraw from the customary activities of living in the modern world.

It is hardly surprising that these old texts, representing a tradition older still, should contain much that to modern eyes appears unscientific, superstitious, incomprehensible, magical, bizarre, and outmoded. The language is at times exaggerated, and as with so much of this type of literature, scholars have fun disputing among themselves over what was intended to be taken literally and what symbolically. Much of the instruction today's readers will wish to discard: for example, the injunction to rub the ashes of dried cow's dung on the skin.

SANSKRIT – CLASSIC LANGUAGE OF YOGA

English belongs to an extensive family of languages that includes most of the languages of Europe and of India, and so is given the name Indo-European. A subfamily of the Indo-European group is the Indo-Iranian, or Aryan. The people who spoke these languages thought so highly of themselves that they called themselves Aryans, or 'noble ones'. The Aryans seem to have invaded India from the north-west, from Afghanistan or Iran. The oral tradition of their ancient Vedic hymns in time gave way to a form of language called Sanskrit, and this was standardized about 300 BC. It is the language of the sacred texts of Hinduism and the classic texts of Yoga. Its place in Indian learning could be said to correspond to that of Latin in Europe.

The relationship between English, Latin, Greek, and Sanskrit can be gathered from these few examples:

Mod. Eng.	Old Eng.	Gothic	Latin	Greek	Sanskrit
Father	Fnder	Fadar	Pater	Pater	Pitar
Three	Thrie	—	Tres	Treis	Trayas
Six	Siex	Saihs	Sex	Hex	Sas·
Nine	Nigon	Niun	Novem	Ennea	Nava

Sanskrit words abound in Yogic literature – the many postures (*asanas*), for example, have Sanskrit names. But English speakers should restrict their use of Sanskrit to the written word: otherwise they may receive a nasty shock one day on hearing a native Indian pronounce the Yogic terms correctly.

BENEFITS FROM THE YOGA OF BREATHING

Mr Archie J. Bahm, in his book *Yoga for Business Executives* (5), devotes no less than sixty-two pages to discussing the immediate, long-range, and comparative values of Yoga. Not even a summary of the benefits will be offered here. They are touched upon here and there in this book, and will be detailed further in dealing with each group of controls and exercises. It may have been necessary a few years ago to 'sell' Hatha Yoga, but it is not necessary now. The West has got the message – *Yoga works*.

This book will tell the reader what it is that Yoga asks him to do – in a word, *practice*. As the *Hatha Yoga Pradipika* (77) says:

Whether young, old or too old, sick or lean, one who discards laziness, gets success if he practises Yoga. Success comes to him who is engaged in the practice; for by merely reading books on Yoga, one can never get success. Success cannot be attained by adopting a particular dress. It cannot be gained by telling tales. Practice alone is the means of success.

II Yogic Relaxation

CORPSE POSTURE (*Savasana*)

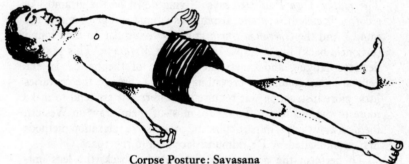

Corpse Posture: Savasana
The Yogin's head, shoulders, back, buttocks, leg and feet must rest on
the ground in this posture of relaxation.

All techniques of Yoga aim to produce tranquillity. Postures, breath
controls, mind-stilling meditation, the bodily, mental, and spiritual
purifications – all have a relaxing influence that is widely
acknowledged as probably Yoga's greatest advantage for Western
man. For he lives at a pace unknown to his forefathers and his
nervous system has to cope with a bombardment of stimuli that
would have been intolerable to earlier generations. Those who
embrace Yoga practice in its full range – that is, Yoga of Breathing,
Yoga of Posture, and Yoga of Meditation – will achieve the maximum body-mind harmony and relaxation. But even those men and
women who practise only the postures, perhaps at evening classes
or at home, report: 'I am more relaxed,' 'My emotions are under
control,' 'My nerves are calm,' or 'I feel more tranquil.' This
frequently is acknowledged after only a few weeks of Yoga practice.

Among the postures are several which aim directly at relaxation. Here we will describe only one – but far and away the most important: the strangely-named Corpse Posture (*Savasana* or *Mrtasana*). It is customary to spend a few minutes 'playing dead' in this posture immediately before and immediately after a programme of *asanas*. Readers fully involved in the hurly-burly of modern civilized living should ensure that a few minutes relaxation are taken in this pose each day, because of its great restorative powers.

HOW TO RELAX

The *Hatha Yoga Pradipika* says: 'Lying down on the ground like a corpse is called *Savasana*. It removes fatigue and gives rest to the mind.' And the *Gheranda Samhita* says: 'Lying flat on the ground (on one's back) like a corpse is called the *Mrtasana*. This posture destroys fatigue, and quiets the agitation of the mind.' In the general living conditions prevailing in India through the centuries little more instruction was required. Western writers tend to make more of the technique. To do so, most of them draw on Western medical knowledge, in particular the progressive relaxation methods first promulgated by Dr Edmund Jacobson in the 1920s.

To perform the posture, lie flat on your back, the legs outstretched so that the heels are a little apart and the feet have fallen limply outwards. The arms lie alongside the body, resting on the floor, the palms of the hands turned up, with the fingers limp and slightly curled. Thin cushions may be placed below the neck and each knee.

Now observe your breathing, which should be through the nostrils, not the mouth. Do not interfere with the in-and-out flow of the breath: just observe. Take two successive deep abdominal breaths, fully exhaling. The abdomen swells out on the inhalation and draws back towards the spine on the exhalation. Then let go with the abdominal muscles and return to observing the rise and fall of respiration. Soon you will notice that your breathing has become quiet, smooth, and of even rhythm. Occasionally during relaxation you may experience an involuntary deep intake of breath, followed by a sighing exhalation. This should be welcomed as a sign that tension is being dissolved somewhere in the musculature.

Having established your breathing in a quiet, smooth, and rhythmic pattern, you next employ your attention like a torch beam to play over your body from feet to scalp, looking for tension, and letting go from it. Relaxation is a letting go from tension. The postures and breathing exercises of Yoga will help to put you on intimate speaking terms with your body muscles in a way you are unlikely to have experienced since childhood. Look upon the various sections of your body listed below as listening muscles ready to obey your silently spoken command – which is simply two words: 'let go.' As a muscle or muscle group lets go, you should instantly feel it become heavier: like the sleeping baby or cat, it rests with its full weight. Think of tension draining away like a dangerous poison from the muscles and body parts listed below. Note carefully the feeling of relaxation.

STAGE BY STAGE RELAXATION

Stage by stage, the relaxation sequence is as follows:

  i.   Lie flat on your back in the Corpse Posture.

  ii. Observe your breathing, without seeking to control it, for a few minutes.

  iii. Make two successive deep inhalations and exhalations, swelling out the abdomen on breathing in and drawing it in towards the backbone on breathing out. Relax the abdominal wall fully at the conclusion of the second breath.

  iv. Observe your breathing again. When it has become quiet, smooth, and of even rhythm, direct your attention like a torch beam in sequence over the parts of the body listed below. Look for tension in each part and let go from it, so that the muscles rest with their full weight. Note carefully the sensations of tension, then of absence of tension (relaxation). The sequence is: left foot; left calf; left thigh, front and rear; right foot; right calf; right thigh, front and rear; pelvis; abdomen; lower back; chest; upper back; left hand; left forearm; left upper arm, front and rear; left shoulder; right hand; right forearm; right upper arm, front and rear; right shoulder; throat; neck; jaw; lips; tongue; eyes; brow; scalp. In relaxing the feet and hands, do not forget the toes and fingers, each one of which should be drained of tension and feel limp.

  v.   Observe your breathing again for a minute or two; then

repeat the sequence of letting go with the muscles from feet to scalp.
Continue in the manner just described for as many minutes as you
are giving to relaxation. Fifteen to thirty minutes is a good average.

At the conclusion of each wave of relaxation from feet to scalp,
the whole body should rest with its full weight and feel drained of
tension. The mind also should be at peace.

RELAXING THE FACIAL MUSCLES

In view of the importance of relaxing the facial muscles, I suggest
a few aids that will be found effective:

To help relax the jaw: yawn slowly, resisting evenly all the way
with the muscles of the jaw. Hold the contraction for six seconds;
then let go, close the mouth, and let the jaw sag.

To help relax the lips: purse and push forward the lips as though
to kiss, taking note of the sensations of tension. Hold the kiss
position for six seconds; then relax the lips fully.

To help relax the tongue: keeping the teeth together, touch the
roof of the mouth as far back as you can with the tip of the tongue.
Keep the tongue immobile in that position for six seconds; then let
go fully, so that the tongue 'floats' in the mouth with its tip behind
the lower teeth.

To help relax the eyes: without moving the head, look as far to
the left as possible; as far to the right as possible; as far upwards as
possible; as far downwards as possible. Thinking of this in terms of
the Clock Exercise, you look at nine o'clock; three o'clock; twelve
o'clock; and six o'clock. Take note throughout of the sensations of
tension in the muscles that move the eyeballs; then give equal
attention to the feeling of relaxation as you let go and close your eyes.

To help relax the brow: frown strongly, contracting the muscles
of the brow. Hold the contraction for six seconds; then let go fully.
This is a useful technique to combat worry, which registers in
forehead tensions.

To help relax the scalp: without moving your head, move the
scalp forwards and backwards a few times by conscious control.
Then let go fully with the scalp muscles.

AIDS TO RELAXATION

Many imaginative techniques are suggested by writers on Yoga to aid relaxation in the Corpse Posture. One idea is to imagine that you are lying on a beach, listening to the soothing sound of the sea and feeling the caress of a gentle breeze and warm sunlight on your flesh.

Another suggestion is to imagine a tiny hole in the small of the back from which tension drains away. This has the effect of flattening the back along the floor and encourages lying with the full weight.

Yet another imaginative technique could be described as the Water Method. You think of a current of water slowly flowing through the body, cleansing it of all tensions and impurities. You think of it flowing through the neck, in the shoulders and along the arms, into the chest, on to the abdomen, down the spine, through the buttocks, filling the thighs, knees, calves, and feet. Finally the purifying water – which is best thought of as warm – trickles away from the fingers and toes. This can be imagined as happening several times.

As skill in relaxation develops, you will find that you are able to let go from tension in sitting as well as in supine positions.

All Yogic practice counters stress, recognized by doctors as one of the greatest threats to health and life faced by modern man. So the Corpse Posture, being specifically intended for relaxation, should not be neglected by any Western practitioner who wishes to protect himself (or herself) from this contemporary killer.

III   Yogic Posturing

THE YOGI AS A FREAK

During the winter of 1896–7 Bava Luchman Dass, a Punjabi, described as 'a Brahmin of the highest caste,' performed the postures or *asanas* of Hatha Yoga in a side-show at the Westminster Aquarium in London, giving between sixty and seventy performances a day for forty days. Outside the show was displayed a framed cheque for £500 'which anyone can claim who emulates the Yoga's [*sic*] fearful and wonderful contortions.'

The performances evoked merriment and humorous comment from the paying viewers. When the Yogi adopted a Kneeling Lotus Posture, a Cockney voice remarked: 'It's a fine mode of pedomotion for a man cursed with corns.' Reporters from newspapers and magazines quoted such remarks, and had their own more sophisticated fun in commenting on the Brahmin's 'contortions,' his diet of goat's milk and dried fruit, and his strange appearance – he was dressed in a woolly leotard and large baggy drawers to meet the requirements of Victorian modesty.

If the Yogin had been a yeti, he could not have occasioned more astonishment or rude and ignorant comment from the general public and journalists alike. No understanding was shown of the lofty aims of Yoga or of the significance of the postures so expertly performed (there is the evidence of photographs) by the unfortunate Punjabi. Unfortunate, because he had been brought to England under false pretences. Thinking he was to demonstrate the ancient art and science of Hatha Yoga exercise, held in almost sacred regard in his own country, to leading citizens of London who might have an interest in perfecting body, mind, and spirit, he found himself stranded in a foreign city, thousands of miles from his homeland, and being *exhibited as a freak*.

The editor of the *Strand Magazine*, (**168**), who adopted a humorous style in a report of the Yogi's performance, observed:

> From what I gathered, I came to the conclusion that when the ghastly consciousness that he was a side-show dawned upon the Yoga [*sic*], he didn't like it at all, and nothing would induce him to go through his sixty or seventy performances a day but the near prospect of a return to his own native land.

THE CURRENT POPULARITY OF YOGA POSTURING

For today's counterparts of Bava Luchman Dass it is a different story. They can set themselves up as respected teachers of Yoga in London, Paris, Amsterdam, New York, and even the smaller cities in Europe and America, and instruct men and women, drawn from multifarious walks of life, in body control – that same body control which was mocked and occasioned such merriment in the London of 1896–7. Yoga continued to attract more mockery and derision than respect and understanding in Western countries until the rapid acceleration of its acceptance which began in the 1950s. Today there is a waiting list for membership of classes in Yoga posturing. What was once thought by many to be a short-lived craze has been established unshakeably for more than two decades. Only one conclusion can be drawn from this: Yoga posturing is worth doing – it brings worthwhile results.

THE AIMS OF POSTURING

'There is not a single *asana* that is not intended directly or indirectly to quiet the mind,' wrote Dr Theos Bernard, an American who underwent in India the most austere and far-reaching disciplines of Hatha Yoga, which he mastered to a remarkable degree. He continued (**7**):

> The teacher emphasizes that the primary purpose of the *asanas*, is the reconditioning of the system, both mind and body, so as to effect the highest possible standard of muscular tone, mental health, and organic vigour. Hence stress is put upon the nervous and glandular systems. Hatha Yoga is interpreted as a method that will achieve the maximum

results by the minimum expenditure of energy. The various *asanas* have been devised primarily to stimulate, exercise, and massage the specific areas that demand attention.

A balanced programme of postures works upon every muscle, nerve, gland, and organ in the body. 'Being the first accessory of Hatha Yoga, *asana* is discussed first,' says the *Hatha Yoga Pradipika* (**77**). 'It should be practised for gaining steady posture, health and lightness of body.' This quotation points out the rewards accurately and succinctly, and is free from the fantastic claims of occult and magical powers found elsewhere in this and other classic texts.

THE UNIQUE CHARACTER OF THE *ASANAS*

You will find nothing like the *asanas* in Western systems of body-culture, and they are also distinct in character from other Eastern exercises. They are not movements, but postures to be adopted and held; most are relaxing rather than effortful, refreshing rather than fatiguing; they are non-competitive; they require no special equipment or clothing; they can be performed by men and women, and persons in all age groups. They take into account the well-being of the whole human organism; their aim is to bring body, mind, and spirit into harmony and equilibrium.

THE ORIGINS OF THE *ASANAS*

Asana is a posture or pose. It is pronounced with the emphasis on the first 'a' – really ā, diacritical marks having been omitted in the printing of this work. The original purpose seems to have been to provide rock-like steadiness in sitting for meditation, for *asana* originally meant 'seat.' The forest sages of old sat immobile for hours, and modern masters do the same. Naturally a compact stable sitting position was needed, in which one would not sway about or fall asleep. A straight back and a low centre of gravity, just below the navel, with unimpaired deep abdominal breathing, were also found to be essential. It looks as though out of this beginning developed a great system of postures, to be held for seconds, minutes, or hours, whose aim was bodily mastery and health. Some *asanas* are copies of the characteristic movements or poses of the

animals, birds, reptiles, and insects after which they are named.
The *Surya Namaskars* group (see *Yoga of Posture*) would appear to
have been originally salutations or prayers to the sun. The term
asana, which began as the name for one of the sitting postures, is
now applied also to standing, supine, prone, and balancing postures.

Yogic postures are depicted in the earliest Indian carvings, and,
later, members of the army of Alexander the Great wrote of the
gymnastic philosophers they saw in India.

PRE-REQUIREMENTS OF POSTURING

A few commonsense rules should be observed before performing a
group of postures. Let at least three hours go by after a main meal,
and one hour following a light snack. Empty the bladder, and the
bowels too if you can, shortly before exercising. Sponge over the
face and body to give a feeling of freshness. Wear loose-fitting
clothing, or none at all. Posture in a room that is well-ventilated and
free from extremes of temperature. Posture on a firm level floor
covered with several thicknesses of blanket.

THE MOST POPULAR CLASSIC *ASANAS*

A study of the now considerable literature of Yogic posturing
reveals that of the several hundred Yoga poses, there is a central
group of traditional *asanas* held in high regard which can form the
base or foundation on which to build varied programmes. We will
describe them concisely here, so that a start to posturing can be
made without delay; for further development the reader should
refer to *Yoga of Posture*. Over four hundred postures are described,
including the warm-up exercises and the modifications and simplifications of *asanas* that most Western practitioners find essential.

SITTING POSTURES

It is necessary that the student should become acquainted with some
of the sitting postures at an early stage. Besides being valuable
exercises in themselves, limbering the legs, hips, and pelvis,

strengthening the back and improving posture, they provide the sitting position for practising breath control (*pranayama*) and meditation. One cannot start too early learning to sit immobile for several minutes with the back straight and the head poised in line with the spine. The vital energies are gathered and conserved.

The Easy Posture can be adopted immediately by most occidentals; the Egyptian (or Chair) Posture by all. The more difficult sitting postures may take some months to master, but provide maximum seated stability. In these meditative postures the centre of gravity should be felt in the abdomen, a little below the navel. Breathe freely and deeply, using the lower lungs, diaphragm, and abdomen. The postures facilitate deep breathing.

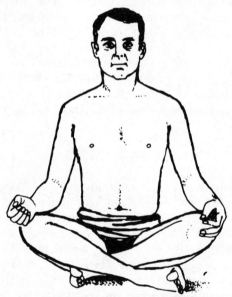

Easy Posture: Sukhasana

Easy Posture (Sukhasana)
This is the most practical cross-legged posture for beginners. The ankles are crossed, tailor's fashion, and the knees taken down as low as possible – in time the knees may actually touch the floor. The most important thing is that the head, neck, and spine should be held in a straight vertical line. Vary the ankle crossing, sometimes right over left, sometimes left over right. The right hand should rest

on the right knee and the left hand on the left knee. Breathe freely.

Every opportunity should be taken to sit for several minutes in the Easy Posture – watching television, listening to the radio or records, sewing, feeding baby, and so on.

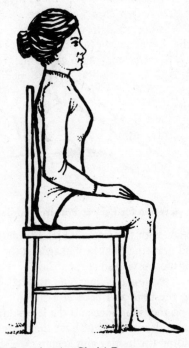

Egyptian (or Chair) Posture

Egyptian Posture

Even simpler than the Easy Posture is the Egyptian (or Chair) Posture, but it should only be employed if the Easy Posture proves too uncomfortable.

Sit on a straight-backed chair, the head and spine in vertical line, the feet and knees together, the palm of the right hand flat on the right thigh and the palm of the left hand flat on the left thigh. Breathe freely.

Preparation for Perfect Posture (Siddhasana)

This limbers the ankle, knee, and hip joints for performance of Perfect Posture (*Siddhasana*).

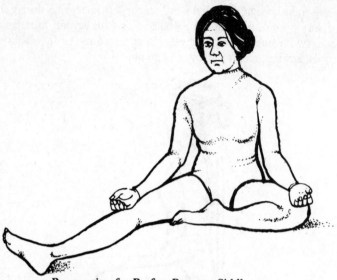

Preparation for Perfect Posture: Siddhasana

Sit on the floor with the legs outstretched and well apart. Fold the right leg and draw the right heel in against the crotch so that the sole of the right foot rests against the inside of the upper left thigh. The right knee rests on the floor and the left leg remains fully extended. Keep the head and back in a straight vertical line. Rest the right palm on the right knee and the left palm on the left knee. Breathe freely and deeply. Stay at least thirty seconds in the pose; then repeat, folding the left leg and keeping the right leg extended.

Perfect Posture (Siddhasana)
Siddha means 'adept' and *siddhas* are 'perfected' Yogins.
    As in the preceding Preparation, the right leg is folded and the heel brought in against the perineum (the soft flesh between genitals and anus). But this time the left leg is also folded, the left heel is pulled back against the pubic bone, and the outer edge of the left foot, sole upturned, is inserted in the fold between the calf and thigh of the right leg. The thighs and knees of both legs are kept flat on the floor. Place the right palm on the right knee and the left palm on the left knee. Sit firmly on the buttocks and legs, keeping the head and backbone poised in a vertical straight line. Breathe

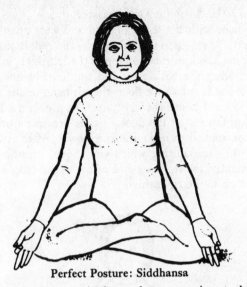

Perfect Posture: Siddhansa

freely and deeply. Stay motionless at least one minute; then repeat, reversing the roles of the legs. The pose has great stability and is frequently used for sitting in meditation by master Yogins.

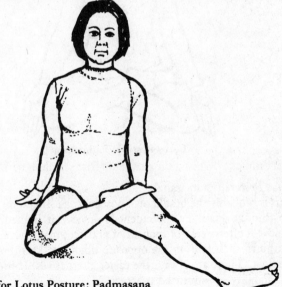

Preparation for Lotus Posture: Padmasana

Preparation for Lotus Posture (Padmasana)

Sit on the floor with the legs extended and wide apart. Bend the right leg at the knee, grasp the right ankle, and pull in the right foot so that it rests, sole upturned, on top of the left thigh, as high up it as possible. Keep the back erect and the head in line. Place the palms of the hands flat on the floor, the left hand beside the left hip and the right hand beside the right hip. The problem is likely to be that the right knee is off the floor – gentle pressure from the right hand may be applied to make the knee lower. After at least thirty seconds in the pose, during which you should breathe freely and deeply, straighten the right leg and repeat to the other side, lifting the left foot on to the right thigh.

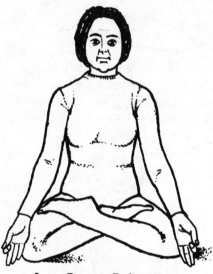

Lotus Posture: Padmasana

Lotus Posture (Padmasana)

This is probably the best known pose in Yoga. It is sometimes called the Buddha Pose. Few occidentals achieve it immediately; some achieve it after weeks or months of practice; many never do manage to upturn each foot on the opposite thigh and keep both knees on the floor. There are always the easier alternatives. It provides rock-like stability for advanced practice.

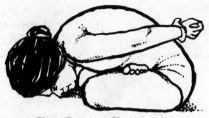

Yoga Posture: Yogasana

Yoga Posture (Yogasana)

The Lotus Posture has a role in several advanced postures. We give one example here. In Yoga Posture you sit in the Lotus Posture, exhale, bend forward, and lower the forehead to the floor. Stay in the pose at least twenty seconds, breathing freely. The hands may be clasped behind the neck or the back.

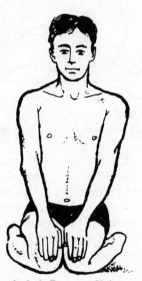

Thunderbolt Posture: Vajrasana

Thunderbolt Posture (Vajrasana)

This is worth learning now, for it provides the starting position for many beneficial postures. It is a favourite sitting position of the Japanese. Kneel on the floor with the knees together and sit back on the inner edges of the upturned feet. To do this the toes may be together, but the heels should be spread apart to support the outer edges of the buttocks. Place the right palm on the right knee and the left palm on the left knee, and keep the head and back erect. Breathe freely and deeply. Stay motionless in the pose for at least one minute.

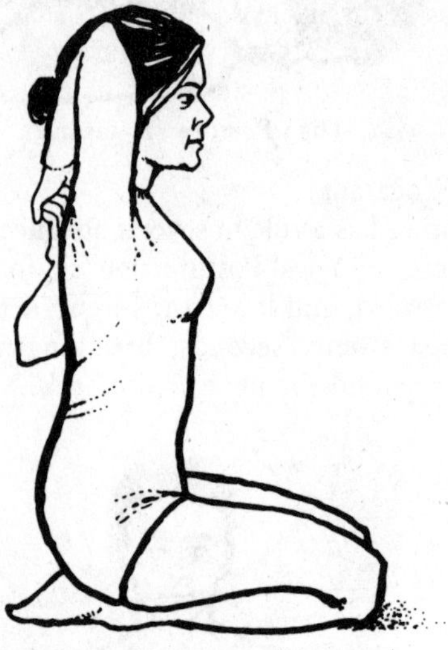

Cowface Posture: Gomukhasana

Cowface Posture (Gomukhasana)
This is one of several poses based on the preceding Thunderbolt Posture.

Keep the back erect as you sit on the inner edges of the heels and soles of the feet. Now flex the right arm, raise the right elbow high and lower the right hand down the centre of the back. At the same time bend the left arm and bring the left hand up the spine from below until the fingers of the right hand and those of the left hand hook together. The palm of the right hand faces the back and the palm of the left hand faces outwards. Breathing freely, stay in the pose at least six seconds. Reverse the arm positions and repeat.

If you find that you cannot lock the hands together, hold a handkerchief, towel, or belt so that it is pulled taut, shortening the grip as suppleness increases.

Viewed from the back the pose is said to resemble a cow's face. It improves posture, limbers the shoulder joints, and strengthens and tones the muscles of the shoulders, upper back, and rear upper arms.

A TYPICAL PROGRAMME OF POSTURES

Corpse Posture (Savasana)
First, spend a few minutes lying quietly on the back in the Corpse
Posture, fully described in the chapter on Yogic Relaxation. You
should commence the programme of postures feeling relaxed and
composed. Each of the poses should be given total attention, an
essential feature of Yogic posturing.

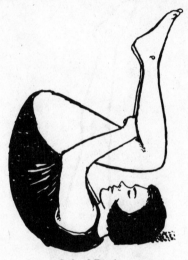

Spinal Rock

Spinal Rock
In *Yoga of Posture* you will find forty-four warm-up or limber-up
exercises, from which several should be selected to prepare the body
for the main postures to follow. The muscles and joints benefit
greatly from these few preliminary movements. The Indian Yoga
masters tend to omit them, but for the majority of occidental
students they are important. Many of the warm-ups are valuable
exercises in themselves. This could be said of the one selected for
inclusion here – the Spinal Rock, also known as the Limbering-up
Rock.

   Lie flat on the back, bend the legs, and bring the knees together
against the chest. The ankles may be together or crossed. Clasp the
hands behind the knees or on top of the knees. Now rock gently

forwards and backwards on the rounded back: on the forward rock
the heels should almost touch the floor and on the backward rock
the upper back touches the floor. Breathe in as you rock forward and
breathe out as you rock backward. Continue for at least thirty
seconds.

A useful variation can be added. Rock gently *from side to side* for
at least thirty seconds. This is called the Cradle Rock.

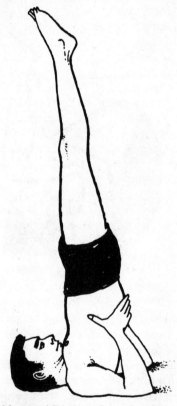

Shoulderstand Posture: Sarvangasana

Shoulderstand Posture (Sarvangasana)
The point behind Yoga's inverted poses is that they enable venous
blood to flow easily to the heart, brain, scalp, and facial tissues; at
the same time blood flows out of the legs and lower abdomen, which
tend to become congested. The effect of reversing the normal

directional pull of gravity on the body is refreshing.

The Shoulderstand is suitable for beginners, whereas the full Headstand Posture (*Sirsasana*) needs to be worked up to in stages, as taught in *Yoga of Posture*. Even then, the full unsupported Headstand is not for everyone – it is too severe for many persons. The Shoulderstand is the simplest and least strenuous of the inverted poses of Yoga.

Lie flat on the back, the legs outstretched together. Bend the legs and bring the knees backward over the chest. Using the elbows and the backs of the upper arms as props, support the lower back with the palms of the hands, the thumbs outspread. The elbows should not be wider than the shoulders. Now raise the trunk to a vertical position and straighten the legs together so that the trunk and legs form a straight vertical line. The chest is brought against the chin, never the chin to the chest. Breathing freely and deeply, stay steadily in the pose for at least twenty seconds.

The Shoulderstand is unsuitable for persons suffering from high blood pressure or ailments of the neck and head.

Incline-board or Tilt-chair

The benefits of the topsy-turvy poses can be combined with those of relaxation by lying full length on an incline-board placed securely at an angle of thirty-five to forty-five degrees. A sturdy ironing board will serve. For a milder effect one may purchase and use a 'Relaxator' chair, manufactured at West Molesey, Surrey, England, which can be adjusted so as to place the feet higher than the head, at the same time supporting the curvature of the spine in a hammock-type structure. For incline relaxation, follow the stage-by-stage method taught in the chapter on Yogic Relaxation.

Plough Posture (Halasana)

This graceful posture can be performed as an extension of the Shoulderstand. Keeping the legs straight, lower the feet overhead from the Shoulderstand position until the toes rest on the floor. The legs should fall to the floor of their own accord: if they do not at first, they soon will with practice. Breathe freely. This is the Supported Plough Posture. More advanced versions are described in *Yoga of Posture*.

This is a superb exercise, stretching the whole body, activating the circulation, and toning the abdomen, hips, and legs. It is said to

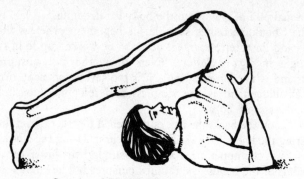

Supported Plough Posture: Halasana

improve the health of the endocrine glands, liver, spleen, and reproductive organs. It is not suitable, however, for persons with weak vertebrae.

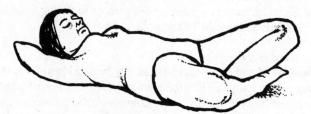

Modified Fish Posture: Matsyasana

Fish Posture (Matsyasana)

This is a complementary position to the Plough as the spine is stretched in the opposite direction. In the advanced version the legs are crossed and locked in the Lotus position, but the Fish Posture can also be performed in a simpler version with the ankles crossed in the Easy Posture.

Lie flat on the back and cross the legs. Keep the knees spread wide apart and held low to the floor. Now cross the wrists behind the neck and rest the head on the arms. Breathe deeply into the abdomen and hold the pose for at least thirty seconds.

In the full version, the legs are crossed in the Lotus position, the back is arched, and the head is thrown back so that the crown of the head is on the floor and the shoulders and back are off the floor. The right hand grasps the left foot and the left hand grasps the right foot. Breathing freely and deeply, stay in the pose for fifteen to thirty seconds. The position is a good one for floating easily in water – hence the name Fish Posture.

In this posture the legs and hips are limbered, the thorax is expanded, the pelvis and abdominal viscera are toned, the spine is strengthened, and the spinal nerves are nourished with blood.

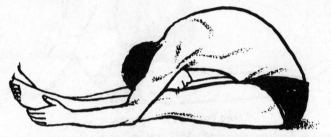

Back-stretching Posture: Paschimottanasana

Back-stretching Posture (Paschimottanasana)
Sit on the floor with the legs fully extended together. Take a deep breath; then, exhaling, lower the face towards the knees, at the same time reaching out and down to grasp either the ankles or the feet, as suppleness permits. In advanced practice the face may actually touch the knees and the chest press down on the thighs. Stay down for ten seconds, and then sit up slowly.

The muscles of the back, arms, and legs are stretched, and the spine is stretched and strengthened. The hamstring muscles at the backs of the thighs may protest at first, but they let go and lengthen with practice. The abdomen is massaged as you bend forward, aiding digestion and correcting constipation.

Cobra Posture (Bhujangasana)
Following the Back-stretching Posture, you now turn over and bend the spine in the opposite direction in the Cobra Posture, which resembles a cobra rearing to strike.

Lie full length on the floor, face down, legs together. Bend the arms, keeping the elbows in against the sides, and place the right palm flat on the floor five or six inches in front of the right shoulder (beginners' version) or underneath the shoulder (advanced version). Place the left palm similarly in relation to the left shoulder. In the beginners' version the fingertips are in line horizontally with the chin, which rests on the floor. Inhaling, slowly raise the head, neck,

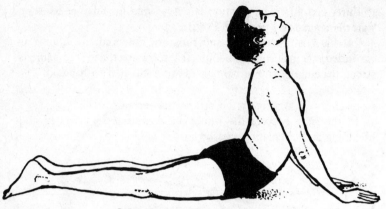

Cobra Posture: Bhujangasana

and upper back successively, slowly straightening the arms. Rely as far as possible on the lower back muscles. Hold the pose for at least ten seconds, the pelvis and legs staying in contact with the floor. Return slowly to the starting position, exhaling.

The Cobra Posture exercises the spine vertebra by vertebra, nourishing the spinal nerves with blood. The front of the body is stretched and the circulation stimulated.

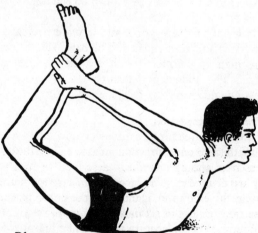

Bow Posture: Dhanurasana

Bow Posture (Dhanurasana)
In the Bow Posture the head and trunk are raised up and back as in

the preceding Cobra Posture, but the arms are stretched back so that the right hand grasps the right ankle and the left hand grasps the left ankle. The arms are pulled taut like a bow-string. The beginner will need to spread the knees apart to raise them off the floor; the advanced practitioner brings the knees together. The spine, trunk, and legs take the shape of a bow. Balance on the stomach, breathing freely, for at least six seconds.

In the Bow Posture the whole body is strongly stretched and breathing and circulation are stimulated.

Corpse Posture (Savasana)
Complete the programme, as you began, with a few minutes' relaxation in the Corpse Posture.

PROGRAMME PLANNING

The above short programme is based on some of the most highly regarded Yogic *asanas*, each with a history going back for centuries. The sitting postures may be practised separately. The programme may be summarized as consisting of:

Corpse Posture (*Savasana*), for relaxation
Spinal Rock, a warm-up exercise
Shoulderstand Posture (*Sarvangasana*)
Incline-board or tilt-chair
Plough Posture (*Halasana*)
Fish Posture (*Matsyasana*)
Back-stretching Posture (*Paschimottanasana*)
Cobra Posture (*Bhujangasana*)
Bow Posture (*Dhanurasana*)
Corpse Posture (*Savasana*)

Readers should go on to plan individual and carefully graduated programmes from the 418 postures described in *Yoga of Posture*, where they are divided into Warm-ups, and Groups A and B. The two groups are based on the difficulty of the postures, and each of the three sections is subdivided into standing postures, sitting and kneeling postures, supine postures, prone postures, inverted postures, and muscular locks. The advanced Group B has an additional section on balancing postures. Each of the three sections – Warm-ups, Group A and Group B – concludes with instructions on how to plan programmes to suit individual needs. Many variations on the main traditional poses are given and an additional section summarizes the therapeutic powers claimed for the *asanas*.

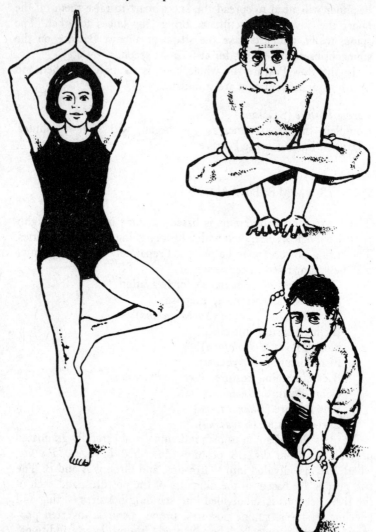

Three advanced poses, whose performance is described in Yoga of Posture: Tree Posture: Vrkasana; Cock Posture: Kukutasana; Shooting Bow Posture: Akaran Dhanurasana.

IV Yogic Hygiene

THE SIX CLEANSING ACTS

If any reader needs convincing that the men who devised the system of bodily, mental, and spiritual perfecting that is Yoga brought a thoroughness to their experiments that resulted in unique, strange, but effective practices, let him look at the six main cleansing duties (*kriyas*) or acts (*shatkarmas*) of the Hatha Yogins. Even if he does not wish to practise them all – at least not in their traditional form – he will have to admit that here is personal hygiene carried to astounding lengths and displaying a remarkable knowledge of the human body.

A warning must be given. Only a few Westerners perform the more severe of these purifications in their traditional form, and then always under the personal supervision of a teacher. But modern adaptations are possible in several cases, and these readers may wish to try. Certainly there is no need to miss *Nauli* and *Kapalabhati*, the last two of the six hygienic duties. The former, with its preliminary muscle control of *Uddiyana Bandha*, has a chapter to itself, and *Kapalabhati* is included in the chapter on Yogic Breath Control (*Pranayama*).

The six hygienic duties (*kriyas*), as given by the *Hatha Yoga Pradipika*, are *Dhauti*, *Basti* (or *Vasti*), *Neti*, *Trataka*, *Nauli*, and *Kapalabhati*. The *Gheranda Samhita* substitutes *Lauliki* for *Nauli*. The duties are used as preparatory cleansing to ensure the full benefits of the breathing exercises (*pranayama*) and to improve health by removing impurities, phlegm, and excess fat. The breathing exercises have themselves a purificatory role, and *Kapalabhati* is itself a respiratory exercise. The six *kriyas* cleanse the respiratory, digestive, eliminatory, and nervous systems. To quote Sir Paul Dukes (21): 'In the last analysis physical health depends on the efficient working of the following four processes: elimination, alimentation, respiration, and relaxation. These are referred to in esoteric schools as the Sacred Physical Arts.' Alimentation (nourishment), respiration, and relaxation are in this book given their own chapters. We will be mainly concerned in this chapter with cleansing by elimination of toxic material.

DHAUTI (WASHING)

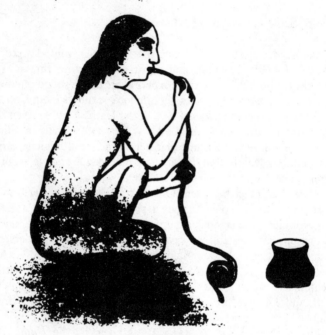

Dhauti (Washing)

A long strip of cloth – surgical gauze can be used – three to four inches wide, is soaked in warm water or milk. It is then swallowed slowly and carefully and allowed to rest in the stomach for ten to fifteen minutes before being pulled out slowly. If you leave the strip of cloth in the stomach longer than twenty minutes it begins to pass through the body. Dr Bernard swallowed the whole strip, and had to retrieve it with an emetic of salt and water. A tendency to retch during first attempts passes with practice. At first only two or three feet should be swallowed; this may increase gradually to fifteen feet or more as the lining of the throat becomes accustomed to the practice.

In *Dhauti* (which means 'to wash') the swallowed cloth soaks up phlegm, bile, and other impurities in the stomach. The process is taught at Yoga therapy centres in India, and is said to cure many diseases. The *Hatha Yoga Pradipika* says (77): 'There is no doubt that cough, asthma, enlargement of the spleen, leprosy, and twenty kinds of diseases born of phlegm disappear by the practice of Dhauti Karma.'

An alternative, with somewhat similar benefits, is to drink several glasses of warm water in which a teaspoonful of salt has been dissolved, until vomiting empties the stomach. This is called *Vamana Dhauti*. Some Yogins develop the ability to vomit at will and cleanse the stomach. Houdini, the famous escapologist, taught himself this art, regurgitating a key that enabled him to unlock a trunk inside which he seemed trapped.

The *Gheranda Samhita* describes four kinds of *Dhauti*: *Antar-dhauti* or internal washing (itself divided into four parts); *Danta-dhauti* or cleaning the teeth; *Hrd-dhauti* or cleaning the chest or throat; and *Mula-sodhana* or cleaning the rectum.

Antar-dhauti (Internal Washing)
The four parts of *Antar-dhauti* are *Vatasara* or air purification, *Varisara* or water purification, *Vahnisara* or fire purification, and *Bahiskrta* or cleansing the intestines.

Air Purification (*Vatasara*): contracting the mouth into the shape of a crow's beak, draw in air slowly, until the stomach feels comfortably full. Move the air in the stomach for a short time, and then release it slowly from the rectum. The *Gheranda Samhita* says (90): 'The *Vatsara* is a very secret process, it causes the purification of the body, it destroys all diseases and increases the gastric fire.'

Water Purification (*Varisara*): take a mouthful of water, and then drink it slowly. Move the water in the stomach; then take it downwards, and release it through the rectum. The *Gheranda Samhita* says (90): 'This process should be kept secret. It purifies the body. And by practising it with care, one gets a luminous or shining body.

The *Varisara* is the highest *Dhauti*. He who practises it with ease, purifies his filthy body and turns it into a shining one.'

Fire Purification (*Vahnisara*): 'Press the navel knot or intestines back towards the spine for one hundred times.' In Yogic physiology the region behind the navel is a place of fire or heat, which is kindled by this instroke. A beginner should commence with five instrokes to one exhalation, and increase gradually over several weeks until he is performing ten. Digestion is aided and the abdominal viscera are massaged. The *Gheranda Samhita* says (90): 'This is *Agnisara* or fire process. This gives success in the practice of Yoga, it cures all the diseases of the stomach [gastric juice] and increases the internal fire. This form of *Dhauti* should be kept very secret, and it is hardly to be attained even by the gods. By this *Dhauti* alone one gets a luminous body.' (*See also* the chapter on Abdominal Retraction.)

Intestinal Purification (*Bahiskrta*): here again we are brought up with a jolt at the lengths to which Yogins go to cleanse the body internally. Readers should *not* attempt this hygienic practice, which has two parts. First, the stomach is filled with air, drawn in by the crow's beak method described for Air Purification. The air is held in the stomach for an hour and a half, and then moved down to the intestines. The second part brings the jolt. Standing in water up to the navel, the Yogin draws out the long intestine (*saktinadi*) and washes it with both hands – the *Gheranda Samhita* says (90): 'wash it with care, and then draw it in again into the abdomen. This process should be kept secret. It is not easily to be attained even by the gods. Simply by this *Dhauti* one gets *Deva-deha* [godlike body.]'

Danta-dhauti (Cleaning the Teeth)
This includes cleaning the gums, the tongue, the ears, and the frontal sinuses.

Teeth Cleansing (*Danta-mula-dhauti*). the teeth and gums are rubbed every morning with catechu plant powder or pure earth.

Tongue Cleansing (*Jihva-sodhana*): the *Gheranda Samhita* says (90):
    Join together the three fingers known as the index, the middle and the ring finger, put them into the throat, and rub well and clean the root of the tongue, and by washing it again throw out the phlegm. Having

thus washed it rub it with butter, and milk it again and again; then by holding the tip of the tongue with an iron instrument pull it out slowly and slowly. By so doing, the tongue becomes elongated.

The text says earlier: 'The elongation of the tongue destroys old age, death and disease.' Lengthening the tongue also has a role in some esoteric practices in which the passing of air through the nostrils is blocked by curling the tongue back in the mouth.

Ear Cleansing (*Karna-dhauti*): the text (90) is concise: 'Clean the two holes of the ears by the index and the ring fingers. By practising it daily, the mystical sounds are heard.'

Cleansing the Frontal Sinuses (*Kapalarandhra-dhauti*): the *Gheranda Samhita* directs (90):
Rub with the thumb of the right hand the depression in the forehead near the bridge of the nose. By the practice of this Yoga, diseases arising from derangements of phlegmatic humours are cured. The vessels become purified and clairvoyance is induced. This should be practised daily after awakening from sleep, after meals, and in the evening.

Hrd-dhauti (Cleansing the Chest or Throat)
Three methods are employed:

With a Stalk (*Danda-dhauti*): a stalk of plantain, turmeric or cane is slowly pushed into the gullet and then drawn out slowly. Thereby, says the *Gheranda Samhita* (90): 'phlegm, bile and other impurities are expelled out of the mouth.' The practice is also considered good for the heart.

With Water (*Vamana-dhauti*): the *Gheranda Samhita* directs (90): 'After meal, let the wise practitioner drink water full up to the throat, then looking for a short while upwards, let him vomit it out again. By daily practising this Yoga, disorders of the phlegm and bile are cured.' This is an example of the ambiguity of much instruction in the old texts. Professor Wood (94) interprets this as 'cleansing by gargling,' but the word 'vomit' would seem to indicate that water is filled 'up to the throat' from the stomach upwards, and this is indeed the way Theos Bernard was taught – an alternative to swallowing surgical gauze.

With a Strip of Cloth (*Vaso-dhauti*): this is the first method described under *Dhauti*.

Mula-sodhana (Cleansing the Rectum)
The rectum is cleaned internally with water, 'over and over again', using the middle finger of one hand or a stalk of turmeric (yellow sandal).

BASTI OR VASTI (COLONIC IRRIGATION)

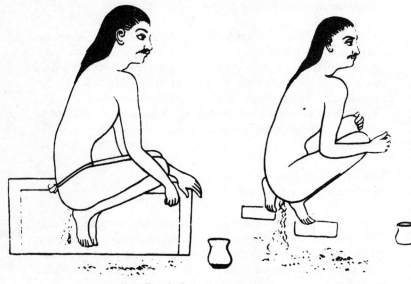

Basti (Colonic Irrigation)

The *Gheranda Samhita* gives two kinds of *Vasti*: *Jala-Vasti* (Water *Vasti*) and *Suska Vasti* (Dry *Vasti*). The first is performed squatting on the heels in water up to the navel and contracting and dilating the sphincters of the anus, letting water into the colon, holding it there for a time and churning it about, and then releasing it by opening the anal sphincters. A vacuum in the colon is created by performing an Abdominal Retraction (*Uddiyana Bandha*) on squatting, and the water is churned about by means of Recti Isolation (*Nauli*). These two abdominal controls are given a chapter to themselves. A greased enema nozzle may be inserted by persons who have not yet mastered the control of the sphincters. Yogins hold their natural method of colonic cleansing to be superior to the use of the modern enema. Western writers on Yoga are divided as to whether or not use of natural colonic irrigation or an enema is desirable. Some take the view that the practices of Yoga ensure regular bowel evacuation and that nothing more need be done. The present writer has so far belonged to this group, those 'playing safe', though he is conscious that he (and his readers) may be missing out on a valuable cleansing practice no more 'unnatural' than brushing the teeth. Sir Paul Dukes, a strong advocate of the Yogic enema, gives detailed instructions for its use in his book *The Yoga of Health, Youth, and Joy* (21). The *Gheranda Samhita* says (90): 'The body becomes free from all diseases and becomes as beautiful as the god Cupid.'

In Dry *Basti* or *Vasti* you begin by adopting the Back-stretching Posture (*Paschimottanasana*). Sit on the floor with both legs fully extended together, locked at the knees. Then lean slowly forward from the waist and lower the head as far as you can towards the knees (experts bring the face against the knees), at the same time reaching forward to grasp either the ankles or the feet. Now press the intestines down and squeeze tightly the muscles of the anus. This is called *Asvini* or Horse *Mudra*, as it imitates the staling of a horse. The *Gheranda Samhita* says (90): 'By this practice of Yoga, constipation never occurs, and it increases gastric fire and cures flatulence.'

BLADDER IRRIGATION

This is more difficult than colonic irrigation by muscle control. Water is drawn up the urethra to cleanse the bladder. Some Hatha Yogins can manage it.

NETI (NASAL CLEANSING)

This is a practice for clearing the nostrils and the head sinuses. There are two techniques: one using a catheter and the other using water.

A thin catheter, lubricated with antiseptic jelly, should be passed up one nostril until the end appears in the throat, when it is gripped

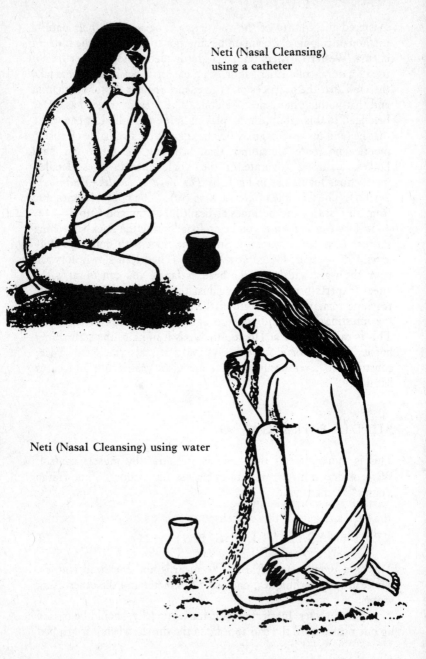

Neti (Nasal Cleansing)
using a catheter

Neti (Nasal Cleansing) using water

between the thumb and forefinger of one hand and drawn out through the mouth. With one end protruding from the mouth and the other from the nostril, gently and slowly draw the catheter to and fro a few times before finally pulling its full length out of the mouth. The traditional method is to use a soft cord, but a catheter is the modern, and safer, device. Clear first one nostril, and then the other.

Many readers will prefer the alternative method, using water, though an uncomfortable sensation in the nostrils has to be overcome by repeated practice. Lukewarm water (previously boiled), to which a teaspoonful of salt has been added, is sniffed from a cup, a saucer, or the cupped hand up both nostrils and then expelled from the mouth. This is called *Vyut-krama*. You can also fill the mouth with water and expel it through the nostrils. This is called *Sit-krama*. A nasal douche may be found more comfortable for cleansing the nostrils.

The *Gheranda Samhita*, with characteristic exaggeration, says (90), 'by this practice of Yoga one becomes like the god Cupid. Old age never comes to him and decrepitude never disfigures him. The body becomes healthy, elastic, and disorders due to phlegm are destroyed.' The practice also has a reputation for improving the vision and bringing a concomitant *claritas* to consciousness.

TRATAKA (CLEANSING VISION)

In this practice an object is gazed at without blinking until the eyes begin to water. Do not stare – *look*. This means looking *through* the eyes, rather than staring *from* them. This exercise is also found in the Yoga of Meditation – a candle flame or a flower is a favoured focus of attention. The practitioner is instructed to sit calmly with the back straight for this concentration, which steadies the mind as well as the body and the gaze.

An occult tradition says that *Trataka* induces powers of clairvoyance, which is perhaps why an old text says the practice 'should be kept secret carefully, like a box of jewellery.'

Stop *Trataka* immediately the eyes begin to water. Bathe them with cold water, and then move them about in the Clock Exercise. You imagine a large clock face about three feet in front of the face and, without moving the head, look up at twelve o'clock, down to six o'clock, up to one o'clock, diagonally down to seven o'clock, up to two o'clock and across to eight o'clock, and so on round the clock face. Repeat in an anti-clockwise direction.

NAULI (RECTI ISOLATION)

For this exercise, see the separate chapter devoted to it.

LAULIKI (ABDOMINAL ROLLING)

The *Gheranda Samhita* (90) substitutes *Lauliki* for *Nauli*. They are on similar lines, though *Lauliki* can be used by students who have not yet mastered *Nauli*. 'With great force move the stomach and intestines from one side to the other. This is called Lauliki-Yoga. This destroys all diseases and increases the bodily fire.'

This is a general rolling of the abdomen, instead of isolation of the vertical recti muscles (as in *Nauli*). *Nauli* is superior, and one should endeavour to master it, first attaining perfect performance of the preliminary Abdominal Retraction (*Uddiyana Bandha*).

KAPALABHATI (CLEANSING BREATH)

For a description of this exercise, see the chapter on Yogic breath control (*pranayama*).

HYGIENIC ACHIEVEMENT

Some Westerners find some of the practices described above grotesque and distasteful, perhaps associating them with the self-mortification of Indian fakirs and so-called 'holy men' – beds of nails, withered limbs, and so on. The comparison, if made, is totally unjust. The purification processes described show a mastery of the body and a regard for cleanliness that should make the average occidental shamefaced. However, readers are free to ignore or use any of the *kriyas*. But whatever the decision, it would be unfair not to recognize them as a remarkable hygienic achievement.

In conclusion, it should be noted that *all* the practices of Hatha Yoga are purificatory. Yogic postures, breath controls, and diet all remove impurities from the body and cleanse the bloodstream; and the practice of meditation is a mental hygiene, making consciousness more lucid and, in Blake's phrase, 'cleansing the doors of perception.'

V Abdominal Retraction and Recti Isolation

ABDOMINAL RETRACTION (*UDDIYANA BANDHA*)

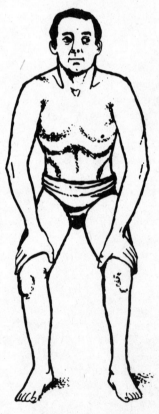

Abdominal Retraction: Uddiyana Bandha

'*Uddiyana Bandha* is a blessing to mankind; it brings health, strength and long life to those who practise it. For abdominal exercises nothing can compete with *Uddiyana* and *Nauli*. They stand unique, unrivalled and unprecedented, amongst all systems of physical exercises in the East and West.' So wrote Swami Sivananda, whose *ashram* is in the foothills of the Himalayas.

In *Uddiyana* the abdominal wall is retracted on empty lungs, creating a deep hollow. 'Make the abdomen look quite hollow just like a tank,' says the *Gheranda Samhita*. After mastering this muscle control, the two recti muscles can be isolated in the centre of the abdomen (*Nauli*). An even more advanced control is the isolation of the left rectus and the right rectus alternately, creating a wave-like motion across the abdomen from side to side.

The two muscle controls are treated in the classic texts as purifactory practices, but here we utilize them as matchless exercises for abdominal health.

Bandha means 'binding', and *Uddiyana* comes from the Sanskrit roots *ut* and *di*, and means 'to fly upwards'. *Prana* or life-force is said to fly upwards via the *sushuma nadi* or main channel of the subtle body. 'To fly' implies speed, but in this esoteric tradition it usually takes several hours of intense concentration and breath and muscle control to take the internal energies upwards to the crown of the head.

To the onlooker, the spectacle of this muscle control is either impressive or revolting. Women are more likely to show disapproval than men, who usually rush home to practice before a mirror – though Arthur Koestler, in *The Yogi and the Commissar*, described it as 'fascinating and faintly nauseating.' The visual impression is, however, of no great importance – what *is* important is the health value of the control.

Technique

i. *It is found that control is facilitated in early practice by standing with the legs a little apart and slightly bent at the knee, the kneecaps directly above the toes* – the skiing position. *The palm of the right hand is placed on top of the right thigh and the palm of the left hand on top of the left thigh, the fingers spread a little and pointing inwards. The arms are fully stretched, the trunk leans forward slightly from the waist, and the back is rounded a little. Later you should be able to perform* Uddiyana *and* Nauli *in other standing and sitting positions. The Lotus Posture and other sitting postures are often used by Yogins for these two muscle controls.*

ii.   *Empty the lungs thoroughly. Success depends on this. The lungs are kept empty throughout the control.* In pranayama *the emptying is usually performed slowly and smoothly through the nostrils, but here you should empty the lungs as fast as possible through both nostrils and mouth. If you take too long over this stage you will have to fight an urge to take an inbreath, which disturbs performance of the control.*

iii.   *Relax the abdominal wall, keeping the lungs emptied of air. Now expand the thoracic cage as though to make a thoracic inspiration – but actually only go through the motions of expanding the ribs, without taking in air. A slight lift of the thoracic cage is usually found helpful.*

iv.   *The diaphragm will now move up into the thoracic cavity and the stomach will travel inwards, as though being pulled by a wire attached to the base of the backbone. Hold the retraction for a few seconds, and then release the abdominal wall smoothly. If you let it spring back with a jerk, the inrush of air will be explosive, which is faulty Yoga practice.*

What happens is that emptying the lungs and expanding the thorax causes the abdomen to move back to fill the vacuum created. This should be effortless. A deep hollow appears, in which both fists could be placed. Fat stomachs make *Uddiyana* and *Nauli* difficult, and women, with their extra fat, find these controls, especially *Nauli*, more difficult than men. The Abdominal Retraction is demonstrated by Lady Dukes (21). In classic performance, when the abdomen is fully retracted, the *oblique* muscles stand out like cords. Those of the Yogin observed by Arthur Koestler did. An exceptionally lean abdomen is needed to display this crowning touch, and few book illustrations show it. It is Dr Theos Bernard, an American, who depicts it best in Plate xxxiii of his *Hatha Yoga*. He also shows cleanly-executed central isolation of the recti, and the left rectus and the right rectus separately. Some Indian experts, though remarkably supple, show a surprisingly large amount of waistline flab – though it must be pointed out that the hard 'wash-board' effect cultivated by Western weight-training body-builders is neither aimed at nor thought desirable in India.

Developing Skill
Yoga's Abdominal Retraction is unique: no other exercise comes near to matching it for squeezing and kneading the viscera – intes-

tines, spleen, pancreas, liver, kidneys, transverse colon – or for toning the supporting muscular 'corset'.

The exercise should be performed on an empty stomach. This means that immediately after rising in the morning is the best time for practice. Two methods should be employed. The first is to hold the retraction for five seconds, and then release the abdomen and breathe normally for a few seconds. Exhale again and repeat the retraction. Perform five times to make up a cycle. The second method is to perform five fast retractions and releases on one emptying of the lungs. This counts as one cycle. Perform as smoothly as possible, taking no air into the lungs. During the first month perform three cycles, during the second month four cycles, and during the third month and thereafter five cycles. This applies to both methods. Later you may wish to include an extra session of practice daily, and to add Recti Isolation.

Agnisari Dhauti
This means literally 'purification through fire' – the digestive fire, that is. It is really the first of the two methods of practice described above, but prolonged. It is only recommended for advanced practitioners. A series of retractions is performed on one exhalation of air. As soon as the maximum hollowing has been achieved, the abdominal wall is released, and immediately drawn back again. The viscera are powerfully massaged and the digestive fires are fanned. Under *ashram* conditions, Yogins may perform as many as 1,500 retractions in one day, but readers should never exceed a number that feels comfortable and beneficial. (*See also* Fire Purification (*Vahnisara*) in the chapter on Yoga Hygiene.)

RECTI ISOLATION (*NAULI*)

The recti abdominis are the straight muscles of the abdomen, lying side by side in vertical strips down the centre of the abdomen from chest bone to pubic bone. The ability to isolate them consciously is another of Yoga's remarkable discoveries about the human body. Success in *Nauli* will not come until you have mastered *Uddiyana* to the extent that a very deep hollow is effortlessly created. Keeping the lungs empty of air, you then isolate the recti by pushing them forward, as though they have stepped forward from a deep cave to

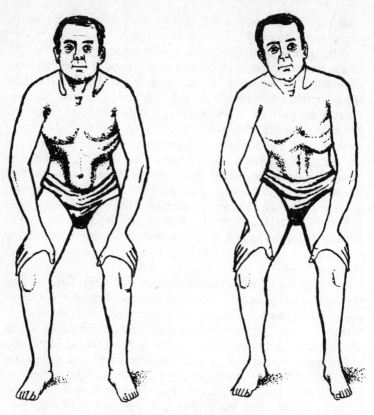

Recti Isolation: Nauli

stand motionless at its entrance. Practising before a mirror helps in the early stages, and slight pressure downwards of the palms of the hands is another aid. Later, both these aids can be dropped.

As soon as you are proficient in *Nauli*, add its practice to that of *Uddiyana Bandha*, performing it in the two ways indicated for *Uddiyana* and with the same number of repetitions.

Lateral Abdominal Rolling
This is the acme of Yogic control of the abdominal muscles. The right rectus is isolated by itself; then the left rectus isolated; then right; then left; and so on in a continuous wave-like motion that crosses the abdomen from right to left and from left to right. Good

form is essential; speed can be worked up gradually. The number of successive 'waves' will depend on how long you can comfortably suspend breathing. Always stay within the borders of comfort.

Recti rolling gives the abdominal muscles and viscera the maximum churning, squeezing, and kneading.

BENEFITS

No exercises superior to these have been devised for what F. A. Hornibrook called 'culture of the abdomen'. Even if you do not progress to Recti Isolation or Lateral Abdominal Rolling, all the benefits described are obtained to some extent by retracting the abdomen (*Uddiyana Bandha*).

In Kundalini Yoga these controls are used to awaken the body's dormant electro-magnetic energies. On a practical level, they firm, tone, and trim the abdomen; massage the viscera; clear congestion caused by sedentary habits and the upright stance; correct constipation; improve digestion; and stimulate the liver, pancreas, kidneys, spleen, and adrenal glands. They are linked with sexual vigour and the overcoming of sexual disabilities. The diaphragm is encouraged to move, to become more mobile, and thus to perform better the up-and-down piston-like movement that operates deep and healthful breathing. The important solar plexus region is stimulated. Elasticity of the lungs is improved, and the heart is said to receive a gentle massage obtainable in no other way. The abdominal muscles and internal organs receive a kneading and squeezing superior to what could be got from the hands of an expert masseur. The viscera are lifted and squeezed against the spine. Repeated uplift prevents prolapse. Metabolism, circulation, and digestion are stimulated.

The controls are unrivalled as aids to natural and regular bowel action. Constipation is corrected long-term, not momentarily treated as by taking a laxative. An Indian doctor, Vasant G. Rele, who made a study of the physiological effects of Hatha Yoga practices, wrote (70):

Excessive activity of the sympathetic nervous system inhibits peristaltic activity of the intestines and produces constipation. On the other hand, an excessive activity of the parasympathetic increases the movements of the intestines, and produces looseness of the bowels. . . . By the practice of *Uddiyana Bandha* the excessive activity of the sympathetic nervous system is controlled without exciting the parasympathetic, overstimulation of which would create a vicious circle. . . . The sudden retraction of the relaxed abdominal muscles, particularly the two recti (straight front muscles of the abdomen), against the spine after their preliminary contraction in the full expiratory effort in the practice of *Uddiyana Bandha*, drags the intestines upwards and downwards to their utmost limit. This stretches with them the sympathetic fibres curbing any tendency towards overactivity of the solar plexus – the brain of the sympathetic nervous system – without the stimulation of the parasympethetic.

Abdominal Retraction (*Uddiyana Bandha*) and Recti Isolation (*Nauli*), in common with other forms of Yoga practice, are thus seen to have a beneficial influence on the nervous system and, through it, the functioning of the whole psycho-physical organism.

THE BREATH OF LIFE

Many physiological processes are essential to human life: the functioning of the heart, the regulation of the temperature, and so on. All must work together for us to survive. But one physiological function seems to us most intimately connected with life – *breathing*. 'Breath is life,' the Yogins say. And few treatises on *pranayama* omit to mention that we can survive for weeks without food, and for days without water, but that our survival without air has to be measured in seconds.

The dominion of breath over the senses is expressed in many old Sanskrit texts, and perhaps most poetically in the *Brihadaranyaka Upanishad* (155):

The senses, when quarrelling together as to who was the best, went to Brahman and said: 'Who is the richest of us?' He replied: 'He by whose departure the body seems worst, he is the richest.'

The tongue [speech] departed, and having been absent for a year, it came back and said: 'How have you been able to live without me?' They replied: 'Like unto people, not speaking with the tongue, but breathing with breath, seeing with the eye, hearing with the ear, knowing with the mind, generating with seed. Thus we have lived.' Then speech entered in.

The eye [sight] departed, and having been absent for a year, it came back and said: 'How have you been able to live without me?' They replied: 'Like blind people not seeing with the eye, but breathing with the breath, speaking with the tongue, hearing with the ear, knowing with the mind, generating with seed. Thus we have lived.' Then the eye entered in.

The ear [hearing] departed, and having been absent for a year, it came back and said: 'How have you been able to live without me?' They replied: 'Like deaf people, not hearing with the ear, but breathing with the breath, speaking with the tongue, seeing with the eye, knowing with the mind, generating with seed. Thus we have lived.' Then the ear entered in.

The mind departed, and having been absent for a year, it came back and said: 'How have you been able to live without me?' They replied: 'Like fools, not knowing with the mind, but breathing with the breath, seeing with the eye, hearing with the ear, generating with seed. Thus we have lived.' Then the mind entered in.

The seed departed, and having been absent for a year, it came back and said: 'How have you been able to live without me?' They replied: 'Like impotent people, not generating with seed, but breathing with the breath, seeing with the eye, hearing with the ear, knowing with the mind. Thus we have lived.' Then the seed entered in.

The [vital] breath, when on the point of departure, tore up these senses, as a great, excellent horse of the Sindhu country might tear up the pegs to which he is tethered. They said to him: 'Sir, do not depart. We shall not be able to live without thee.'

PRANAYAMA DEFINED

Pranayama, the Yogic science of breath control, is at the very heart of Hatha Yoga practice. Basically, Hatha Yoga is mastery of body and of breath. Sir Paul Dukes, who studied and taught Yoga in India, says (21) that purification is the keynote of Hatha Yoga, and the foremost practice of purification is *pranayama*. For this reason, breath control is more important than the *asanas* or postures, though ideally both should be an integral part of the Hatha Yoga system. Breathing exercises are considered essential for the preliminary purification whereby the cells and nerve channels are cleansed and made ready for advanced control of subtle inner energies.

The Sanskrit word *hatha* has associations with breathing. In Yogic tradition the flow of breath through the right nostril is controlled by the sun, and that through the left nostril by the moon.

The Sanskrit *ha* means 'sun' and *tha* means 'moon'. The air that travels through the right nostril (*pingala*) is positive ('sun breath') and that which travels through the left nostril (*ida*) is negative ('moon breath'). The word *yoga* means 'union'. Hatha Yoga thus unifies the positive and negative, male and female, sun and moon universal principles within the human organism. This balancing of energy currents is subjectively experienced as a state of inner poise and equilibrium. Controlled breathing (*pranayama*) is the key practice for attaining this desirable physiological and psychical state.

In the eight 'limbs' (*angas*) of classical Yoga as mapped out by Patanjali, breath control comes after bodily poses (*asanas*), and before withdrawal of the senses from external objects (*pratyahara*), the first step in turning the attention inwards for concentration (*dharana*) and its extension as contemplation (*dhyana*), leading to the superconscious experience of *samadhi*.

Yogic breath control operates at several levels, from the exoteric boosting of vitality and health to esoteric approaches to mystical states of consciousness. A multiplicity of benefits accrue from raising the level of general health and from having rich reserves of energy. The mind benefits from the calming and toning of the nervous system, and the tone and texture of consciousness itself is influenced by the rate and rhythm of respiration and by pausing between inhalation and exhalation and between exhalation and inhalation. *Pranayama* prepares the mind for the meditative practices of Raja Yoga, and breathing may itself become the object of concentration and contemplation. Breathing meditation is found in the practices of Hindu, Taoist, Buddhist, Zen, and Sufist mysticism.

The term *pranayama* is made up of two parts. One meaning of *prana* is 'breath'. *Yama* belongs to the ethical foundation of Yoga practice: it means 'restraint' or 'control'. *Pranayama* is therefore in one sense 'breath control'. The breath flow into and out of the lungs is regulated, and made smooth and slow in most exercises. Sometimes first one nostril is used while the other is closed, and then the roles of the nostrils are reversed. Breathing is suspended at the end of each inhalation or exhalation. For normal purposes this should only be for a few seconds – holding the breath to the point of discomfort or strain could be damaging to health, whereas controlled breathing well within capacity enhances health. Readers should not anticipate essaying any remarkable feats in this direction.

Yama has another related meaning, given by Archie Bahm (5) as: 'persisting disposition or enduring nature or tendency to retain strength,' to which definition he adds a rider in keeping with our practical approach: 'to interpret *yama* as sustained relaxation, and *pranayama* as a way of sustaining unanxious living through healthy breathing habits, would not be inappropriate.' Yogic breathing relaxes body and mind. But this is a peripheral definition.

We have given one definition of *prana* – 'breath'. *Prana* has also wider connotations, described below.

PRANA

Translating *prana* as 'life breath' rather than 'breath' goes some way towards indicating its broader dimension. *Prana* is the power within breath and 'the vital force in every being'. As cosmic energy, it pervades everything. It is a vital substance not yet covered by scientific classification, though it should be noted that the modern physicists' discovery that 'all is energy' recalls statements on the origins of the universe and its evolution made by Yogic philosophers many centuries ago. *Prana* is the life-force within and about us. It operates in the working of our respiration, circulation, digestion, and other body processes, and is at the same time the universal life-force in which we share. An ocean of energy is at our disposal and through Yoga we can learn how to tap it.

Vivekananda, in his *Raja Yoga*, expressed this concept with characteristic eloquence:

> In an ocean there are huge waves, then smaller waves, and still smaller, down to little bubbles; but back of all these is an infinite ocean. The bubble is connected with the infinite ocean at one end, and the huge wave at the other end. So, one may be a gigantic man, and another a little bubble, but each is connected with that infinite ocean of energy which is the common birthright of every animal that exists. Wherever there is life, the storehouse of that infinite energy is behind it.

Air is strongly charged with *prana*, and it is potently present in sunlight and in the foods we eat, especially those that are sun-ripened. Air being the most vital of all foods, improved breathing methods mean a richer supply of *prana*, that is, of life itself. Disease is unlikely to gain a hold in a body whose tissues and organs are charged with *prana*.

Apart from the *prana* absorbed from air and food, Hatha Yogins say that there are concentrations of *prana* stored within the body. These, coiled and latent, are sources of physiological and psychic power, which *pranayama* helps activate. This comes within the practice of Kundalini Yoga, also called Laya Yoga, which will be discussed in a later section.

In Yogic breathing, *prana* – both as breath and as vital cosmic force – is gathered and utilized to physiological, mental, and spiritual advantage. The spiritual side is only a peripheral concern of Yoga of Vitality, but one is reminded of it by Tennyson's words, 'Closer is He than breathing, and nearer than hands and feet.' The poet was referring to the personal God of Christianity, but for the pure Yoga of the *upanishads* one must substitute *Brahman*, the impersonal Absolute, in pure consciousness the ground of Being.

In breathing we make our most intimate contact with the cosmic life force, which is why the Yogins consider breath control to be of primary importance, and why breath is given dominion over the senses and other physiological processes in Yoga's classic texts and in the sublime *upanishads*.

FAULTY BREATHING

Only a minority of adults in civilized countries breathe with full efficiency and for maximum healthful effect. Young children, unless they have some bodily defect, breathe more effectively than adults, but once they are subjected to social pressures and tensions they develop the faulty respiratory habits of their parents, principally shallow high-chest breathing.

If great numbers of people have lost the technique of using their respiratory muscles and lungs with adequate elasticity, the result can only be destructive to health. The bloodstream is not being fully purified and oxygenated, nor is food being adequately burned in the body to provide energy. It also goes a long way to explaining the prevalence of fatigue, headaches, and neurasthenia in civilized life.

Breathing deeply, for great numbers of people, has to be re-learned, and shallow upper-chest inhalation replaced by diaphragmatic and abdominal breathing, of the kind visible in sleeping infants.

To understand the physiological basis of what is involved in breathing deeply and healthfully, it is helpful to acquire knowledge of the basic facts of the anatomy and physiology of respiration. Readers wishing to extend their knowledge beyond the summary given here can find suitable textbooks on anatomy and physiology in bookshops and libraries.

MAN'S NEED FOR OXYGEN

Scientists believe that several hundred million years ago all living organisms on our planet lived in the sea. Later the first amphibian managed to live in both water and air. Even now only fifteen per cent of living organisms exist on land and breathe the earth's oxygen-charged atmosphere. For man's living on dry land he has to thank his hard-working lungs, which take in oxygen, process it, and transfer it to the blood.

The earth's atmosphere contains twenty-one per cent oxygen. On it consciousness itself depends: if the oxygen level in the atmosphere surrounding us falls, we rapidly become unconscious.

Our billions of body cells need to breathe; more exactly, they need to receive oxygen and to return carbon dioxide, the waste product of metabolic activities within the cells. The lungs pass oxygen from the air we breathe into the blood, which is carried to the cells. The circulating bloodstream also carries the waste gases, and the lungs expel carbon dioxide on our outgoing breaths.

Oxygen could be described as our most essential food. It is essential for the metabolic processes on which our vitality depends. Burning up food produces energy in much the same way as burning up petrol in the engine of an automobile provides power. A large and constant supply of oxygen is needed for the combustion of food products (oxidation). The amount we absorb through the skin is insufficient for our needs, so we must depend on the efficient functioning of our respiratory muscles and organs.

THE RESPIRATORY TRACT

The main components of the respiratory tract are the nostrils, the pharynx, the larynx, the trachea (windpipe), the bronchi, and the lungs.

Yogic (and healthy) breathing uses the nose and not the mouth. The nasal passages are lined with fine hairs, which act as filters and trap dust and bacteria, and with mucous membrane, which warms and moistens the incoming air. The nose is divided by the septum into two narrow passages. In some *pranayama* exercises alternate nostrils are used: this tends to produce a relaxing effect.

Inhaled air, having been drawn up the nostrils, passes into the pharynx, the cavity behind and communicating with the nose, mouth, and larynx. The vocal cords normally are not vibrated in *pranayama* (though they are in Mantra Yoga, which is based on vocalizing), but there are one or two Yogic breathing exercises in which the glottis, which modulates the voice, is half-closed.

The windpipe or trachea is about four and a half inches in length and one inch in diameter. The word 'trachea' derives from the Greek *trakhus*, meaning 'rough'. The roughness, which can be felt in the throat with the fingertips, is caused by alternate rings of cartilage and fibrous tissue.

The windpipe enters the thoracic cavity at the neck and divides into the right bronchus and the left bronchus, which supply air to the right and left lungs respectively. Trachea and bronchi are hollow tubes which stay open due to the cartilaginous rings in their walls. The unpleasant bronchitis is an infection of the bronchi. From each bronchus radiate smaller branches, which ramify into a bronchial tree composed of fine bronchioles, ending in clusters of air-filled sacs called alveoli, which contain blood vessels. There are about 750 million air sacs or alveoli in the lungs, an indication of their tiny size.

The lungs are not of equal size: the right lung is slightly the larger of the two and has three lobes to the left lung's two. If a diseased lobe is removed, the others carry the extra work. Adult lungs weigh from two to two and a half pounds, and if the lining could be spread out flat it would cover about a hundred square yards of ground. Healthy lungs that have enjoyed nothing but fresh air are pink; those of heavy smokers are purple-black.

The mucous membrane lining the respiratory tract has goblet cells and hair-like cilia. The mucus keeps the windpipe and bronchi moist. The cilia, moving always in one direction, trap particles of dirt and sweep them up towards the mouth. If the cilia are faced with too much work, a spasm of coughing is triggered, in the same way that too much dust or dirt in the nostrils sets off a sneeze.

Each lung is enveloped by a double layer of smooth membrane, which prevents any friction that might arise from movements of the lungs against the rib-cage. The inner layer of this protective membrane is called the visceral pleura and the outer layer the parietal pleura. Pleurisy is inflammation of the pleura, and pneumonia is inflammation of the lungs.

THE THORACIC CAGE

The bony thoracic cage, which houses the heart and lungs, is of intricate construction and quite narrow at its apex, though the shoulders to each side give an impression to the contrary. At the front is the breastbone or sternum; at the back are the twelve thoracic vertebrae of the spinal column; on each flank are the ribs – twelve pairs, whose interstices are filled by the intercostal muscles, nerves, and blood vessels. The top seven pairs are known as the true ribs; the eighth, ninth, and tenth pairs as false ribs, joining up with the ribs above and in the breastbone; and the two pairs of short bottom ribs which join into the abdomen are called floating ribs.

It is the expansion of the ribs that initiates the act of breathing.

THE BREATHING PROCESS

The act of breathing is a complex muscular performance, whose co-ordination is directed by a respiratory centre in the medulla or hindbrain. Among its nerve cells one group is responsible for inhalation and another for exhalation. Inhalation is an active process; exhalation is a passive process, a recoil or letting go.

The muscles called into action in filling and emptying the lungs are those of the diaphragm, the walls of the chest, and the floating ribs. The diaphragm is the most powerful muscle, acting in a piston-like up-and-down movement. We can see it operating, flattening down and rising again, vigorously in athletes panting after exertion, and gently in a sleeping baby.

During inhalation the dome-shaped diaphragm flattens, pressing down on the ciscera below and bulging out the abdomen in deep breathing; at the same time the thoracic cage expands and the atmospheric pressure outside the body fills the lungs through the nasal passages (or mouth), pharynx, windpipe, and bronchi.

During exhalation, there is a passive recoil. The chest cage relaxes (rather like an umbrella closing), the abdominal wall recoils, and the diaphragm, which was lowered by the pressure of the inflowing air, rises by its own elasticity. During this process, air is expelled from the lungs. Exhalation is a letting-go from the tension of expansion.

Ordinarily, the lungs inflate and deflate some fifteen to twenty times each minute. They have elasticity, but are not muscular organs. They rely for expansion and contraction on the muscles of the thoracic cage and the diaphragm. When the muscles surrounding the lungs expand, a partial vacuum is created, and atmospheric pressure sees to it that air flows into the lungs. The natural elasticity of the lungs and the chest wall, on their recoil, pushes air out of the lungs. The so-called 'iron lung' used in hospitals does not operate by pumping air into the lungs, but by increasing and reducing the air pressure on the outer walls of the chest.

The expansion of the lungs depends on the chest walls providing an air-tight compartment; if the wall is punctured, as in stabbing, air will rush in and collapse the lungs. Occasionally doctors admit air to one side of a patient's chest so as to collapse and rest a diseased lung.

The respiratory centre in the brain operates from nerve feedback information from the lungs and body muscles, and from the oxygen-carbon dioxide balance of the blood passing through the brain. The chemical and nerve controls can be triggered by the emotions, a factor taken into account in Yoga.

RESUSCITATION

Until recently the most widely-used method of artificially stimu-lating the mechanical process of breathing was to place the patient face downwards, kneel at his side or astride him, facing his head, place one's hands flat against his lower ribs at each side of the spinal column, and then every four or five seconds throw the bodyweight forward onto the hands, between thrusts sitting up and relaxing the pressure without removing the hands from the lower ribs.

But now the most popular method of artificial respiration is mouth-to-mouth, the resuscitator exhaling air from his own lungs into those of the patient, whose head is held back. Air should be transmitted in this way every four or five seconds.

A BEAUTIFUL SYSTEM

Analysis of inhaled and exhaled air shows the former to be composed of 20.95% oxygen, 0.05% carbon dioxide, and 79% nitrogen; and exhaled air of 16.5% oxygen, 4.0% carbon dioxide, and 79.5% nitrogen. Behind these figures is a neat physiological process.

In describing the lungs we mentioned the alveoli, the millions of tiny air sacs, like miniature balloons, around which the blood flows. On an inbreath, by the Law of Gaseous Diffusion, oxygen moves from the area of higher pressure in the air sacs to that of lower pressure in the red blood cells, specifically in the haemoglobin, the colouring matter of the red corpuscles. The blood transports the oxygen to the body cells. The medical term for what then happens is osmosis. Oxygen and nourishment from the food we have eaten, now in liquid form, is handed over to the tissues, and the cells hand over in return their waste (carbon dioxide), which the blood carries back to the lungs. The red blood cells act somewhat like bottles on an assembly line. On their reaching the lungs, the Law of Gaseous Diffusion operates again, but this time with the reverse effect: the pressure of carbon dioxide in the veins being higher, the waste gases move into the air sacs and are expelled from the body on the outgoing breath.

It is a beautiful system, and worth making the most of through Yogic breathing.

RESIDUAL AIR

The air that remains in the body after the bulk has been processed is called the residual volume. Some of this air remains in the lungs, and there is also air in the 'dead space' between the lungs and the nostrils. There can be an increase in the volume of residual air in persons with diseased lungs or in those who have been inactive for a long time. Even the master Yogins must have residual air, but the breathing pauses of *pranayama* are thought to give fresh air the opportunity to diffuse healthfully with static air in the respiratory passages and the lungs.

VITAL CAPACITY

The vital capacity is the maximum volume of air that can be exhaled following a deep breath. Vital capacity for an average person is estimated at 3,800 cubic centimetres, but variations occur due to differences in physical build, or through exercising the muscles of respiration, as in Yoga. The figure of 3,800 cubic centimetres is made up as described below.

In normal breathing at rest the average person takes in about 600 cubic centimetres of air. A further 2,000 cubic centimetres can be drawn in by making an effort to inflate the lungs as fully as possible. 600 cubic centimetres is the average expiration under normal conditions, but this too, with an effort, can be increased by about 1,200 cubic centimetres. Add the three together – they are known respectively as tidal air (600), complemental air (2,000), and supplemental air (1,200) – and we see that the maximum volume of air that can be expelled by this average person (a non-athlete, and untrained in Yogic and other deep breathing) is 3,800 cubic centimetres. This is his vital capacity.

Arthritis and certain other diseases can restrict the capacity of the chest muscles to move, leading to extremely shallow breathing and eventually very often to lung infections. Asthma is a spasm of the bronchial muscle, making exhalation difficult: what is normally a passive act becomes effortful.

OXYGEN DEBT

An oxygen debt occurs when the proportion of oxygen in the bloodstream is less than it should be. A familiar indication of this is a yawn. The debt can be incurred as you read these words by holding your nose firmly for a few seconds. Another indication is that the lungs have to work faster after running or other effortful activity. The amount of carbon dioxide in the bloodstream acts as a trigger: when it exceeds a certain level, a centre in the brain orders faster breathing.

The long-distance runner builds up his oxygen debt slowly. As he runs he breathes more deeply, his heart beats more rapidly, and the exchange of oxygen and carbon dioxide in the body speeds up. But if the long-distance runner has trained properly, this combination of faster and deeper breathing with more rapid blood circulation enables him to cover several miles (in the marathon over twenty-six miles) without great respiratory distress. The sprinter has a somewhat different experience. He makes an all-out effort over a hundred metres. His metabolic demands during this explosive effort are such that there is no natural way of giving the blood cells the oxygen they need: about six quarts in ten seconds or less. So the body makes what might be called a gentleman's agreement with the runner's mind and says: 'All right, run like a hound of hell for a hundred metres, go into oxygen debt for ten seconds or less, and recoup your shortage at the end of the race.' The mind agrees, and the athlete goes 'into the red' for almost the whole requirement of oxygen. But once he has crossed the winning line and pulled up, his mouth is drawn wide open and his lungs dilate and contract like a fast-working bellows until the oxygen debt has been repaid.

So one way to stimulate deeper breathing is to exercise vigorously the body's main muscle masses, as in running or in active sports and games. Another method is that of standing or sitting still and voluntarily breathing deeply. The latter is the way of *pranayama*. Because the large muscles are not worked and because lactic acid does not therefore have to be converted into glycogen in the muscles, this kind of deep breathing is of a different nature to the athletic effort we have just described. The Yogin breathes deeply through a conscious decision that controlled breathing fulfils certain aims.

BREATHE BETTER

Through the practice of *pranayama* the respiratory muscles and the lungs function more effectively, and in a short time this becomes habitual, to the great betterment of psycho-physical well-being. Yogic breathing increases bodily vitality, improves air processing in the lungs, purifies the blood, calms and tones the nervous system, and fosters mental poise and equanimity. It relaxes body and mind.

To dissolve tension, sit poised, back straight, head level; let tension go, open up, and for several minutes breathe smoothly, slowly, and deeply. Influencing the mind through the body muscles is a practical aim which Yoga has made a valuable part of the system. Rhythmic breathing inculcates feelings of lightness and buoyancy felt both in the muscles and in emotional tone. *Pranayama* practice is therefore enjoyable – so much so that one has to guard against going on too long with it, and perhaps inducing giddiness.

The action in shallow breathing is restricted to the upper chest. (Women tend to suffer from shallow breathing more than men.) Only a meagre amount of air enters the lungs, and thus only a small amount of oxygen permeates the blood vessels of the air sacs. Correct breathing enriches the blood, stimulates the circulation, and feeds life-force to the blood, tissues, and organs.

On average the shallow breather is found to inhale about 500 cubic centimetres of air, but the conditioned deep breather can draw in about 4,000 cubic centimetres. Thus deep breathing takes in about eight times as much air as shallow breathing, which fails adequately to aerate the alveoli of the lungs. The air we breathe is composed of approximately 21% oxygen and 79% nitrogen. This oxygen-nitrogen balance is maintained and we cannot increase the proportion of oxygen; but we can improve the ability of the lungs to take in more air and to process air. The volume of air a person can inhale is dependent on the amount of space his chest muscles can create for the lungs to expand into and for them to contract into on the recoil. Running, brisk walking, jogging (alternating running and brisk walking), active sports and games, and deep breathing exercises improve the tone, mobility, elasticity, and strength of the respiratory muscles and increase vital capacity. Vital capacity, as mentioned earlier, is the measured amount of air exhaled in a deep breath. But even in a trained deep breather, vital capacity is only about 75% of the total lung capacity. The condition and sizes of the lungs themselves are factors in the amount of air that can be processed. The sizes of the lungs are normally proportionate to the physical build of the individual.

Dr Kenneth H. Cooper, a major in the United States Air Force Medical Corps, recently led a team which studied the physiological condition of thousands of airmen before and after physical fitness training. The study showed that the trained man can push twenty times his vital capacity through his lungs in one minute, whereas an out-of-condition man has to struggle to force ten times his vital capacity through his lungs. However, six weeks' training was

usually enough to enable young airmen who were out of condition
to rise from the lower figure to the higher.

Dr Cooper says (112):

Getting oxygen to the body tissues is the rockbottom basis of conditioning, and it's convenient to think of the systems that process and
deliver oxygen as one huge, magnificent, wondrous assembly line,
complete with receiving lines to dispose of wastes, and the most
beautiful engine ever conceived to keep all of it moving.

He also says that conditioning

produces more blood, specifically more hemoglobin which carries the
oxygen, more red-blood cells which carry the hemoglobin, more blood
plasma which carries the red-blood cells, and consequently more total
blood volume. In our laboratory and others, tests have repeatedly
shown that men in good physical condition invariably have a larger
blood supply than deconditioned men of comparable size. An average-
size man may increase his blood volume by nearly a quart in response
to aerobic conditioning. And, of this amount, the red cells may increase
proportionately more.

SLIMMING

People who take up Yogic breathing may be surprised to find
superfluous fat melting away from the waistline, hips, and other
places where it is prone to gather. It seems likely that the link
between breathing and burning up foodstuffs for energy partly
explains this result. *Pranayama* improves metabolic efficiency. The
combined practice of *asanas* and *pranayama* also fosters a muscular
feeling tone (kinesthesis) that finds the physical effects of overeating
uncomfortable and somewhat reprehensible. This too has a bearing
on the way Hatha Yoga slims and reshapes the figure. The postures
also break up fatty deposits and streamline the body.

WHY WE NEED TO *LEARN* TO BREATHE

That Yoga masters insist we need to learn to breathe correctly
puzzles many people. 'What have I been doing with my lungs from
the moment of birth?' you may ask. 'Surely the act of breathing is
instinctive? I am breathing every minute of my life, am I not?

Otherwise I would be dead in a minute or two. Why, then, should I be told to "learn" to breathe?'

The Yoga master replies something like this: 'Of course you have been breathing all your days. But there is a world of difference between breathing shallowly and incorrectly and breathing well for health and vitality. Left to our natural animal instinct, it is true that we would breathe efficiently: after all, we nearly all manage to do so when babies. But Man is both animal and something more. His glory, and most of his problems likewise, dwell in this mystery of his being naked ape plus much more – one foot solidly on earth, but the other itching to stride the heavens, god-like. Animals in their natural habitat instinctively select those foods which are good for them. Can the same be said of Man? And when it comes to the most fundamental act of all, we find that great numbers of men and women, through faulty and shallow breathing habits, fail to gain the maximum benefit in purification and vitality freely available from the air they inhale.

'The quality of your breathing as a baby – deep, abdominal, relaxed – is almost certain to have been superior to what it is now. Inhibitions and restraints, moral, social, physical (poor posture and bands of muscular tension), and environmental (stuffy rooms and so on) all destroy the growing child's ability to breathe deeply and healthfully. Without our being aware of it, the passing of the years is often accompanied by a deterioration in the efficiency and effectiveness of respiration. Western society, based on competition and results-orientated, contracts the respiratory muscles, and lack of exercise after the end of the schooldays exacerbates a loss of mobility and elasticity in the thoracic muscles and the diaphragm. Breathing becomes shallower and more restricted, resulting in the drawing in of less air and less oxygen, the most vital of all foods.

'Yes, you are breathing now – breathing in a way. You are getting by. You are managing to survive. But if you train yourself to breathe healthfully, Yogic style, you will soon discover that the way you breathed before was a travesty of the real thing, shallow and inadequate. Now you are being asked to breathe *correctly*. Through controlled Yoga breathing you will raise your level of vitality, clarify consciousness, tone your nervous system, brighten your eyes, put bounce in your step, feel light and buoyant, and float along with the flow of life, in harmony with Nature and the Universal Energies.'

SURELY CONTROLLED BREATHING IS UNNATURAL?

The answer to this question is 'No', because the human organism is equipped for both automatic and consciously-regulated breathing. If anything is unnatural, it is the kind of inferior, inadequate breathing habits so often acquired once the carefree years of early childhood have passed.

AUTOMATIC CONTROL

Co-ordination of the act of breathing is operated from a respiratory centre in the medulla or hindbrain. This collection of nerve cells has two parts, one part being responsible for inhalation and the other part for exhalation. The centre operates on the basis of nervous feedback information from the lungs and muscles, and from the oxygen–carbon dioxide balance of the blood passing through the brain. This is automatic machinery on which we depend for staying alive. Yet, unlike most physiological processes, we can also exercise some degree of voluntary control. This also is a necessity for survival, as when we hold our breath under water.

Inspiration comes from an impulse through the vagus nerves and expiration from its inhibition. Inhalation of air is thus an active process, and exhalation a passive process – a recoil or letting go.

Inflating the lungs stretches the sensory nerve endings, a signal for the expiratory part of the respiratory centre in the brain to inhibit the action of inspiration through an impulse along the vagus nerves. When exhalation ends, the vagus action returns, and the in-and-out flow of the life breath continues.

A slight rise in the content of carbon dioxide in the blood results in an immediate command from the respiratory centre for more air to be drawn into the lungs, and the muscular activity necessary for inspiration is triggered off. A gentle example of this is an involuntary yawn; a vigorous example is the panting of the sprinter at the end of a race. A progressive accumulation of carbon dioxide in the body leads to convulsions and an agonizing death. A fall in oxygen, on the other hand, leads to a slow loss of consciousness.

When the haemoglobin is insufficiently oxidized, the blood takes on a bluish tinge. This may occur because heart disease has slowed down the circulation; through lung disease; or because of a low oxygen content in the atmosphere at high altitudes.

Overbreathing when at rest so successfully removes carbon dioxide that respiration may actually cease for several minutes.

CONSCIOUS CONTROL

Along with these automatic functions we have been describing, there is also a measure of voluntary control of breathing. By means of this dual control, Man achieves many of the things that make him distinctively human.

'Considering that our life depends upon our breathing, it is remarkable that we have as much conscious control over it as we do,' says Benjamin F. Miller and Ruth Goode in *Man and His Body* (154).

Our automatic controls keep us breathing, fortunately, whether or not we are paying attention, or we would not be able to go to sleep. If we had only automatic controls, we would not perform many of our most highly developed acts of skill. Nor would we be capable of those most human forms of expression, laughter, song, and speech. (Animals make their sounds by the same physiological mechanisms, but the controls are instinctual or reflex rather than voluntary. . . .)

Probably our survival, or rather the survival of our evolutionary forebears, also depended upon a thousand unforeseen adaptations and co-ordinations in attack and defence that were more skilfully managed with the breath held or expelled at will. And so we have the wonderful gift of dual control, part voluntary, part automatic, of the very breath of life.

Breath control is brought to its most extraordinary development, though not one we should seek to emulate, in burial alive, success in which depends on slowing down the heartbeat by conscious control and surviving on a modicum of air in a trance state. If levitation is possible, it also must be based on breath control. Fully authenticated is the art of engendering body heat through breath control (*tumo*). By this means Yogins in the Himalayas and in Tibet sit for hours, naked or scantily clad, in sub-zero temperatures.

Levitation, burial alive, and *tumo* will be discussed further in a later chapter. It is more important to move on now to a more practical function of the 'wonderful gift of dual control' we all possess – as regulator of the four stages of the act of breathing.

VI   Yogic Breath Control

THE FOUR STAGES OF BREATHING

In *pranayama* one is aware that the act of breathing has four distinct stages. We normally think in terms of only two, inhalation and exhalation, forgetting the brief pauses after each before we change gear and go into reverse, as it were.

The four stages are:

i.   Inhalation, or puraka. *This in Yoga is a continuous process, evenly controlled.*

ii.   A pause in breathing, called kumbhaka, *retaining the air in the inflated lungs. When distinguishing this from stage iv, which is a pause on empty lungs, we will call this stage full pause. B. K. S. Iyengar calls it* antara kumbhaka (35), *and Archie Bahm calls it* abhyantara kumbhaka (5).

iii.   Exhalation, or rechaka. *Again, this should be a smooth and continuous process, a recoil or letting go from the inflation of the lungs, the expansion of the thoracic cage, and the pressing down of the diaphragm. In Yoga special care is taken to make sure outbreathing is thorough.*

iv.   A pause in breathing again, this time on empty lungs. This is an effortless breath suspension (kumbhaka), *at the end of which a slow smooth inflow of air through the nostrils commences, and we return to stage i. Archie Bahm calls stage iv* bahya kumbhaka (5).

In *pranayama* there is a measured timing ratio for the stages, especially for the first three stages. This ratio is carefully observed. We will return shortly to this matter of timing; meanwhile we will discuss the stages in more detail.

INHALATION (*PURAKA*)

In Yogic breathing this consists of the muscular action detailed earlier when describing the act of breathing. The movement has two parts, working together. In the first part the thoracic cage expands to make room for the lungs to inflate. In the second part the dome-shaped diaphragm flattens out and descends, swelling out the abdomen and, incidentally, massaging beneficially the abdominal viscera.

At this point it needs to be pointed out that Yogic breathing is not a competition to see how much air we can cram into our lungs. Competition is alien to the spirit of Yoga, and here it could be dangerous. The criterion should always be *comfort*. Breathe deeply, pour air into the lungs – but the point at which the inflation and expansion ends should be just before the point at which discomfort intrudes. If you sit easily, with the back straight and the head level, the respiratory muscles will be free to expand and recoil in comfortable *pranayama*.

False reasoning is behind the temptation to cram the lungs with air. For it is a mistake to think that beyond a certain point (which is a comfortable threshold, easily attained), the more air you take in the more oxygen you will absorb, to the benefit of the billions of body cells. The fact is that a point is reached after a short period of deep breathing when optimal oxygen is being received, and a surplus is then exhaled on the outgoing breath. If the deep breathing follows intense physical activity – as in running a sprint race – then huge amounts of oxygen will be needed and the chest will automatically heave and the mouth gape and gasp for air. But the immobile sitting Yogin is at the opposite end of the activity scale from the sprinter. Though vital capacity is improved, other factors than quantity of air are the Yogin's prime concerns: smoothness, and the length of inspiration and expiration and the in-between pauses. In a word: *control*. The minimum amount of air needed in Yogic practice is during the quiescence of meditation.

SUSPENSION (*KUMBHAKA*)

Holding the breath is a conscious act which checks the mechanism, described earlier, whereby our respiration is automatically regulated. We explained then that inspiration comes from an impulse through the vagus nerves and expiration from its inhibition, and that inflating the lungs stretches the sensory nerve endings, a signal for the expiratory part of the respiratory centre in the brain to inhibit the action of inspiration through an impulse along the vagus nerves. At the end of exhalation, the vagus action returns.

Now, with conscious suspension of breathing, we are switching from 'automatic' to 'manual', as it were. This requires some practice for smoothness and ease. And this means, as mentioned in discussing inhalation above, refraining from forcing, and making comfort the criterion. When *kumbhaka* follows filling the lungs, the thoracic 'umbrella' must stay open and the diaphragm down and the abdomen out during the immobile breathing pause. One has to inhibit an initial tendency of the ribs and diaphragm to recoil during the full pause, and to expand and rise respectively during the empty pause. However, after some weeks of training, inhibition becomes effortless as long as *kumbhaka* is not prolonged to a point of strain.

Once you have supplied the body richly with oxygen through deep breathing – the Yogin, unlike the athlete, is not making excessive calls for supply – you will find that the breath can be held longer without discomfort. In advanced practice Yogins may check their breathing for several minutes, but it would be prudent for most practitioners to suspend breathing for only a few seconds. Experiment will disclose your comfortable limits. The longer you have been breathing deeply, the more relaxed and poised is your sitting position, the more easily will air be retained in the lungs or and empty pause be sustained.

If after retention the air bursts out noisily, the suspension has been over-prolonged: the air should be released in a steady smooth stream from the nostrils. Similarly, following the empty pause, the air should unhurriedly and quietly begin its ascent of the nostrils. Do not push the muscles and lungs beyond comfortable capacity. The ease and comfort of performance should be reflected in the serenity of the facial expression.

During *kumbhaka* with full lungs or empty lungs, one should resist the temptation to let a little air through the nostrils or mouth to keep the suspension going comfortably. The abdomen should not change tone by contracting or relaxing.

THE IMPORTANCE OF SUSPENSION

Every day we perform numerous little *kumbhakas;* but few people give any thought to how much control of breathing is tied up with the diurnal pursuit of being a human. We suspend breathing to listen intently; to concentrate; to cry, sob, laugh, sing; when we are surprised; when we are waiting 'with bated breath'; when we need to be very still or very silent.

But what does Yogic breath suspension achieve? Why is it so important in *pranayama*?

There are esoteric answers, connected with the arousal and channelling of latent inner powers: but this aspect will be discussed in a later section of this book. The direct benefits from *kumbhaka* are both physiological and psychological.

A possible physiological benefit from *kumbhaka* is that the pause gives time for a better mixing of fresh air with the stale residual air in the air sacs of the lungs. The fact that some residual air remains in the 'dead space' between the nostrils and the bronchi and in the lungs was mentioned several pages back, in our account of the anatomy and physiology of respiration. Several writers on Hatha Yoga have pointed out that a suspension of breathing on filled lungs can have a cleansing and purifying effect on residual air. One of these is Professor Ernest Wood. The figures for residual air vary somewhat according to which textbook one consults, but the principle Professor Wood posits remains valid (94):

While the inflow and outflow of air should be 'regular', still an occasional practice of inner suspension (*kumbhaka*) has a cleansing value. We can see how this works, especially with reference to the alveolar air in the lungs. The lungs may be considered in three parts – the wider channels (the bronchi), then the narrower passages (the bronchioles), and lastly the very fine, even hair-fine, clusters of branchlets (the alveoli). A standard intake of breath by the average person occupies approximately two seconds. If it is 'shallow' it does not satisfactorily aerate the alveoli. Now, shallowness is not a matter of time or length of the inhalation, but of lack of strength and decisive action of the chest muscles, so that there is here an important point to be considered by shallow breathers, and to be acted upon by means of some decisive muscle-toning and habit-forming exercise. . . .

It must be understood that after full expiration the lungs are by no means empty of air. There will be, let us say, in a given person (for cases differ) 150 cubic centimetres of air in the space from the nostril to and including the bronchioles, which is termed 'dead space' because the air therein does not penetrate the relatively thick walls and produce any interchange of gases with the blood. After the expiration there will be, say, 200 cubic centimetres of air remaining in the lungs. Now, in inhaling let us say that 500 cubic centimetres of new air comes in, 150 cubic centimetres of the mixture will still be in the 'dead space', and 350 cubic centimetres will join the unexpired alveolar air, which is higher in carbon dioxide content and lower in oxygen content than the incoming air. A standard figure is that inhaled air contains 21% oxygen and exhaled air about 12%. The aeration of the blood is a big business, since the whole of the blood flows through the lungs in about 3 minutes, and amounts to one fifth of the entire weight of the body.

It is in the manner in which this incoming air arrives in the aureoles that one finds reason for the *kumbhaka* exercise. Experiments have been made which indicate that the diffusion or mixing of the inspired air (with its higher oxygen content and its lower carbon dioxide content) with the static air takes a little time. Further, the new air enters in the form of a cone in the centre of the duct, so that the old air still forms a layer on the inside walls of the tube until that diffusion takes place. . . .

I take it that the *kumbhaka* allows of more perfect diffusion than would occur when the exhalation begins immediately at the cessation of the inhalation. The ratio of inbreathing (1 unit of time), holding (4 units), and outbreathing (2 units) which is generally followed and taught by the *hatha-yogis* must, however, have been arrived at empirically, with a view to maximum benefit and operational economy, although it is thus seen to be scientifically sound.

In advanced Yoga practice 1:4:2 is indeed the timing ratio followed, but it must be understood at this point that 1:1:1 or 1:1:2 is a more realistic and less potentially harmful timing for the beginner or intermediate student. We will come to the timing of inspiration, retention, and expiration shortly.

'All forms of Yoga aim at producing a state of tranquillity in the subject,' says Aubrey Menen in *The New Mystics*. Yogins speak of *kevala kumbhaka*. *Kevala* means 'perfect', 'pure', 'whole'. *Kevala kumbhaka* refers to the practice of respiratory pause, either at the end of inbreathing or outbreathing, when it has become effortless and refined, so that the experience is one of inner peace and tran-

quillity, a freedom from anxiety, fear, and negative emotions of all
kinds, at its highest 'the peace that passeth all understanding'. The
benefits of repeated short peaceful respiratory pauses in *pranayama*
is cumulative. The nervous system is soothed and calmed, and
something of the tranquillity of Yoga practice is carried into everyday living. Combined with the postures, with mind-stilling meditation, and with the many other techniques of Yoga, breath regulation
and breath suspension make their large contribution to conducing
to equanimity of mind, in Sanskrit *samatwa*. To paraphrase Mr
Menen, all techniques of Yoga aim at producing a state of
tranquillity in the subject.

LOCKS (*BANDHAS*)

Various muscular restraints, seals, or locks are employed in advanced
pranayama. The Sanskrit term is *bandha*, related etymologically to
the English 'band', 'bind', 'bond', and 'bound'. *Bandhas* are part of
a larger grouping called *mudras*, which are muscle controls or exercises devised for special attainments, usually of an esoteric nature,
and for more specific results than the general postures (*asanas*).
There are 'seals' relating only to the control of energy currents
within the body – such as *mula bandha* and *asvini mudra*, which are
associated with the sexual energies, and the bizarre *khechari mudra*,
which requires that the tongue be cut loose from its attachment to
the floor of the mouth, so as to be free to curl back and block off the
passage of air from the nostrils to the windpipe. These esoteric
controls will be brought up again later, but a few locks employed in
holding the breath steady will be described now – though in my
opinion their use is best put to suspending breathing for durations
in excess of the moderate *kumbhakas* advocated in our practical
approach. The reason I say this is that each in some way creates
muscular tensions and pressures that disturb the sense of lightness,
buoyancy, and psycho-physical freedom that should be an exhilarating and liberating reward of Yogic breathing. It is true that they
are recommended in a number of works on Hatha Yoga, including
some written for the popular market. Readers may wish to experiment, and some may find the locks useful and without the discomfort experienced by this writer, who admittedly has a dislike of
unnecessary restraints and muscular tensions. The use of the

muscular locks is conceded if you are holding the breath for longer than, say, one minute – an exact time is impossible to give, for individual capacities vary. In advanced practice breath suspension may be sustained for several minutes, with profuse sweating and trembling; locking is then clearly essential. But our practical approach does not include *pranayama* carried to such lengths.

Stopping air from entering the nostrils requires some practice. Some people acquire the ability to pinch the nostrils by mental control, and also to dilate them to inhale air. Closing the mouth is a primary seal, and should be employed by all readers; this is combined with keeping the air steady in the lungs and in the passages ('dead spaces') between the nostrils and the lungs. This air can be used as a kind of 'ball' (metaphorically, not literally) to block any intrusion of external air into the body. A further control is essential: the muscles of respiration – the thoracic cage, the diaphragm, the abdomen – must, like the air in the lungs and passages, be held immobile.

The technique just described this writer finds adequate, but other methods are suggested in Yogic literature, and these some readers at least may wish to try out. Each, as mentioned above, involves some kind of muscular contraction or pressure.

One of these techniques is to lift the soft palate against the roof of the pharynx. Another is to close the glottis. Whether you know what the glottis is or not, you use it every time you swallow, and it can be dilated at will to modulate the tones of the voice. Italian operatic tenors sometimes employ what is known as the glottal stop to give a high note a cutting edge and a faintly explosive effect – the great Caruso was not immune from this gimmick. We have reflexes that command the glottis to open again after each swallow, so that the trick of keeping the glottis closed for some seconds has to be worked on. It is achieved by starting to swallow, and then freezing the movement at the point when the trachea or windpipe has closed.

Both the techniques described in the preceding paragraph I find unpleasant, imposing a suffocating feeling that defeats the purpose. Some readers, however, may find either one or both of the techniques helpful and not uncomfortable. But I repeat, in moderate *kumbhaka* bodily immobility plus the 'ball of air' method described above should prove adequate and have no tension-producing drawbacks. However, the two most frequently recommended *bandhas* have yet to be described. Their use in prolonged *kumbhaka* is probably essential, though not, I say again, in moderate breath suspension.

Chin Lock (Jalandhara Bandha)

Jala means 'a net'. The neck is stretched up and the chin lowered until it is pressing into the jugular notch between the collar bones and high up on the breastbone. The position is very similar to the one you should've already experienced in performing the Shoulderstand. In that posture you could not do otherwise, for the chest is brought against the chin in elevating the legs, pelvis, and trunk to a candle-straight vertical. But in the Shoulderstand one should always breathe as freely as possible, whereas *Jalandhara Bandha* is a way of firmly suspending breathing.

As with the soft palate and glottal controls, I experience a constricted and suffocating feeling during the Chin Lock. B. K. S. Iyengar considers *Jalandhara Bandha* essential; otherwise, he says, pressure is felt on the heart, behind the eyeballs, and in the ears, and the head feels dizzy. This may be so for prolonged breath control, but my experience is the reverse in moderate *kumbhaka*, when the contraction of the throat and neck causes a build-up of pressure. I am not alone in feeling this, for other students of Yoga report similar experiences; and my experience agrees with that of Archie Bahm, who finds the Chin Lock more valuable in sustaining a pause on emptied lungs than on filled lungs. He says (5): 'This position proves more useful in holding an empty pause, for the pressure of the chin against the chest pushes the base of the tongue and the larynx up into the pharynx and against the palate, thus providing aid in resisting the pressure caused by the vacuum in the lungs.' This account of what happens during *Jalandhara Bandha* reveals why I experience a choking effect and discomfort in the Chin Lock similar to that in lifting the soft palate against the roof the pharynx or in closing the glottis. It may be, of course, that persisting with practice of any of these three methods would eventually lead to a dissolving of my discomfort and psychological resistance.

Abdominal Uplift (Uddiyana Bandha)

Uddiyana means 'flying up'. This muscle control was described earlier. The lungs are emptied, the diaphragm is drawn up into the cavity of the thorax, and the abdominal wall and viscera are pulled back towards the spine, creating a deep hollow. The diaphragm is immobilized and a lock put on breathing action until the diaphragm and abdominal wall are released. The lock applies only to the empty pause, and clearly would be harmful on full lungs. Deep retraction is possible only on a full exhalation and an empty stomach. An instroke of the abdomen expels air and would be counterproductive following an inhalation. *Uddiyana* and the Chin Lock can be combined effectively.

Abdominal Uplift is effective for its purpose on emptied lungs, but it is based on a muscular contraction and it is not necessary for breath suspension of moderate duration. A drawback to its use, in my opinion, is the difficulty of releasing smoothly the retraction of the abdominal wall and diaphragm following a breath suspension: a sharp recoil causes an involuntary jerked inrush of air into the nostrils, whereas in skilled *pranayama* there should be a smooth, gentle start to inhalation or exhalation. Here again, some readers may not find this a problem.

Uddiyana Bandha is included among the cleansing processes in the classic texts, for reasons given in the section on that aspect of Yoga practice. We repeat what we said then - that the Abdominal Uplift is a superb muscle control in its own right, massaging and toning the diaphragm, abdominal wall, and abdominal organs (viscera), and is probably the greatest discovery ever made for achieving and maintaining intestinal and abdominal health and stimulating peristaltic action in the intestines, leading to more efficient absorption of nourishment from food and to regular natural emptying of the bowels.

The expression 'flying up' has also an esoteric reference. *Prana* or cosmic energy 'flies up' the main *nadi* or subtle nerve of the astral or subtle body. We will return to this in a later section.

In very advanced *pranayama*, *kumbhaka* may be prolonged for several minutes, until the subject sweats profusely, trembles, and even (we are told in the *Siva Samhita*) starts making short hops on the buttocks along the ground. When breath suspension is pursued to such lengths, suitable locks and seals are obviously essential.

WARNING

No more than momentary pauses between inhalation and exhalation are safe for persons with lung, heart, eye, or ear troubles, or for

persons with high blood pressure. Inhalations and exhalations should
be only of moderate length, and the vigorous breathing exercises,
the Cleansing Breath and the Bellows Breath described below,
should be omitted. Persons with low blood pressure may pause
briefly after breathing in, but should make no deliberate pause after
breathing out. The breath should not be deliberately held during
pregnancy.

If you have any doubts as to the suitability of any breath control,
consult your doctor.

EXHALATION (*RECHAKA*)

In *pranayama*, usually twice as much time is allocated to emptying
the lungs as to filling them – a result of the importance given to
thorough exhalation in traditional Yoga.

Carbon dioxide, the waste product which the cells exchange for
fresh oxygen every three minutes, is expelled from the body on the
outgoing breath. Some residual air, as we have seen, remains; but
the more complete and efficient the exhalation, the more efficient
the purification, and the greater the lung expansion and inflow of
fresh air and oxygen on the following inspiration.

The Austrian psychotherapist Wilhelm Reich, a pupil of Sigmund
Freud, found that his neurotic patients had developed muscular
blockages against thorough expulsion of stale air. The ability of
persons who have advanced far in Yogic self-mastery to respond
calmly in situations which would before have evoked an excited
response – anxiety, anger, flight, or fight – is in large part due to
mastery over breathing. Yoga psychology says that all ideas have
attendant emotions and that these play upon the respiratory processes. Excited emotions mean jerky breathing; smooth breathing
means calm emotions. Reich's work confirms this.

Full exhalation is a central technique in the psychotherapy of the
Reichian School. Reich himself wrote (163):

There is no neurotic individual who is capable of exhaling in one
breath, deeply and evenly. The patients have developed all conceivable
practices which prevent *deep expiration*. They exhale 'jerkily', or, as
soon as the air is let out, they quickly bring their chests back into the
inspiratory position. Some patients describe the inhibition, when they

become aware of it, as follows: 'It is as if a wave of the ocean struck a cliff. It does not go on.'

The sensation of this inhibition is localized in the upper abdomen or in the middle of the abdomen. With deep expiration, there appear in the abdomen vivid sensations of pleasure or anxiety. The function of the respiratory block (inhibition of deep expiration) is exactly that of avoiding the occurrence of these sensations. As a preparation for the process of bringing about the orgasm reflex, I ask my patients to 'follow through' with their breathing, to 'get into swing'. If one asks the patients to breathe deeply, they usually force the air in and out in an artificial manner. This voluntary behaviour serves only to prevent the natural vegetative rhythms of respiration. It is unmasked as an inhibition; the patient is asked to breathe without effort, that is, *not to do breathing exercises*, as he would like to do. After five to ten breaths, respiration usually becomes deeper and the first inhibitions make their appearance. With *natural* deep expiration, the head moves *spontaneously* backwards at the end of expiration. Patients are unable to let their heads go back in this spontaneous manner. They stretch their heads forward in order to prevent this spontaneous backward movement, or they jerk their heads violently to one side or the other side; at any rate, the movement is different from that which would come about naturally.

With natural respiration, the shoulders become relaxed and move gently and slightly forward at the end of expiration. Our patients hold their shoulders tight just at the end of expiration, pull them up or back; in brief, they execute various shoulder movements in order not to let the spontaneous vegetative movement come to pass.

TIMING

Yogic breathing is based on rhythm, and rhythm is life.

Strain can be avoided by keeping to a ratio between inhalation, retention, and exhalation of 1:1:1 for beginners, and later of 1:1:2. A few people may care to go on, whenever it is comfortable, to 1:2:2, but I do not recommend, without long preparation and personal supervision, the traditional ratio of 1:4:2.

Start breathing again after retention immediately the onset of any strain is discerned – at the first faint warning tickle, like the intimation of a sneeze; but in normal practice you should resume breathing action a little before that point. There are sound commensense grounds for sticking to 1:1:1 or 1:1:2; and the person who thinks that increasing the duration of breath retention will bestow on him occult powers is playing a dangerous game.

If you are unable to practise breathing with evenness, you need to shorten the duration of the stages. Remember that evenness of breathing is conducive to evenness of mind.

Few Yoga instructors teach more than a brief pause on empty lungs. The timing ratio quoted in Yoga literature is nearly always three figures rather than four. Archie Bahm (5) is an exception, for he considers that a longer empty pause is conducive to relaxation.

Counting seconds silently is the most straightforward method of timing. Some practice at inwardly repeating 'one'; 'two'; 'three'; or 'hundred-and-one'; 'hundred-and-two'; 'hundred-and-three;' and so on, with a watch before you, matching up the count with the seconds, will produce a skill useful in *pranayama* and also in activities outside Yoga. (I have always used it, with no loss of efficiency, in timing photographic enlargement exposures, and have never purchased a darkroom clock.)

Another method of timing is to repeat silently the Sanskrit words for inspiration, suspension, and expiration – *puraka*, *kumbhaka*, and *rechaka*. To accord with a 1:1:2 ratio, one would therefore silently pronounce '*puraka*' once, '*kumbhaka*' once, and '*rechaka*' twice as the basic timing units. Each word, it is true, has three syllables, but Sanskrit words do not come easily to Western lips and it can be embarrassing to compare your own pronunciation with that of an Indian.

Some Yogins listen to and count their heartbeats, but this is a technique not everyone can acquire.

There is another traditional method which uses a *matra* as the measure. Vachaspati, in his gloss on the *Yoga Sutras* of Patanjali, says: 'A *matra* is the time which is taken up by thrice turning up one's hand over one's knee and then snapping the fingers once. Measured by thirty-six such *matras* is the first attempt (*udghata*), which is mild. Twice that is the second, which is middling. Thrice that is the third, which is intense. This is the *Pranayama* as measured by number.' Theos Bernard says that a *matra* 'is generally considered to be equivalent to our second.'

Learning to count seconds silently seems the most practical approach.

SITTING FOR YOGIC BREATHING

The postures of Hatha Yoga, by stretching the muscles and by toning, relaxing, and strengthening the muscles of the chest, diaphragm, and abdomen, and improving their mobility and elasticity, encourage deep and efficacious breathing. The nature of many of the *asanas* is to trigger off naturally deep abdominal breathing. Stretching stimulates circulation and respiration, and by lifting bands of tension from the chest, diaphragm, and abdomen, sets free the muscles of deep breathing. Smooth deep breathing is an integral part of the performance of many postures.

But for Yogic breathing proper (*pranayama*) an immobile poised sitting posture is invariably adopted. This means sitting cross-legged on the floor with the back kept straight, the head held level, and the head, neck, and backbone in a vertical line, though always without rigidity. The sitting postures used for *pranayama* are the same as those used for meditation. Here, for Yogic breathing, we must be able to sit easily and without movement (other than respiratory) for fifteen minutes.

The experienced Yogin probably will sit in either the Perfect Posture or the Lotus Posture, both of which were described in the section on the *asanas*. But beginners may use the Easy Posture, which is as simple as its name implies. If you carried out the advice to start using it as soon as it was described earlier in this book, by now you will probably be able to sustain it comfortably for fifteen minutes of breath regulation. If not, sit with the head and spine in a vertical line on a straight-backed chair, or on a stool with your back and the back of your head against a wall.

When the head, neck, and spine are kept in poised vertical line, the internal organs are not cramped in any way: the ribs are free to expand and recoil to their limit of mobility, the lungs have space to inflate and deflate within the thoracic cage, and the abdomen is free of pressures either from below or from above, so long as no tight clothing, belt or girdle is worn. The diaphragm, between the thoracic cage and the abdomen, is unconstrained in performing its natural piston-like down-and-up action during inhalation and exhalation respectively. There is a sense of freedom and poise, and deep smooth *pranayama* is closely associated with both.

HAND POSITIONS

You can cup your hands in your lap, the back of the top hand resting on the palm of the hand below, the thumbs touching; or rest the right palm on the right knee and the left palm on the left' knee. But if you wish to observe good traditional form, you should straighten the arms until they are locked at the elbows and rest the back of the left wrist on the left knee and the back of the right wrist on the right knee. Hold your fingers in the Symbol or Seal of Knowledge (*Jnana Mudra*), which means bringing the tips of the thumbs and forefingers together and holding the other fingers out straight. The index finger here symbolizes the individual spirit (*Atman*) and the thumb the cosmic spirit (*Brahman*). The gesture thus represents the Union that is Yoga.

The only break from these positions is when one hand is raised to manipulate the nostrils with the fingers during the Alternate Nostril Breath. This technique is described and illustrated in the account of that exercise.

HOW OFTEN, AND FOR HOW LONG?

If you join an *ashram* in India you may be expected to practise *pranayama* four times a day: soon after rising in the morning, at noon, in the early evening, and shortly before retiring to bed for a night's sleep. But here we recommend once a day, morning or evening, or twice a day if you are very keen, morning *and* evening. If you practise once a day devote fifteen to twenty minutes to *pranayama*, and if twice a day, give ten minutes on each occasion.

PRE-REQUIREMENTS

Certain commonsense pre-requirements need to be observed before starting a session of breath controls.

Practise *pranayama* at a different time from postures. There should be an interval of at least one hour between finishing breath controls and starting postures, or between finishing postures and starting *pranayama*. There are several good reasons for this separation of the two programmes. Deep rhythmic breathing is an integral part of the postures, and you spend the whole of the fifteen minutes of Yogic breathing sitting in one of the postures. If combined, the programmes could produce fatigue by the end, instead of the customary refreshment. Moreover, starting the postures with the lungs highly ventilated and the organism highly vitalized is not the ideal approach: in some *asanas*, such as the inverted poses, it could produce dizziness. And, lastly, joining the two programmes together makes it more difficult to sustain the special kind of awareness and total attention that Yoga exercise requires.

Allow at least two hours to pass after a main meal, and one hour after a light snack, before starting *pranayama*.

Sit in a clean, well-ventilated, pleasant room; better still, sit out of doors when the weather and temperature permit.

Wear a minimum of slackly-fitting clothing, or no clothing at all if conditions permit, so enabling your skin to join fully in the breathing.

Empty the bladder just before practice and evacuate the bowels if you can. The former is always possible; the latter can be achieved regularly if you make a habit of going to stool at this time every day.

Pranayama is a process of purification. It is traditional before breathing practice to wash the hands and face with tepid or cold water, to gargle and rinse out the mouth, and to massage the tongue and gums gently with the fingers for a minute or so. Some Yogins also clean the tongue by scraping it carefully and gently with the back of a spoon.

Blow each nostril sharply a few times to clear it. One nostril is likely to remain partly blocked, but opens further during exercise. Some Yogins use the traditional nasal cleansing method of drawing water up the nostrils and expelling it from the mouth: this clears the nostrils and is said to prevent colds, though not everyone finds it easy to become accustomed to the strange sensation.

According to Hatha Yoga teaching, the flow of *prana* normally changes from one nostril to the other every two hours, and one nostril is usually partially or totally closed. You can clear a nostril by lying on that side with the arm strongly pressed against the body, or alternatively by pressing down the armpit on the active side on top of a chair-back or a similar narrow firm object. The Hatha Yogins actually use a piece of equipment which looks rather like a crutch for this purpose; the lower end rests firmly on the ground and the Yogin presses down his armpit on the handle.

PERFORMANCE

Sit in one of the meditative cross-legged postures or on a straight-backed chair or a stool with your back against a wall. Head and backbone must be in a straight vertical line.

Close the eyes to help the mind focus sharply on the breath flow. In the stable sitting posture there should be no overbalancing or swaying.

Breathe through the nostrils, not the mouth, unless instructed to the contrary in the description of the exercise. Yogins point out that the mouth is for eating and the nostrils are for breathing. Blood circulating in the nasal passages heats the inhaled air so that it is warmed before entering the lungs. The nostrils also perform two more valuable services: dry air is moistened in the passages, and the hairs in the nostrils trap dust or any foreign matter in the atmosphere that could be harmful if it reached the lungs. Many Yogins develop an ability to dilate the nostrils to produce a silent and automatic inflow of air.

Never force any of the stages of breathing. Especially is this true of suspending the breath (*kumbhaka*). Never cram the lungs with air to what feels like almost bursting point. Start the breath flowing again before reaching the point of discomfort or strain in the suspension.

If the tongue is kept still, saliva should not be a problem; but if it does gather, you should swallow it, though not while holding the breath or exhaling it.

Powerful practice causes profuse sweating and muscular trembling, but this should rarely result from the moderate practice advised here. If it does, bring the session to an end with a few minutes relaxation, lying on the back in the Corpse Posture.

There is a right attitude of mind for performing Yogic breathing, and that is one of calmness, quietness, and total attention. Concentration is complete, yet never effortful. The Buddhists call such rapt and effortless attention 'mindfulness'. When turned to *pranayama*, one becomes unsure whether one is directing a breathing activity or being breathed, just as brilliant ballroom dancers cease to be conscious of which of them is the leader and which the led.

Some treatises advise harnessing the considerable powers of the imagination during breath controls, visualizing the expulsion of fatigue toxins and impurities on exhalation, and the intake of purity, oxygen, vitality, and *prana* on the inhalation.

PREPARATIONS FOR THE TRADITIONAL *PRANAYAMAS*

The inadequacies of shallow high upper-chest breathing have already been stressed, and so has the importance of breathing deeply and diaphragmatically. It was also explained how the diaphragm, the key and largest muscle in the act of breathing, acts like a piston, flattening out and moving down on inhalation, and rising and regaining its dome shape on exhalation. With each inspiration and expiration during deep breathing there is a concomitant action on the abdominal wall, which swells out on the inspiration and subsides and moves back towards the spine on the expiration. It is important to experience this combined diaphragmatic and abdominal movement, to feel it clearly and to memorize that feeling, and to acquire the habit of deep breathing in this way for life.

Supine Abdominal Breathing
One effective way of acquiring this experience and habit in the early stages of learning is to lie flat on the back, the legs fully extended, the arms bent, and the palms of the hands flat on the abdomen so that the tips of the longest fingers meet over the navel. The backs of the upper arms rest on the floor, and the forearms are held in against the ribs.

Only the thoracic cage, the diaphragm, and the abdomen will be in action, so relax the rest of the body muscles. The full length of the back should be flat against the floor. If the legs are relaxed, the feet should naturally fall out to the side, with the inside edges of the heels staying in contact, or almost so. If the lower back stays down flat on the floor, the muscular sensations of the widening of the thoracic cage will be more strongly felt.

Now inhale slowly, taking a deep unhurried breath, though without cramming the lungs with air to the point of discomfort. Concentrate your attention fully on the muscular movement: the ribs expanding outwards, pushing against the forearms, the diaphragm flattening and moving down, the abdomen swelling out and rising below the palms of the hands (*see* illustration). Breathe slowly and smoothly, through the nostrils, not the mouth.

Pause for two or three seconds at the comfortable limit of inspiration; then start releasing air slowly and steadily from the nostrils. The reverse muscular process to that of inhalation will now be experienced. Note the sensations carefully, as you did during inbreathing. The ribs subside like an umbrella being closed, the forearms move inwards in sympathy with the thoracic cage, the diaphragm rises, the abdomen flattens and moves back towards the spine below the palms of the hands (*see* illustration). Make a thorough exhalation; pause for two or three seconds; then start another inhalation.

Breathe slowly and evenly in this way – inspiration, brief pause, expiration, brief pause, inspiration, and so on – for about three minutes. Give your full attention to memorizing the muscular sensations of deep breathing – the thoracic, diaphragmatic, and abdominal movements, the pressures against the palms of the hands and the forearms, and those of the back against the floor.

After four weeks of daily practice you should record the muscular sensations with the palms of the hands and the forearms only during the first minute of Supine Abdominal Breathing. During the following two minutes keep the palms of the hands flat on the floor and the arms relaxed along the sides of the body, and with muscular (kinesthetic) sense, without the aid of the palms or forearms, concentrate on the now subtler sensations of deep breathing as you slowly and smoothly inhale and exhale. Again take careful mental note of the rise and fall of the abdomen, the down-and-up movement of the diaphragm, and the out-and-in, umbrella-like expansion and recoil of the rib-cage.

One important further operation is necessary. So that deep healthful breathing becomes an established habit, from now on, as long as it proves valuable, for a minute or two several times each day – while standing, sitting, walking, or lying on your back – move the beam of your attention to your breathing and re-create the sensations of abdominal breathing anew.

Pumping
This is a useful associate exercise to Supine Abdominal Breathing. It is an abdominal rather than a breathing exercise, but it focuses attention on the rise and fall of the abdomen, as the preceding

breathing exercise does, though it is more localized and powerful. At the same time it beneficially massages the abdominal viscera.

Lie flat on the back, the arms by the sides with the palms of the hands turned up, the legs fully extended together. Relax fully, and concentrate all your attention on the abdomen – the head, neck, shoulders, arms, and legs all stay relaxed. The back should be flat against the floor along its full length. Take a rapid deep breath through the nostrils, so that the abdominal wall swells out; then immediately pull the abdomen back towards the spine with a sharp instroke and expel air from the nose in an exhalation as rapid as the preceding inhalation. It is important that the shoulders, the upper and lower back, and the pelvis stay in firm contact with the floor. All the action is centred in the abdomen, except for the inevitable piston action of the diaphragm and the expansion and recoil of the rib-cage – but this being an abdominal and not a breathing exercise, all your attention should be brought to bear on the swelling out and pulling in of the abdominal wall.

Each out-and-in movement of the abdomen should take one second, and ten successive out-and-in movements should be performed. Relax for about twenty seconds, breathing normally; then perform another round of Pumping.

Pumping should be performed daily during the period of establishing the habit of abdominal breathing, and may be continued afterwards by those readers who find its deep massage beneficial.

The Complete Yoga Breath
This differs from Supine Abdominal Breathing only in being a fuller sensation, and always being performed with the back and head held erect. You are conscious that you draw more air into the lungs and empty them more thoroughly. The upright posture makes possible a greater vital capacity than is practicable when lying flat on the back. But this should not be taken to mean the filling of every nook and cranny of the lungs, which is physiologically impossible, or the emptying out of every scrap of air from the same organs, which is again physiologically impossible. It does, however, mean an inhalation carried to the point of a feeling of fullness without strain, and an exhalation carried to the point of full subsidence of the abdomen, full raising of the diaphragm, and full recoil of the ribs, accompanied by the feeling of having emptied the lungs completely. *Complete* Yoga Breath is the customary description of this exercise, and only

pedants will cavil at the use of the word 'complete'. The movement is complete in that you are conscious of all the respiratory muscles working and have a feeling first of fullness, and then of emptiness in the lungs.

Sit on the floor in one of the cross-legged postures, or on a straight-backed chair, keeping the back and head erect, the hands cupped in the lap, or right and left hand on right and left knee respectively. Kneeling and then sitting back on the heels with the spine straight and vertical also encourages natural deep breathing. Inhale and exhale through the nostrils.

In the Complete Yoga Breath you fill the lungs to a point of fullness without strain or discomfort. A key part of the 'completeness' of this exercise is to think of the lungs as having three parts – this is a ruse, a visualization, an employment of imagination, but it serves a purpose. Think of the lungs as being composed of lower, middle, and upper spaces. The lower lungs are visualized and imagined as being filled first; then the middle lungs; and finally the upper lungs: the accompanying muscular movements are the act of breathing described above – thoracic cage expanding, diaphragm lowering, abdomen swelling out – divided into three stages, and reaching the limit of expansion at the conclusion of the third stage, filling the upper lungs and broadening the chest. Some instructors advise lifting the collar bones at the very end of the inspiration, in addition to the diaphragmatic and intercostal action. There is a tendency for shallow high-chest breathers to lift their shoulders, and it is therefore undesirable, in my opinion, in daily habit or in practising the Complete Yoga Breath.

The Complete Yoga Breath fills and empties the lungs very efficiently, richly oxygenating the blood during filling and removing waste gases during emptying. Though the exercise is visualized as having three stages, there should be one continuous smooth movement. Do not strain – when the lungs feel comfortably full, stop the movement and the intake of air. Exhale in a controlled smooth continuous movement, the air streaming steadily out of the nostrils. Employ imagination to think of and visualize an inflow of universal energy (*prana*) and an outflow of impurities and fatigue toxins.

Make four or five complete in-and-out breaths in a minute. Rest for twenty seconds, and then perform four or five more Complete Yoga Breaths. Include pauses between inhalation and exhalation, and between exhalation and inhalation, lasting two or three seconds.

The Complete Yoga Breath vitalizes; removes phlegm; tones and steadies the nervous system; purifies and enriches the blood; improves appetite; aids digestion; broadens and strengthens the thorax; massages the abdominal organs; and makes consciousness lucid and alert. Once it has been mastered, deep, even, and rhythmical breathing can be produced at will. It will be found valuable at times when instant vitality is required. It has the power to lift anxious, fearful, and melancholy moods.

Walking Breath Control
Professor Wood (94) suggests that beginners may start regulating respiration by taking a brisk early-morning walk, breathing in for eight paces, and then breathing out for the following eight paces; and that the beginner takes such walks for two weeks to a month before starting *pranayama*.

I see no need for such a preliminary, but recommend Walking Breath Control at any time of day for students at any stage of experience. As the student introduces breath pauses, these can be included in the breathing rhythm of walking also. But avoid excesses. It would not be sensible to employ breath control throughout a walk of several miles: rather, perform five or six in-and-out breaths, and then breathe freely for two or three minutes; then repeat the rhythmic controlled breathing for five or six in-and-out breaths. Three rounds of such regulated breathing will be sufficient for the beginner, increasing gradually to ten on longish walks.

THE TRADITIONAL *PRANAYAMAS*

The preceding controls – Supine Abdominal Breathing and the Complete Yoga Breath – are preparations for the traditional *pranayamas*, eight in number. The *Hatha Yoga Pradipika* says (77):
Brahma and other Devas [gods] were always engaged in the exercise of *Pranayama*, and, by means of it, got rid of the fear of death. Therefore, one should practise *Pranayama* regularly. So long as the breath is restrained in the body, so long as the mind is undisturbed, and so long as the gaze is fixed between the eyebrows, there is no fear from Death. When the system of the *Nadis* becomes clear of the impurities by properly controlling the *prana*, then the air, piercing the entrance of the *Sushumna* [spinal channel], enters it easily. Steadiness of mind

comes when the air moves freely in the middle [of the *Sushumna*].
This is the *manomani* condition [*samadhi*], which is attained when the
mind becomes calm. To accomplish it, various *Kumbhakas* are performed by those who are expert in the methods; for, by the practice
of different *Kumbhakas*, wonderful success is attained. *Kumbhakas* are
of eight kinds, viz. *Surya Bhedana, Ujjayi, Sitkari, Sitali, Bhastrika,
Bhramari, Murchha,* and *Plavini.*

The *Gheranda Samhita* says (90): 'The *Kumbhakas* or retentions
of breath are of eight sorts; *Sahita, Surya-bheda, Ujjayi, Sitali,
Bhastrika, Bharmari, Murchha,* and *Kevali.*' The substitutes *Sahita*
and *Kevali* are controls belonging to esoteric *pranayama* and need
not concern us now.

To the eight main traditional controls we will here add a ninth,
Kapalabhati, which is included with the purification (hygienic)
practices in the classic texts, but which is now usually listed as
pranayama.

Cleansing Breath (Kapalabhati)

'When inhalation and exhalation are performed very quickly, like a
pair of bellows of a blacksmith, it dries up all the disorders from the
excess of phlegm, and is known as *Kapalabhati*,' says the *Hatha
Yoga Pradipika* (77). *Kapala* means 'skull' and *bhati* means 'light'.
This is the only major Yogic breathing exercise that does not
include a breath retention (*kumbhaka*), though the somewhat similar
Bellows Breath (*Bhastrika*) includes an apoenia only on the last
breath of each round.

Kapalabhati is one of the *shatkarmas* or purifying techniques,
and its purpose is not deep breathing but a cleansing of the frontal
air passages. It should therefore be performed immediately before
practice of the main *pranayamas*. The Bellows Breath (*Bhastrika*)
may be used as a substitute, and is slightly more vigorous.

To perform *Kapalabhati*, you breath in and out rapidly,
contracting the stomach muscles and pulling them back towards
the spine on each sharp expulsion of air, and immediately letting go
from the contraction so that the natural recoil of the abdominal wall
brings an automatic inspiration. The Pumping exercise described
above will strengthen the abdominal muscles for the repeated
instrokes required for the Cleansing Breath.

Use diaphragmatic breathing, swelling out and drawing in the
abdomen, and concentrating on the exhalations, which should be

one a second at the start, speeding up to two exhalations a second after three or four weeks' practice. Begin with a round of ten exhalations, and add to this gradually until you are comfortable with twenty to a round. Perform three rounds, with rest pauses between first and second, and second and third, lasting from a few seconds up to a minute, as comfort allows.

Rhythm of performance is important. One tradition gives the durations of inhalation and exhalation as equal, but another tradition says that outbreathing should take only half the time taken by inbreathing. The former is the easier rhythm for beginners; the latter may be acquired later, if you wish.

Dr Behanan (6) says that any of the meditative postures is good enough as long as *kapalabhati* is practised for a short time, say, four or five minutes. When practised for a longer period, however, the lotus-posture is the only one available. The reason is that when the breathing is carried on over long periods certain vibrations are started all over the body and this, coupled with a feeling of exhilaration, results in a lessening of the motor control over the limbs. But in the lotus-posture the legs are formed into such a firm lock that it is impossible to undo them without the help of the hands, and hence [the legs are] not likely to be disturbed by the lessening motor control.

This shows why the Lotus Posture is considered essential for advanced Yogic practice, but we do not recommend that the home practitioner, using book instruction, should prolong either *Kapalabhati* or *Bhastrika* to the point, mentioned by Dr Behanan, where there is a loss of motor control.

The Cleansing Breath and Bellows Breath are not suitable for persons suffering from high blood pressure, or from eye or ear, complaints.

The benefits of the Cleansing Breath are to clear the nasal passages, purify the blood, cleanse the sinuses, remove phlegm, improve circulation, generate *pranic* vitality, tone the nervous system, stimulate the liver, spleen, and pancreas, improve digestion, facilitate evacuation, strengthen and tone the abdominal muscles, and massage the abdominal organs (viscera).

Bellows Breath (Bhastrika)

Bhastrika means 'bellows'. Dr Behanan says (6): '*Bhastrika* is a *pranayama* which is held in high esteem by yogins. This type of breathing is claimed to be best among all the yogic *pranayamas* for arousing the spiritual forces and for preparing the practitioner for concentration (*dharana*) and meditation (*dhyana*).' The Bellows Breath resembles the Cleansing Breath in its first part, and Dr Bernard, when training in Hatha Yoga in India, was taught the former in place of the latter breath control as a purificatory practice.

There are several varieties, but all use the rapid bellows-like breathing of *Kapalabhati*. Each version, however, unlike *Kapala-bhati*, concludes with a long deep breath, a suspension, and a long slow exhalation – a Complete Yoga Breath, or *Ujjayi* with wide-open glottis.

Version I.   This is the most straightforward version, and as efficacious as any. In the first stage, perform the preceding Cleansing Breath ten to twenty times, using both nostrils for inhalations and exhalations. In the second stage, after the final rapid breath, take one slow smooth deep breath through both nostrils, hold it comfortably for a few seconds, and then let it out of the nostrils in a slow smooth continuous flow. This completes one round. The early bellows-like breathing should be vigorous and noisy, though always with rhythmic timing, and the second stage a model of smoothness and control.

Version II.   The first stage is as given for version I, but the second stage, like *Ujjayi*, uses a tradition in which one breathes in through the right nostril, keeping the left nostril closed, and then out through the left nostril, keeping the right nostril closed. During retention, both nostrils are closed by the fingers and thumb as will be described and illustrated when we come to the Alternate Nostril Breath. The right hand is not raised at all during the first part of the exercise.

Version III.   During the first stage, which is like *Kapalabhati*, inhale and exhale through the right nostril while keeping the left nostril closed. Then immediately take your customary number of rapid breaths (ten to twenty) through the left nostril while keeping the right nostril closed. Follow with *Ujjayi*, using both nostrils and keeping the glottis open.

Version IV.   Proceed as in version III, except that you use the traditional *Ujjayi* in which you inhale through the right nostril and exhale through the left nostril, as described for version II.

Version V.   Breathe rapidly in and out during the first stage, using only the right nostril. In the slow deep complete breath which follows, again use the right nostril only, keeping the other nostril closed. For the second round use the left nostril only for both stages. For the third round use the right nostril only for both stages. Return to keeping the right nostril closed and the left nostril open for the fourth and final round. Odd numbers – right nostril. Even numbers – left nostril.

Version VI.   This is similar to version V; but in the slow final stage breathe in through the nostril which was kept open in the fast early stage, and breathe out through the nostril which was kept closed.

Version VII.   During the *Kapalabhati* stage, inhale through the right nostril and exhale through the left nostril during rounds one and three, and breathe in through the left nostril and out through the right nostril during rounds two and four. Procedure in the second stage, the single complete breath, remains the same: inhale through the right nostril and exhale hrough the left nostril.

Version VIII.   The first stage is as in version VII, but in the second stage the use of the nostrils corresponds to that in the preceding round of fast breathing. This means that during rounds one and three the *Ujjayi* breath is inhaled through the right nostril and exhaled through the left nostril, but during rounds two and four the roles of the left and right nostrils are reversed.

This by no means completes the number of variations, for some teachers favour the use of the slightly closed glottis during stage one or stage two, or even during both. This produces a sort of sobbing sound in the throat. A somewhat similar effect is produced by the use of the Chin Lock (*Jalandhara Bandha*) during either the *Kapalabhati* or the *Ujjayi* stage, or during both stages.

By first introducing the slightly closed glottis into the eight versions given above; then the Chin Lock; and finally the glottal contraction and Chin Lock in combination, the permutations of *Bhastrika* can be made enormous. Fortunately, I feel we can dispense with both techniques. Slightly closing the glottis serves a purpose in slowing down and introducing a greater element of control into *Ujjayi*, and *Jalandhara Bandha* has its value in advanced *kumbhaka*, but both methods may be omitted without real loss of effect in the Bellows Breath. And as the traditional *Ujjayi* practice of inbreathing with the right nostril and outbreathing with the left nostril is not insisted upon in most modern instruction, our choice of versions to make up four rounds can be made from versions I, III, V, VI, and VIII. In performing four rounds, you can concentrate or combine as you wish, though it is probably desirable that version I should be included at least once.

The benefits are as given for the Cleansing Breath (*Kapalabhati*), though more intense, since a greater intake of air and oxygen results from the complete breath that terminates each round. There are also different physiological effects due to the retention of air between inbreathing and outbreathing during the second stage.

AlternateNostril or Sun and Moon Breath (Anuloma Viloma Pranayama)

Anuloma and *viloma* mean 'with the hair' and 'against the hair' respectively, or, as we might say, 'with the grain' and 'against the grain'.

This is given as a cleansing *pranayama* in the old texts, and makes a gentle alternative for those who find *Kapalabhati* or *Bhastrika* too vigorous. You breathe slowly, smoothly, and deeply through one nostril, the other nostril being held closed, either with the thumb (right nostril) or the ring and little fingers (left nostril) of the right hand. It has the effect of purifying the *nadis* or nerve channels, and its ability to soothe the nervous system and to calm the mind will be apparent from even early practice. This is a most valuable breath control by any criterion.

Before describing the respiratory procedure, it is important to learn the technique traditionally used for closing and releasing the nostrils. No special magical or occult significance need be attached to this particular use of the fingers, but it has been found effective for many centuries.

The index and middle finger of the right hand are folded over and pressed against the palm. The thumb is used to close the right nostril, and the ring and little finger together close the left nostril. Some authorities say that the fingers and thumb should be kept straight; others say that they should be bent at the top joint. Use whichever technique feels most comfortable. To close a nostril, press against the fatty tissue below the nasal bone so that its inner surface rests against the septum that divides the nose into two passages, blocking the nostril on that side. Only gentle pressure need be applied. Keep your fingernails clear of the tissue (*see* illustration).

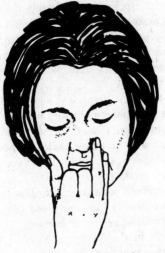

The traditional Yogic method of closing the nostrils during single nostril breathing

Left-handed people may, if they wish, use the left hand, closing the left nostril with the thumb and the right nostril with the ring finger and little finger of the left hand.

For once the classic texts give straightforward and unambiguous instruction for practice of this breath control, and are in accord. It is given as a purification process, prior to the naming and describing of the main *pranayamas*. A similar type of single-nostril breathing *is* included among the main *pranayamas*. This is the Sun Piercing Breath, so named because the right nostril or 'sun tube' is used invariably for inhaling.

The *Hatha Yoga Pradipika* gives a straightforward and clear description of the Alternate Nostril or Sun and Moon Breath (77):

Sitting in the *Padmasana* [Lotus] Posture the Yogi should fill in the air through the left nostril (closing the right one); and keeping it confined according to one's ability, it should be expelled slowly through the right nostril. Then, drawing in the air through the right nostril slowly, the belly should be filled, and after performing *Kumbhaka* [suspension] as before, it should be expelled slowly through the left nostril. Inhaling thus through the one, through which it was expelled, and having restrained it till possible, it should be exhaled through the other, slowly and not forcibly. If the air be inhaled through the left nostril, it should be expelled again through the other, and filling it through the right nostril, and confining it, should be expelled through the left nostril. By practising in this way, through the right and the left nostrils alternately, the whole of the collection of the *nadis* of the *yamis* [practitioners] becomes clean, i.e. free from impurities, after three months.

The account in the *Siva Samhita* is equally clear (91):

Then let the wise practitioner close with his right thumb the *Pingala* [the right nostril], inspire air through the *Ida* [the left nostril]; and keep air confined – suspend his breathing – as long as he can, and afterwards let him breathe out slowly, and not forcibly, through the right nostril. Again, let him draw breath through the right nostril, and stop breathing as long as his strength permits; then let him expel the air through the left nostril, not forcibly but slowly and gently. . . . He should practise this daily without neglect or idleness.

The account given in the *Gheranda Samhita* is in accord with that given in the other two texts, but adds visualizations (*yantras*) and recitations (*mantras*).

Blow each nostril before practice, and clear it. Some Yogins sniff water and expel it from the mouth after it has appeared in the throat. If one nostril remains partly blocked, it should clear during the exercise. If it is badly blocked, use it for exhaling only for a few rounds.

If one nostril seems more open than the other, this is not surprising, for according to Yoga teaching one nostril predominates in breathing, and the roles are reversed every two hours. During illness this two-hourly rhythm is impaired and one nostril may stay blocked or partly blocked for much longer.

The stages of the Alternate Nostril Breath are as follows:

Sit cross-legged in one of the meditative postures, keeping the head and back erect.

The left hand may be in one of two positions. In the first position, the arm is straightened and the back of the wrist rests on the left knee; in this case it is customary to have the thumb and index finger joined at their tips and to hold the other fingers out straight (*Jnana*

Mudra). Alternatively, let the left hand rest, palm up, in your lap.

Hold the right hand up to the nose, with the thumb and fingers held in the manner described and illustrated above.

Close both eyes.

Close the right nostril by pressing the thumb against the fatty tissue below the nasal bone until it meets the septum that divides the nose into two passages.

Exhale steadily through the left nostril until the lungs feel emptied.

Inhale slowly, smoothly, and deeply through the left nostril, blocking the right nostril, until the lungs feel comfortably filled. Breathe in deeply in the manner already taught, filling the lower, middle, and upper lungs progressively.

Close the left nostril with the ring and little fingers of the right hand. Both nostrils are now blocked.

Hold the breath steadily and easily in the lungs for a few seconds. The Chin Lock may be used, but it is not essential for a short suspension.

Now open the right nostril by lifting the pressure of the thumb against it, but keep the left nostril blocked. Raise the chin from the chest if you have been using the Chin Lock (*Jalandhara Bandha*).

Exhale slowly and smoothly through the right nostril until the lungs feel emptied.

Pause only a second or two before starting inhaling through the right nostril. The left nostril stays blocked. Fill the lungs comfortably.

Close the right nostril with the thumb. Both nostrils are now blocked.

Retain the air for a few seconds without strain.

Open the left nostril by releasing the pressure from the ring and little fingers of the right hand.

Exhale slowly, smoothly, and continuously through the left nostril until the lungs have been emptied.

That completes a round. Perform three to five rounds.

The facial muscles should stay relaxed during the breath control; ideally, the facial expression should be serene.

The traditional texts advise fixing the attention between the eyebrows. The point where the flow of air first strikes the nasal passages is another favoured focusing spot. The aim of such focusing is to steady the mind. Another way of concentrating the mind is to listen to the hissing sound the air makes as it enters and leaves the nose.

The technique of the Alternate Nostril Breath can be briefly summarized as follows:

Having closed the right nostril, effect a preparatory emptying of the lungs through the left nostril before the breath control proper.
Inhale through the left nostril.
Close the left nostril.
Suspend the breath for a few seconds with both nostrils blocked.
Open the right nostril.
Exhale through the right nostril.
Inhale through the right nostril.
Close the right nostril.
Suspend the breath for a few seconds with both nostrils blocked.
Open the left nostril.
Exhale through the left nostril.
Repeat for a second round.

A number of variations are possible. A few rounds may be performed using one nostril for both inhalation and exhalation, without alternating; or you may inhale through one nostril but exhale through both; and so on. But the basic technique is as given in detail above.

Deep and finely-controlled breathing is possible with the Alternate Nostril Breath. The benefits are that it aerates the lungs richly, cleanses the nasal passages and sinuses, purifies the *nadis* or nerve channels, richly oxygenates and purifies the blood, tones and soothes the nervous system, stimulates the appetite, improves digestion, relaxes and refreshes the body, and calms and steadies the mind.

In Sun and Moon breathing the positive and negative *pranic* currents are harmonized and equalized, and the technique of alternate nostril breathing has a role in esoteric Yoga connected with the arousal and control of latent psychic force and the fluctuations and movements of psychic nerve-force within the body.

If for some good reason you cannot perform your full programme of breath controls, then at least perform this one. It can moreover be employed with advantage at times when you particularly need to relax and to calm the mind.

Sun Piercing Breath (Surya Bhedana)

Surya means 'sun' and *bhedana* comes from the root *bhid*, which means 'to pierce'. The sun features in this *pranayama* because you always close the left nostril and inhale through the right or sun nostril, filling the lungs comfortably. You then close the right nostril, so that both nostrils are blocked, and hold the breath for a few seconds, avoiding strain. Open the left nostril by releasing the pressure of the ring and little fingers, and exhale slowly, smoothly, and continuously through the left nostril until the lungs feel emptied.

This completes one round. Perform five to ten rounds. Concentrate the attention as described for the Alternate Nostril Breath.

To summarize the technique:

Close the left nostril.

Breathe in through the right nostril.

Close the right nostril.

Suspend breathing for a few seconds with both nostrils blocked.

Open the left nostril.

Exhale through the left nostril.

Repeat for a second round.

The *Hatha Yoga Pradipika* describes this control succinctly (77): 'Taking any comfortable posture and performing the *asana*, the Yogi should draw in the air slowly, through the right nostril. Then it should be confined within, so that it fills from the nails of the toes to the tips of the hair on the head, and then let out through the left nostril slowly.'

Compare this with the *Gheranda Samhita* (90): 'Inspire with all your strength the external air through the sun-tube [right nostril]: retain this air with the greatest care, performing the *Jalandhara Mudra*. Let the *Kumbhaka* be kept up until the perspiration burst out from the tips of the nails and the roots of the hair.'

Readers without personal supervision should not attempt such prolonged breath-retention, which is common practice under Indian *ashram* conditions. Theos Bernard (7) mentions holding his breath in this *pranayama* for thirty seconds, using the Chin Lock (*Jalandhara Bandha*), and performing ten rounds at the beginning; he worked up to eighty seconds. He was performing *pranayama* four times a day: morning, noon, early evening, and at midnight. This is an old tradition. But he adds that such intensive *pranayama* 'is quite unnecessary for the beginner,' and that 'I was advised never to hold the breath so long that it caused undue strain. It is the repetition of the practice that is recommended, not the use of a great amount of effort.'

Dr Bernard used the Chin Lock (*Jalandhara Bandha*) between inhalation and exhalation, which is customary procedure, but B. K. S. Iyengar (35) in his descriptions of *Surya Bhedana* and Alternate Nostril Breath says that it should be applied prior to the inhalation and that the chin should be kept down throughout the controls.

The benefits are as given for the Alternate Nostril Breath.

Victorious Breath (Ujjayi)

This is another of the main varieties of *pranayama*, and one of the most important. The most widely-practised version uses both nostrils for inhalation and exhalation, and this we will describe first. An older tradition instructs that the breath, after being held, is released through the left nostril. The glottis is partly closed during inhalation and exhalation, producing an audible sound.

Theos Bernard (7) calls *Ujjayi* 'an easy method of deep chest breathing'. That the chest is here expanded is shown by the naming of this *pranayama*, for *jaya* means 'victory', 'triumph', or 'conquest'. The abdomen is kept slightly contracted, and the thoracic cage is expanded fully – a different emphasis from that of the Complete Yoga Breath taught earlier.

Sit in one of the meditative postures, keeping the spine and head erect. As no manipulation of the nostrils is required in this version, the hands stay cupped in the lap, or the arms are straightened so that the back of the left wrist rests on the left knee and the back of the right wrist rests on the right knee, the thumbs and index fingers together and the other fingers held out straight in the gesture known as *Jnana Mudra* or Symbol of Knowledge.

Exhale fully, using either nostrils or mouth. This is preparatory to the start of the Victorious Breath proper.

Draw air in through both nostrils in a slow and continuous flow, whose evenness is measured by its being made audible by partly closing the glottis, the opening from the pharynx into the windpipe which modulates speech and which can be felt to close in swallowing. This partial closure means that the air enters more slowly, and as well as being felt, it is heard to be regulated by the frictional sound produced. The indrawn air strikes the palate with a cool, soft, brushing effect. Continue the inhalation until the lungs feel full, though not so full that they seem about to burst. The prime mover in making this deep inhalation is a full expansion of the thoracic cage. The abdomen is slightly contracted and drawn slightly back to form a flat surface from breastbone to pubic bone. A slight raising of the chest at the end of inspiration helps this. Note how here the action differs from the more diaphragmatic and abdominal emphasis of the Complete Yoga Breath.

Hold the breath comfortably for a few seconds. The glottis is here closed. Dr Bernard was taught to swallow and then use the Chin Lock (*Jalandhara Bandha*). Again B. K. S. Iyengar differs from most accounts in operating the Chin Lock throughout inspiration, suspension, and expiration, and teaches the use of two *bandhas*, *Uddiyana* and *Mula*, during the *kumbhaka*. In the former the abdominal wall is pulled back towards the spine; in the latter the sphincters of the anus are squeezed tightly. But I repeat that the seals need only be used by advanced students.

Now let the air out slowly, smoothly, and continuously through both nostrils until the lungs feel emptied. The glottis having been partly opened, again we hear the regulated sound as the breath flows. Raise the chin from the chest if you have used the Chin Lock.

That completes a round.

Beginners should take exactly the same length of time for inhalation (*puraka*) and for exhalation (*rechaka*), and also for suspension (*kumbhaka*) if comfort allows – a ratio of 1:1:1. For intermediate students the ratio may be 1:1:2 or 1:2:2. Only advanced students should attempt 1:4:2. This means that if five seconds is taken for inhaling, then beginners may suspend breathing for five seconds and exhale for five seconds. Intermediate students inhaling for five seconds may suspend breathing for either five or ten seconds, and exhale for ten seconds. Advanced students inhaling for five seconds may suspend breathing for twenty seconds, and exhale for ten seconds. The unit of time taken in inhaling may gradually be increased with practice.

In summary, the Victorious Breath (*Ujjayi*) is simply described:
Inhale through both nostrils.
Suspend breathing (without raising a hand to the nose).
Exhale through both nostrils.
The above method was taught to Theos Bernard and to Dr Behanan, and is now taught by leading authorities, though the

performance of the exhalation (*rechaka*) deviates from what is described in the traditional texts. The *Hatha Yoga Pradipika* gives this description (77):

> Having closed the mouth the air should be drawn again and again through the nostrils in such a way that it goes touching from the throat to the chest, and making noise while passing. It should be restrained, as before, and then let out through *Ida* [the left nostril]. This removes *slesma* [phlegm] in the throat and increases the appetite. . . . *Ujjayi* should be performed in all conditions of life, even while walking or sitting.

The right hand has here to be raised to close the right nostril at the exhaling stage. This version is now little used: students are now told to exhale through both nostrils.

Ujjayi may be practised on occasions while walking or lying down, without using a Chin Lock or any other seal. The benefits are that it invigorates and increases vital capacity, richly oxygenates and purifies the blood, removes phlegm, improves thoracic mobility and broadens the chest, improves digestion, tones the nervous system, and can be used at times when courage is needed.

A traditional therapeutic claim is that it prevents and cures asthma and consumption. According to the *Hatha Yoga Pradipika* (77), 'It destroys the defects of the *nadis*, dropsy and disorders of *Dhatu* [humours].' The *Gheranda Samhita* says (90): 'All works are accomplished by *Ujjayi Kumbhaka*. He [the Yogi] is never attacked‧ by phlegm-disease, or nerve-disease, or indigestion, or dysentery, or consumption, or cough; or fever, or [enlarged] spleen. Let a man perform *Ujjayi* to destroy decay and death.'

Hissing Sound Breath (Sitkari)

This *pranayama* is unusual in that inhalation (though not exhalation) is through the mouth. The lips are slightly parted and the tip of the tongue is thrust between the upper and lower sets of teeth. This means that the tip of the tongue is between the lips; enough space is left between the tongue and the upper lip for air to be drawn in, producing a hissing sound. The air strikes freshly on the forepart of the tongue, and has a cooling effect. When the lungs are comfortably inflated, the lips are closed; the breath is held for a few seconds, and then it is exhaled *through the nostrils*. Perform this three times.

Theos Bernard was taught a different method. He was told to bring the teeth together and to 'float' the tongue in the mouth so as not to touch any part, and then to suck air in between the teeth. With this method too there is a hissing sound, and the effect is cooling. Exhalation, following a suspension, is through the nostrils.

Some aspects of the effects described in the *Hatha Yoga Pradipika* will appeal particularly to male readers (77):

Sitkari is performed by drawing in the air through the mouth, keeping the tongue between the lips. The air thus drawn in should not be expelled through the mouth, but by the nostril. By practising in this way, one becomes next to the God of Love in beauty. He is regarded adorable by the Yoginis [female Yogis] and becomes the author and destroyer of the cycle of creation. He is not afflicted with hunger, thirst, sleep, or lassitude. The *Sattva* of his body becomes free from all the disturbances. In truth, he becomes the lord of the Yogis in this world.

Likewise, surely, the Yogini must become 'next to the Goddess of Love in beauty' and be 'regarded as adorable by the Yogis'.

The benefits are that the Hissing Sound Breath purifies the blood, cools the system, appeases hunger and quenches thirst, and prevents and cures diseases, according to traditional claims.

Cooling Breath (Sitali)

Sitali means 'cool'. *Sitali* is closely related to *Sitkari*, inhalation again taking place through the mouth and exhalation through the nostrils. And again the tongue is pushed between the teeth, but this time the outer edges are curled up to form a trough through which the air is drawn. The tongue is kept between the lips, with the tip protruding slightly beyond them. Draw air slowly and smoothly along the folded tongue. This has been compared to drinking air through a straw.

Then draw the tongue back into the mouth and bring the lips together, holding the breath.

Finally, let the air out smoothly and continuously through both nostrils.

Perform three times.

'This *Sitali Kumbhaka* cures colic, [enlarged] spleen, fever, disorders of bile, hunger, thirst, and counteracts poisons,' says the *Hatha Yoga Pradipika* (77). And the *Gheranda Samhita* says (90): 'Draw in the air through the mouth (with the lips contracted and the tongue thrown out), and fill the stomach slowly. Retain it there for a short time. Then exhale it through both the nostrils. Let the

Yogin always practise this *Sitali Kumbhaka*, giver of bliss; by so doing he will be free from indigestion, phlegm and bilious disorders.'

Theos Bernard was taught the method described above, but he was also given an alternative method in which, during inhalation, the tongue was turned back in the mouth until it was touching the soft palate.

The benefits are that the Cooling Breath purifies the blood, cools the system, quenches thirst, stimulates the liver and spleen, improves digestion, and calms the nervous system and mind.

Bee Breath (Bhramari)

Bhramari means 'bee'. This is sometimes called the Droning Beetle Breath. The ears are closed with the thumbs – the right ear with the right thumb and the left ear with the left thumb – and one listens to the air being drawn into the lungs and squeezed out of them, breathing through both nostrils. The smoothness of breathing can be studied in this *pranayama* by listening to the evenness of the sustained and continuous sound.

The description in the *Hatha Yoga Pradipika* makes a distinction between the sounds of inbreathing and outbreathing (77): '*Bhramari* consists in filling the air with force, which makes a noise like a male bee, and in expelling it slowly which makes a noise like a female bee; this practice causes a sort of ecstasy in the minds of Yogindras.'

The mention of ecstasy shows the connection between this *pranayama* and the concentration (*dharana*) and contemplation (*dhyana*) of Raja Yoga practice. The *Gheranda Samhita* makes it clearly a meditative exercise, concentrating and stilling the mind, and lists many internal sounds to be listened to (90): 'The first sound will be like that of crickets, then that of a flute, then that of a beetle, then that of bells, then those of gongs of bell-metal, trumpets, kettledrums, *mrdanga*, military drums, and *dundubhi*, etc. Thus various sounds are cognised by daily practise of this *Kumbhaka*. Last of all is heard the *Anahata* sound rising from the heart.' These sounds are to be heard, and concentrated upon, during the breath-retention or *kumbhaka*. An 'ah' sound may be uttered low in the throat, causing the palate to vibrate.

Swooning Breath (Murchha)

Here we have mystical experience again. The swooning is by the mind, either during breath retention (the attention being firmly fixed between the eyebrows), or as the breath is slowly released.

The *Gheranda Samhita* says (90): 'Having performed *Kumbhaka* with comfort, let him withdraw the mind from all objects and fix it in the space between the eyebrows. This causes fainting of the mind and gives happiness. For, by thus joining the *Manas* [Mind] with the *Atman* [Soul], the bliss of Yoga is certainly obtained.' And the *Hatha Yoga Pradipika* has this to say (77): 'Closing the passages with *Jalandhara Bandha* firmly at the end of *Puraka* [inhalation], and expelling the air slowly, is called *Murchha*, from its causing the mind to swoon and giving comfort.'

Dr Bernard was taught to sustain a suspension of breathing with the air locked outside the lungs in this *pranayama*, in addition to retention until the mind 'swooned' on filled lungs. He warns (7): 'The beginner is advised not to work on this practice during his preparatory period.'

In *Murchha* the Chin Lock (*Jalandhara Bandha*) is used during retention of breath and during exhalation, though beginners are permitted by their *gurus* to use it only for the former.

Floating Breath (Plavini)
This is a most unusual *pranayama*, for it is practised while floating on water. The legs are crossed – into the Lotus position, each foot upturned on the opposite thigh, if you can manage it – and the head is thrown back. The hands are crossed behind the head to support it. You inhale deeply, suspend breathing, and float easily with a light and buoyant feeling.

It is significant that the posture adopted here is called, when transferred to performance on dry land, the Fish Posture (*Matsyasana*).

The *Hatha Yoga Pradipika* is succinct but poetic (77): 'When the belly is filled with air freely circulating within the body, the body easily floats even in the deepest water, like the leaf of a lotus.'

ADDITIONAL BREATHING EXERCISES

We have now described the main traditional *pranayamas*. The concluding two breathing exercises are simplifications of esoteric 'psychic force' controls.

Pranic *Breath*

This is an exercise in imagination as well as in breath control.

Prana, or cosmic energy, is potently present in oxygen. In this breathing exercise, which in mechanical performance is straightforward deep breathing – inhalation, retention, exhalation – one adds visualization and the feeling of rich quantities of *prana* being taken in on inspiration and then being directed to every part of the body, feeding blood, nerves, vital organs, tissues, bones, and hairs, with its life-force.

Prana is the life-enhancing principle pervading the whole universe, moving the stars in their courses, and operating, in progressively finer qualities, on physical, mental, and spiritual levels in Man. Muscular movement is a gross and obvious manifestation, and thought a subtle manifestation. In Yogic meditation the aim is to refine thought itself until it reveals its source.

Solar Plexus Charging

This is more localized and concentrated in its effects than the preceding *Pranic* Breath.

The solar plexus is a complex of nerves at the pit of the stomach, and is connected with the sympathetic nervous system. It has a strategic situation in the centre of the body. This is one 'centre' or *chakra* whose importance occidentals will recognize: some writers identify it with the *manipura chakra* of Kundalini Yoga.

Take deep controlled breaths through both nostrils, and through an act of psychic direction concentrate the drawn-in *prana* in this storage centre in the pit of the stomach. As you hold your breath for a few seconds, stockpile *prana* in the region of the solar plexus, which should become warm.

This is a useful exercise in mind-control, skill in which builds the ability to warm any part of the body by directing the attention to it.

Yogic therapy consists of sending *prana* and warmth by conscious control to damaged or diseased parts of the body, or of directing healing force to another person's body by laying on hands.

AIMS AND USES OF YOGIC BREATHING

We conclude this section by summarizing the various aims and uses of Yogic breathing (*pranayama*), not all of which are completely practical for Western man.

The Daily Programme of Pranayama

Fifteen to twenty minutes should be devoted to *pranayama* each day, selecting exercises from those given above. Of these, *Sitkari* and *Sitali* are somewhat specialized, and most effectively brought into use during hot weather or at times when the practitioner is over-heated; this is certainly true of *Plavini*. The basis of a sound effective programme is Cleansing Breath (*Kapalabhati*) or Bellows Breath (*Bhastrika*), or Alternate Nostril Breath if you find these too vigorous. This should be followed by Alternate Nostril Breath and/or Victorious Breath (*Ujjayi*). The other breath controls may be introduced to provide variety, these form the foundation. If you are short of time – though you must have a good reason for not finding it – Alternate Nostril Breath or Victorious Breath (*Ujjayi*) can be practised unobtrusively at some time during the day, the latter while walking if that is the only real opportunity.

The daily session of Yoga breathing increases vital capacity, energizes, exercises the lungs and the respiratory muscles, oxygenates and purifies the bloodstream, removes phlegm, cleanses the sinuses and the *nadis* or nerve channels, soothes and tones the nervous system, improves thorcacic mobility and broadens the chest, improves digestion, massages the abdominal viscera, and calms and concentrates the mind. In addition, the regular programme of *pranayama* brings success in establishing heathful breathing habits, as detailed below.

Establishing Heathful Habits of Breathing

This results from practice of the daily Yogic breathing programme, and from mastering the Complete Yoga Breath given as additional training. These train the thoracic, diaphragmatic, and abdominal muscles to operate efficiently at all times, the habits established in conscious training being carried over into everyday activities, even during the important hours of recuperative sleep.

In the first few weeks of practice the daily programme should be reinforced by making spot checks on your breathing several times a day – while sitting at an office desk, perhaps, or simply reading at home; while travelling to a place of work; or while lying in bed just before going to sleep. At such times play the beam of your attention over the respiratory muscles and make sure they are not being cramped by poor or awkward posture, or by tight clothing, and that your breathing is deep and relaxing, building up the many benefits to physical and mental health that result from Yogic breathing as a daily habit, some of which have been listed in the previous section.

Pranayama *at Moments of Need*
There are occasions when one needs to be lifted out of fatigue and energized, to let go and relax, or to dispel annxiety or fear and to boost courage. At such times *pranayama* can be brought into use: Alternate Nostril Breath to relax and vitalize, Victorious Breath (*Ujjayi*) to energize and give courage. When you are overheated or during hot weather, *Sitkari* and *Sitali* will cool the system.

Pranayama *for Equanimity and Serenity*
Equanimity has been defined as 'evenness of mind; that calm temper or mental firmness which is not easily elated or depressed.' Serenity is 'calmness; quietness; stillness; calmness of mind; evenness of temper.' To be serene is to be unruffled, like the surface of a quiet lake mirroring the sky. The Latin *serenus* means 'clear', and serene has a poetic meaning as a noun – 'the clear expanse of cloudless sky'.
  Spotting the practical significance of the link between the emotions and breathing was a manifestation of genius on the part of the sages who first developed *pranayama*. We all know how excitement and agitation accelerate the rate of breathing; that nervous breathing is fast, jerky, and shallow; that relaxed breathing is slow, steady, and deep. But these sages saw the potentialities of using slow controlled respiration to calm body, mind, and spirit.

Pranayama *as Preparation for the Yoga of Meditation* (*Raja Yoga*)
Slow, deep, quiet breathing conduces to meditative states of consciousness. In some Yogas it is itself a technique for attaining higher consciousness. And in Buddhist, Taoist, and some other Yogas, the act of breathing becomes a focus for mindfulness. In Raja Yoga *pranayama* may serve to make the breathing so quiet and restful that it can be forgotten, leaving the attention free for one-pointing and concentration (*dharana*).
  Patanjali, the author of the key work systematizing Raja Yoga, treats *pranayama* as one of the eight *angas* or limbs of Yoga, but devotes very few *sutras* or aphorisms to it. Patanjali knew he could leave practical instruction in the breath controls to the *gurus*. The stilling of the mind in his overriding purpose. It is in the classic texts of Hatha Yoga – the *Hatha Yoga Pradipika*, the *Siva Samhita*,

the *Gheranda Samhita* – that we find more detailed instruction, though even here, as we have seen, the information would be inadequate and confusing were it not for the oral teacher – pupil (*guru – chela*) tradition already in operation when they were written, transmitted down through the centuries to our own day.

Closing the eyes and concentrating on the gentle ebb and flow of breath and the rise and fall of the respiratory muscles induces moods and states of consciousness that are indisputably meditative. In some schools of Yoga *pranayama* is itself a form of meditation.

We know that the achievement and maintenance of health and vitality and the unfolding of higher states of consciousness are both goals found in Yoga, and that some Yogins put the emphasis more on one than the other. But even the Yogin who gives his attention almost entirely to the attainment of glowing health cannot fail to become aware of the reciprocal relationship between respiration and movements within the psyche. Even the most complex and subtle emotions have their concomitant breathing tones, and one discovers that Yogic breathing refines the emotions and the textures and vibrations of consciousness itself. In the highest states of consciousness breathing becomes quiescent and imperceptible. In the folklore of many countries the breath is equated with the soul or spirit. In Genesis 2:7 we find: 'And the Lord God formed man of the dust of the ground, and breathed into his nostrils the breath of life; and man became a living soul.' And in the Gospel According to St John 22:21: 'Jesus *breathed* on his disciples and said, Receive the holy spirit.'

Pranayama *as a Technique in the Yoga of Latent Energies* (*Laya or Kundalini Yoga*)
Pranayama – in particular the *kumbhaka* or breath retention – is applied in its most intensive form in the esoteric Yoga concerned with the awakening and control of vital air or currents (*vayu*) within the body. But long breath suspensions are called for, and this is not a Yoga that can safely be taught by book instruction; personal supervision by a qualified instructor is necessary, and difficult to obtain.

Pranayama *as a Healer : Breathing Therapy*
Yogic breath control may be used as a therapy. Here the principle of *prana* or life-force is much involved. Its flow may be directed by

the practitioner to injured or diseased parts of his own body, or by the laying on of hands or psychic concentration to the body of another.

Pranayama *for the Performance of Extraordinary Feats*

Levitation, *tumo* (engendering heat), and burial alive are three bizarre and unusual feats that are linked with mastery over breathing. Exhibitions of remarkable powers are, however, frowned upon by responsible Yogins, and public demonstrations of such powers are usually by fakirs and ascetics who have acquired Yogic mastery over body and mind.

The last two uses of *pranayama* listed above will be given separate chapters. But before going on to these, let us take thought for the quality of the air we breathe.

VII Poisonous Air and Vital Air

AIR POLLUTION

Clean dry air is a mixture of gases: 78.9 per cent nitrogen, 20.94 per cent oxygen, and 0.97 per cent other gases. If breath is life, then it is essential that the air we breathe should be fresh, pure, and adequately oxygenated. Water pollution affects mainly the nation causing it, but air contamination may be spread around the world. When a nuclear device is exploded, people thousands of miles away may receive radio-active fall-out. On the brighter side, strong winds help to disperse dirty air.

Great Britain, with her coal-based economy, has had an air pollution problem since Elizabethan times, when wood for burning was becoming scarce. Queen Elizabeth I prohibited the burning of coal in London while Parliament was sitting, but the citizens had no protection most of the year. John Evelyn, the famous diarist, wrote of London during the reign of Charles II: 'Her inhabitants breathe nothing but an impure and thick mist, accompanied with a fulginous and filthy vapour, which renders them obnoxious to a thousand inconveniences, corrupting the lungs, and disordering the entire habit of their bodies; so that Catharrs, Phthisicks, Coughs and Consumptions, rage more in this one City, than in the whole earth besides.' Evelyn did not just fulminate: he put forward sensible remedies. He advised that industries causing smoke should be moved five or six miles out of London, and that trees and shrubs should be planted in the city.

Killer Smog
The situation became much worse in London, and in other smoky British cities, with the Industrial Revolution. From the time of the

Industrial Revolution until comparatively recently, London suffered periodic attacks from killer smog, a combination of smoke and fog, as its name reveals. The term is sometimes used erroneously for chemical and other air-polluting concentrations that do not combine both smoke and fog. Smog occurs when smoke, fog, and low temperatures coincide with a temperature inversion: a layer of cold air becomes trapped under a layer of warm air and gathers smoke and fumes. This situation recurrently causes ill-health and deaths in areas in many parts of the world.

That London is no longer the city of smog is due to action finally taken to combat it in 1956, when the Clean Air Act was implemented. The spur to action was over four thousand deaths in London caused by five days of acute smog in December 1952. Another smog blanket over the metropolis in 1956 caused more than one thousand deaths. Other British cities suffered fatalities from the same cause in 1952 and 1956.

There is another type of smog that may occur during hot weather. During one week in July 1970, this photochemical smog made many thousands of people ill in Buenos Aires, Los Angeles, Milan, New York, and Tokyo.

Industrial Air Pollution

The main air pollutants produced by industry are carbon monoxide, sulphur dioxide and sulphur trioxide, nitrogen oxides, and hydrocarbons. Winds, fortunately, break up and disperse the poisons to some extent, but under certain conditions there can be a build-up of polluted atmosphere in one area to a dangerous degree. Scientists are still struggling to gain an accurate estimate of the possible long-term effects of chemical atmosphere pollution.

Injury to Health

Newspapers, radio, and television report instances of dramatic injury to health and fatalities caused by concentrations of pollutants; but there is also a continuous and gradual damage to health that goes unreported. Elderly people suffer most. Air pollution causes and worsens bronchitis and emphysema. Chronic bronchitis, at the time of writing, is fourth among the major causes of death in Great Britain. The attack on the body by air pollutants takes different forms. Carbon monoxide is preferentially absorbed by the blood. Sulphur dioxide forms an acid solution that eats into lung tissue – which is also damaged by solid particles. In smoky cities it is rare for doctors carrying out autopsies to see a pink lung; when they do they deduce that the dead person has not been in the city long. Other parts of the body may be damaged; the main effect of photochemical smog is eye irritation.

Governments, somewhat tardily, have been taking action of late, though much remains to be done in many parts of the world. In the USA responsibility remains with individual states, though the Federal Clean Air Act (1963) and the Air Quality Act (1967) mean that the Government can advise and give financial aid to control pollution.

AIR AS FOOD

Yogins hold that air is our most essential food, and that one should seek to breathe air of the highest nutritional value, meaning highly charged with *prana* or life-force. The most vitalizing air, they say, is by the sea, in the mountains, by lakes, and in large open spaces. Modern scientific investigation shows that these areas, which Yogins associate with high concentrations of *prana*, have atmospheres marked by negative ionization. This makes Professor Robert E. Ornstein, a research psychologist at the Langley Porter Neuro-psychiatric Institute in San Francisco, say (158):

> The presence of the minutely charged atmospheric ions may constitute a physical analog of the esoteric 'energy form' of *Prana*. In the Hindu tradition, *Prana* is held to be the 'life force', from which health and creativity flow, the force which aids in physical as well as psychological growth. At this point, we cannot measure precisely how much overlap there is between negative air ions and the concept of *Prana*, but some interesting similarities do exist. The esoteric traditions have long taken advantage of favourable microclimatic conditions for their students. Esoteric psychological schools have often been located on mountain tops, near waterfalls, near the ocean. Some recent biological studies have determined that the ionization of the air in these places is predominantly negative.

> Many aspects of esoteric tradition stress that when breathing exercises are performed, 'time and place' must be taken into account. The 'time' is the acknowledgement of the rhythmic structure of man. The 'place' may refer, in part, to the presence of the favourable

microclimate – negative ionization. The relationship between breathing and consciousness has been little explored by contemporary psychology, but has been stressed in esoteric tradition. As it does for 'body energies', our colloquial language preserves some of the dimensions of this relationship. To note one instance, 'inspiration' refers to both creativity and the process of breathing.

AIR IONS

An ion, *Nuttall's Standard Dictionary* tells us, is 'the electrified particle produced when an atom loses or gains one or more electrons by electrolytic dissociation, or when a molecule of a gas loses an electron through X-ray action.'

In 1899, Elster and Geitel proved that atmospheric electricity depends upon the presence of gaseous ions in the air. Equipment was produced that could indicate the number of ions in the air, and generators were able to produce them. It was found that small air ions are formed when enough energy acts on a gaseous molecule to displace an electron, the latter joining with an adjacent molecule (negative molecular ion), and that the original molecule is positively charged (positive molecular ion).

The number of ions in the air varies from 50 to as much as 10,000 in a cubic centimetre. The number is higher during the day than during the night, higher on unclouded days than on clouded days, higher in summer than in winter. The balance between negative and positive charged ions also varies, depending on several factors. Thunderstorms add to the number of positive ions; so does cloud. Negative charged ions predominate on sunny days, and also on mountaintops. Electricity in the air produces ions, and even the flame from a household fire ionizes. There are large and small ions: the number of large ions increases after sunset, and the number of small ions in the first hours of morning. Investigations show that it is the small ions that have the direct physiological influence, though the large ions have an indirect influence.

Negatively Ionized Air

In a Japanese survey (138), people were asked to give their responses to the atmosphere in rooms with varying quantities of ions and a varying balance between negative and positive ions. When there were few ions the people in the room found the atmosphere 'close'; when positive ions predominated they found the room 'sultry'; 'light and cool' was the response to the introduction of more negative ions, and 'light and fresh' when there was a boost of both negative and positive ions.

The feeling of freshness we experience in the proximity of water-falls and fountains is not just psychological – the air around them is high in negatively charged ions. In Russia, Germany, France, and Italy the ionic content of the atmosphere of spas near waterfalls was studied and found to have a high negative charge. In contrast, positive ions are present in abnormally high amounts in photo-chemical smog, and in those 'winds of ill-repute' (the Mistral, the Khamsin, the Santa Ana, and the Foehn) which raise the incidence of phyiscal and mental ill-health wherever and whenever they blow.

Ions and Air Pollution

Air pollution of the kinds discussed earlier reduce ion levels in the atmosphere: this is found even far out at sea where air pollutants have drifted from the land. Unless we do more to defeat air pollu-tion, mankind faces growing dangers from ion loss as well as from irritation to the lungs and respiratory passages. Professor A. P. Kreuger, a leading investigator of the effects of varying ion levels and balances in the atmosphere, asks (141):

Will the smogs, hazes and invisible pollutants we generate with a lavish hand so reduce the small-ion content of the atmosphere that plants, animals, and man must suffer harmful consequences? Although the early result of ion depletion very likely will be unimpressive compared to the immediate and dramatic action of known toxic com-ponents of polluted air, this alone should furnish little solace. We have every reason to be aware from past experience that adverse effects may follow continued exposure to a small amount of a minor irritant (e.g. organic solvents) or the long-term deprivation of an essential metabolic requirement (e.g. trace elements or vitamins). The ultimate dimen-sions of biological changes produced by air-ion loss conceivably may prove to be as disenchanting as some revealed by Rachel Carson in *The Silent Spring*.

On the brighter side, Professor Kreuger foresees the eventual regulation of negative-positive air ion balances and levels for com-fort in living and working quarters, just as we already have tempera-ture and humidity regulation. There is a potential use for air ions in stimulating agricultural production. Experiments have shown that the growth of plants is regularly accelerated by high concentrations of either negative or positive air ions (141). And additional negative or positive charges have been found to speed up the germination of silkworm eggs and the growth rate of the developing larvae.

But it is the treatment of disease and the enhancement of health that most interests us here.

Ionization and Health

A. P. Kreuger and others have also studied the effect of positively charged and negatively charged air ions on the breathing of some mammals. They found that a positively charged atmosphere was associated with congestion of the bronchial tubes, a reduced flow of mucus, slow working of the cilia of the windpipe, and a disturbed peristaltic reflex. But when the mammals were exposed to negative ions, the bronchial tubes expanded and relaxed, mucus flowed freely, the cilia of the windpipe worked busily, and peristalsis became normal.

In experiments made at the Institute of Hygiene, Prague, men were exposed to air ions for an hour three times a week for eight weeks. It was found that positive ions induced a rise in blood pressure, a drop in blood albumen, and an increase in the globulin content of the blood; whereas exposure to negative ions raised the blood albumen and lowered the globulin.

A. L. Tchijevsky (170), a Russian scientist, reported to an International Conference on Therapeutic Radiation that 'ion therapy can lead to improvement in eighty-five per cent of patients with vascular and cardiac conditions, hypertension, angina, bronchitis, migraine, endocrine disturbances, allergies, burns, bronchial asthma, and stomach ulcers.'

Other reports indicate that treatment by negative air ions relieves headache, dry mucous membrane, nasal blockage, and irritation of the respiratory tract; and also that negatively charged air produces greater relaxation throughout the whole organism, with an increase of haemoglobin, red blood cells, and iron in the blood. But working out the correct amount of increase of negative ions in treating patients has presented problems. Too strong or too frequent a dose can be harmful – like an overdose of some vitamins. And while some persons are very sensitive to negative ions, others show the opposite characteristic.

Raising and lowering ion levels in the atmosphere of a room, and altering the balance between negative ions and positive ions, are known to influence human moods and states of consciousness. Professor Robert E. Ornstein asks (158): 'Could the introduction of negatively ionized air produce results similar to those achieved by difficult and esoteric breath manipulations?' He refers to the breath controls of Yoga, Sufism, and so on. Insufficient evidence is available so far to give a clear answer to the question, but enough is available to justify the raising of the question.

SMOKING AND HEALTH

While the individual person may not be in a position greatly to influence the cleanliness of the air breathed in our cities, there is one concentrated pollution, the commonest and most dangerous, over which he does have full control – he can choose whether or not to inhale cigarette smoke into his lungs.

The link between heavy cigarette smoking, and lung cancer and some other diseases, is indisputable. The first report of a Committee set up by the Royal College of Physicians of London in 1959 was published in 1962, under the title *Smoking and Health*. The 1962 report said that 'diseases associated with cigarette smoking cause so many deaths that they present the most challenging of all opportunities for preventive medicine.' A second report, *Smoking and Health Now*, published in 1971, says: 'The challenge remains. The total number of deaths attributable to cigarette smoking rises year by year and is likely to do so unless there are radical changes in smoking habits,' and adds, 'the suffering and shortening of life resulting from smoking cigarettes have become increasingly clear as the evidence accumulates. Cigarette smoking is now as important a cause of death as were the great epidemic diseases such as typhoid, cholera, and tuberculosis that affected previous generations.'

The reports of the Committee set up by the Royal College of Physicians of London are unequivocal, and the findings are supported by scientific investigations in several parts of the world. The link between smoking cigarettes and disease and death has been clearly established. But here we are concerned not only with deaths from lung cancer and diseases caused by the smoking habit, but with the multiplication of cases – running to millions – of people who are inflicting upon themselves lower standards of health.

Increased Death-risk for Smokers

The nicotine addict says, along with Charles Lamb:

> For thy sake, Tobacco, I
> Would do any thing but die.

But the risk of dying prematurely is exactly the risk that he takes, according to the most influential surveys of the hazards associated with the smoking habit.

The most important of the scientific studies are these: R. Doll and A. B. Hill, 'Mortality in relation to smoking: ten years' observations of British doctors', *British Medical Journal*, 1964. H. A. Kahn, 'The Dorn study of smoking and mortality among US veterans: report of 8½ years of observations', *National Cancer Institute Monograph*, 1966. E. W. R. Best, 'A Canadian Study of Smoking and Health', Department of Health and Welfare, Ottawa, 1966. E. C. Hammond, 'Smoking in relation to the death rates of one million men and women', *National Cancer Institute Monograph*, 1966.

The four investigations came up with similar and unequivocal findings:

Cigarette smokers have a shorter life-expectancy than non-smokers.

The greater the number of cigarettes smoked daily, the greater the death-risk.

Cigar or pipe smoking is less hazardous than cigarette smoking, but still produces an increased death-risk.

There is a link between cigarette smoking and lung cancer, heart disease, arterial diseases, chronic bronchitis and emphysema. Some non-smokers get these diseases, but the risk of having them is much higher in smokers, especially heavy smokers.

These smoking habits increase the hazards to health and life: inhaling tobacco smoke; keeping the cigarette between the lips as you puff; smoking a cigarette down to a tiny stub; and relighting partly-smoked cigarettes.

These investigations also came up with some encouraging news for smokers: give up cigarette smoking and you run a steadily diminishing risk of dying from the effects. Hammond, in his study of one million men and women, found that when light smokers broke the habit, after ten years their death risk was on a par with non-smokers.

A poster published in Britain by the Health Education Council informs us that:

Every time you inhale from a cigarette tiny particles of nicotine and other chemicals are left inside your lungs. These particles gradually build up into an oily tar that irritates your lungs till they become clogged or infected with phlegm and pus. Then, as more of this septic discharge forms, the mixture of tar, phlegm and pus sometimes rises up into the throat and is swallowed. But the rest of it slithers deep into the lungs, where it congeals and festers. It is not surprising that smokers cough, are short of wind, have bad breath, and are more susceptible to crippling incurable diseases.

Breaking the Smoking Habit

The truth about will-power is that the power comes easily when we really want to give up something. Irritating and fouling the lungs with tobacco smoke is totally opposed to the aims of the practices of Hatha Yoga, which are cleansing and health-enhancing. If he practises Yogic breath controls regularly, the smoker loses the craving for cigarettes and usually cuts down, and then finally drops the habit. A relaxed and healthy system has no need for the stimulation provided by nicotine, and blackening the lungs with inhaled smoke becomes unthinkable.

VIII   Yogic Breathing and Health

THE UNIQUENESS OF *PRANAYAMA*

Dr Kovoor T. Behanan, in his still-pertinent scientific evaluation of Yoga first published in 1937, reported a series of experiments measuring the oxygen consumption in *Kapalabhati*, *Bhastrika*, and *Ujjayi*. One would expect all three to cause an increase in oxygen consumption over normal breathing and, from the nature of performance, that *Bhastrika* would induce a greater oxygen consumption than *Kapalabhati*, and *Ujjayi* a greater consumption than *Bhastrika*. This, in fact, proved to be the case, the increased consumption over normal breathing for *Kapalabhati*, *Bhastrika*, and *Ujjayi* being 12.0, 18.5, and 24.5 per cent respectively. It should be remembered that the first two are rapid cleansing breaths, with a different role in *pranayama* from that of *Ujjayi*, which is deep breathing, filling the lungs to comfortable capacity.

That Yogic breathing enhances health and aids healing has been discovered in practice by thousands of people from all walks of life, ranging in age from young to old. Oxygen consumption is increased above that of normal breathing, that much is clear – but so too is it increased by numerous forms of active exercise. Wherein then lies the special merit of *pranayama*?

Here is Dr Behanan's opinion as to what makes *pranayama* unique as bodily exercise (6):

> Increased oxygen consumption, which is characteristic of yogic breathing, in itself does not mark it off as different from other kinds of exercises, because any kind of exertion involves an increase in metabolic rate which is manifested by the greater intake of oxygen. A few details, like the tipping of the head [Chin Lock] during the holding period and inspiration and expiration with half-closed glottis, may

appear to be unique features. Until we have positive evidence concerning the physiological changes introduced by these details, however, it does not seem reasonable to believe that they are a very important part of the system.

This view remains reasonable almost forty years later. D. Behanan continues:

One thing seems rather unique. In yogic breathing, while the respiratory muscles are exercised in the execution of deep cycles, the other groups of muscles remain relatively inactive. Thus it differs markedly from the deep breathing incident to riding a bicycle. Here, although the trunk and arms are rather inactive, they can hardly be relaxed and the lower limbs are called upon to do vigorous exercise.

The different stages of the respiratory act are executed with calculated deliberation. The contraction and relaxation of the respiratory muscles are accomplished slowly, while jerky movements are avoided. It would seem reasonable, therefore, to believe that *the chief purpose of the yogic breathing exercises is to increase the consumption of oxygen with the minimum of physical exertion, under conditions probably favourable to the storage of oxygen.*

(The italics are mine.)

To this I would add that there are significant differences which elevate *pranayama* above not only other forms of physical exercise that activate deeper breathing, but also the other much less well-known systems of breathing exercises for health (such as the Muller method). These are the basic insistence upon rhythm and smooth control; the retention (*kumbhaka*); and the unique regard for the reciprocal relationship between respiration and the mental state. Search as you may, you will find nothing similar in range and depth of importance to *pranayama*. No other system dares to contemplate Yoga's sublime aim: to perfect body, mind, and spirit.

YOGIC BREATHING AS HEALER

Yogins hold that *prana* is the force behind the renewal of the body cells, and that disease is unlikely to gain a hold on a body whose every body cell is permeated with *pranic* energy. Further, a body freshly charged with *prana* can be a source of healing for others, by transmission. It is especially effective with certain specific complaints.

Asthma and Bronchitis

Deep breathing of the Complete Yoga Breath type is widely
employed in physiotherapy throughout the world. Diaphragmatic
and abdominal breathing relaxes the respiratory muscles and gives
relief and therapeutic benefit in ailments like asthma and bronchitis,
where tension adds to the trouble. Some doctors recommend Yogic
breathing exercises for asthmatics. During asthmatic attacks the
muscles controlling the bronchioles go into a spasm and air gets
into the lungs, but has difficulty in getting out. The sufferer adds
to his problem if he gives way to panic and tries to force air into
lungs already distended. Training in Yogic breathing gives the
asthmatic confidence and the ability to relax and control the
respiratory muscles. The Alternate Nostril Breath and the Victorious Breath (*Ujjayi*) may be practised between attacks with
retention, and during attacks without retention. They may also be
practised by people with bronchitis.

Persons suffering from asthma, bronchitis, and other respiratory
complaints tend to avoid physical exercise, so that their general
health suffers. Yoga practice, with its gentle approach, gives them
exercise, greater confidence, and control.

Colds ,Catarrh, and Sinus Trouble

Yogic breathing prevents head colds and is helpful in clearing up
catarrh and sinus troubles. In particular this is true of the Cleansing
Breath (*Kapalabhati*), the Bellows Breath (*Bhastrika*), and the
Alternate Nostril Breath (*Anuloma Viloma Pranayama*).

Nervous Tension

Nervous tension causes muscular contractions and rigidities in many
parts of the body. As there is a close link between the emotions and
breathing, anxiety, fear, and other stresses result in the respiratory
muscles becoming constricted, so impairing free functioning and
deep breathing.

Neurosis

The value of deep breathing as a therapy for neurotic conditions
was mentioned earlier, when we pointed out that psychotherapists
of the Reichian school use deep-breathing exercises to break up the
rings of muscular tension with which the neutoric 'armours' himself
in the upper body, originally to inhibit emotional expression. Such

self-inflicted strait-jacketing of the respiratory apparatus may persist long after any psychological need for inhibiting emotional expression has passed. In particular, Reich attached importance to his patients learning to exhale thoroughly.

Insomnia
Controlled breathing calms the nervous system and relaxes body and mind. Breathing smoothly and rhythmically on first going to bed keeps away the tension and nervous activity so often responsible for sleeplessness or sleep of poor quality.

Headaches
These are often eased by the Alternate Nostril Breath. The practice of Yogic breathing corrects most of those various conditions that are responsible for headaches.

Indigestion
The practice of *pranayama* improves appetite and aids digestion.

Abnormal Weight
Breathing has an important role in metabolism, the process by which the body uses nutritive elements – which provides a clue to the reason why many people who take up Hatha Yoga find the weight of the body normalizing, the obese losing weight and the thin gaining it. Factors other than respiratory control are likely to be involved, but more efficient breathing is thought to play a part.

Constipation
The abdominal massage given by the Cleansing Breath (*Kapalabhati*) and the Bellows Breath (*Bhastrika*) stimulates natural peristaltic action in the intestines and aids regular elimination of waste matter from the bowels. Performance daily of Abdominal Retraction (*Uddiyana*) and Isolation of the Recti (*Nauli*) is a must for persons who tend to suffer from this complaint.

Compulsive Smoking
An increased and sensitive respect for the body develops with Yoga practice, and blackening and polluting the lungs with inhaled smoke is soon seen as an intolerable affront to bodily hygiene. Yogic

breathing exercises have been found to undermine the craving for nicotine that grips smokers so powerfully, so that the smoking habit loosens its hold and fades away without the smoker being aware of any great struggle of the will.

It can be seen that breathing exercises act as a substitute for smoking: air is inhaled, retained, and exhaled, but it is fresh pure air in place of poisonous air that destroys health. And Yogic breathing, and Yogic practice in general, is more successful than smoking cigarettes in combating restlessness and taut nerves.

HEALING OTHERS

The Yogin who wishes to heal should first build up *prana* in his body and become a channel whereby the cosmic life-force can pass into the patient. Healing is preceded by controlled breathing, charging the body with *prana*, which is usually visualized as being stored in the region of the solar plexus. The healer may also think of *prana* flowing in the *nadis* or nerve channels, and of drawing in the energy of the elements – fire, air, earth, and water.

The Yogin about to heal must be fully rested. The patient is told about the universal life-force, whose healing power he is about to receive. The transmission of energy is usually by the healer placing the palms of his hands flat against the patient's spine and drawing them down it while he (the healer) exhales. This, performed from five to ten times, provides a general vitalization, after which the right hand of the healer is applied to the diseased or damaged part of the patient's body.

After the act of passing *pranic* force to the patient, the healer should lie on his back for some minutes in the Corpse Posture (*Savasana*), resting and recharging.

The most direct link between breath and healing is found in Chinese Taoist breathing therapy. In what they consider the most potent of their treatments, the Taoist healers place cotton wool on the body part affected, and the healer breathes rhythmically on it with parted lips, warming the area.

SELF-HEALING

In Taoist Yoga one comes across methods of self-healing and life prolongation on lines similar to Hatha Yoga's control of bodily energy currents. The following account (154) of how breath control and meditation can be combined for self-healing could equally well be a description of the technique of Hindu Yoga.

The cure for specific maladies is thus described:

> One harmonizes the breath, then swallows it and holds it as long as possible; one meditates on the affected part, by thought one pours the breath upon it and by thought makes the breath fight the malady by attempting to force its way through the obstructed passage. When the breath is exhausted, one expels it, then begins again from twenty to fifty times; one stops when one sees sweat running over the affected part. One repeats the procedure daily at midnight or at the fifth watch, until a cure is effected.

A later Chinese text describes the same technique applied in sequence to all the body's vital organs. As Ssu-ma Ch'eng-cheng says in his *Discourse*: 'Those who absorb the breaths . . . must follow them by thought when they enter their viscera, so that the humours [of the viscera] shall be penetrated [by the breaths], each [breath] conformably with the [inner organ] over which it presides, and thus they can circulate through the whole body and cure all sicknesses.'

LONGEVITY AND YOGA

Exaggerated claims for the longevity of Indian Yogins – that they live for hundreds, even thousands, of years – do damage to Yoga's credibility among Westerners, who may on reading this sort of thing be put off trying techniques, physical and psychological, that greatly enhance the quality of everyday living. Such statements are on a par with those that claim that some Yogins can fly like birds across the Himalayas, or at the very least across a troublesome gorge or ravine. What *can* be stated with certainty – and impressive it is – is that some elderly Indian Yogins display a bodily tone and lissomness and a mental alertness that men half their age in any country in the world would be delighted to possess.

It is noteworthy that those living creatures that breathe more slowly tend to live longer than those with rapid breathing rates. A few comparative figures may be pondered:

A monkey	about 30 breaths a minute
A hen	about 30 breaths a minute
A dog	about 28 breaths a minute
A cat	about 24 breaths a minute
A duck	about 20 breaths a minute
A horse	about 16 breaths a minute
A man	about 15 breaths a minute
A tortoise	about 3 breaths a minute

Some writers on Yoga put forward the theory that as master Yogins breathe more slowly (though more efficiently) than the average citizen, therefore they live longer. A corollary of this argument is that the practice of *pranayama* prolongs life. This is difficult to prove – but it can be safely said that Yogic breathing adds life to one's years, whether or not it adds years to one's life. Probably it does both for many people. Indian Yogins measure their lives, it is said, by the number of breaths they take rather than by minute and hours.

All this leads to puzzling problems as to the nature of chronological, physiological, and psychological time; and intriguing hypotheses arise and are presented.

Professor Eliade, an erudite investigator of Yoga, particularly in its philosophical, metaphysical, and metapsychological aspects, relates a personal experience that illustrates our discussion of a possible link between longevity and the practice of *pranayama*, and a certain link between Yogic breathing and youthfulness (119):

I have been struck, at Rishikesh and elsewhere in the Himalayas, by the admirable physical state of the yogins, who took hardly any nourishment. At my *kutiar* at Rishikesh one of my neighbours was a *naga*, a naked ascetic who spent almost the whole night practising *pranayama*, who never ate more than a handful of rice. He had the body of a perfect athlete; he showed no sign of under-nourishment or fatigue. I wondered how it was that he was never hungry. 'I live only by day,' he told me; 'during the night, I reduce the number of my respirations to a tenth.' I am not too sure that I understand what he meant; but may it not simply be that, the vital duration being measured by the number of inhalations and exhalations, which he reduced to a tenth of the normal number during the night, he was living, in 10 hours of our time, only one tenth as long – namely one hour? Reckoning by the number of respirations, the day of 24 solar hours was lived, by him, in no more than 12 to 13 breathing-hours: by the same measure, *he was eating a handful of rice, not every 24 hours, but every 12 or 13 hours*. This is only a hypothesis which I do not insist upon. But so far as I know, no one has yet given a satisfactory explanation of the astonishing *youthfulness* of some yogins.

In the work – *Images and Symbols* – in which this experience is related, Professor Eliade explains how the Yogin advanced in *pranayama* is existing in a different 'time' from that of our ordinary waking consciousness:

Pranayama, by rendering the respiration rhythmic, transforms the yogin, little by little, into a cosmos: breathing is no longer a-rhythmic, thought ceases to be dispersed, the circulation of the psycho-mental forces is no longer anarchic. But, by working thus upon the respiration, the yogin works directly upon the time that he is living. There is no one adept in Yoga who, during these exercises, has not experienced quite another quality of time. In vain have they tried to describe this experience of the time lived during *pranayama* : it has been compared to the moment of bliss that comes when listening to good music, to the rapture of love, to the serenity or plenitude of prayer. What seems certain is that, by gradually slowing down the respiratory rhythm, prolonging the inhalations and exhalations more and more, and leaving as long an interval as possible between these two movements, the yogin lives in a time that is different from ours.

IX Extraordinary Feats

EXTRAORDINARY FEATS

In this section we will look briefly at three of the most extraordinary feats performed by Yogins – each of which depends for success on advanced skill in *pranayama*. Two of them – burial alive and 'resurrection' many hours later, and *tumo* (engendering body heat) – are fully authenticated; the third feat – levitation – cannot be said to have been performed under conditions that would satisfy the scientifically-minded investigator.

BURIAL ALIVE

In 1926 Harry Houdini, the most famous escapologist, did something almost unknown among magicians – he revealed the secret of one of his most mystifying performances.

In 1974 the Mining Enforcement and Safety Administration in Washington found on their files a letter from Houdini that had been put away and (seemingly) forgotten: it revealed, for the benefit of miners who might find themselves trapped underground with a meagre supply of air, the technique Houdini used to survive $1\frac{1}{2}$ hours in a sealed iron coffin at the bottom of the swimming pool of New York's Shelton Hotel. The letter was written four months before Houdini died. 'I know you are doing worthwhile work,' he wrote, 'and as my body and brain are trained for this particular line I am at your service.' He went on to tell how, struggling with heat nausea, hallucinations, and the urge to sleep, he controlled and conserved his breathing so as to live for ninety-one minutes on an air supply that would normally suffice for only five minutes of life.

Houdini, as with the method of swallowing and regurgitating a key mentioned in the chapter on the cleansing processes, had again hit upon a Yogic method of bodily mastery. However, the technique of burial and 'resurrection' displayed on many occasions by Yogins in India is more radical and prolonged than Houdini's, and involves going into a trance state. The performer needs to have full trust in the associates who bury him and who massage him 'back to life'. There have been some fatalities.

Major F. Yeats-Brown, who served for twenty years in the Bengal Lancers, gave one description of burial alive in the *Sunday Express*, London:

Resurrection of the 'dead' is a fairly common exercise in Indian magic. I have seen it done twice. The adept undergoes twenty-four hours of secret preparation, which consists in purgation, fasting, and 'swallowing' air.

Before the trance state is induced, the adept is in a state of oxygen intoxication. Then, pressing his carotid arteries, he passes into unconsciousness.

His disciples bury him.

On one of the occasions when I was present, the adept remained thus for an hour, on the other occasion he remained in the death-trance for only fifteen minutes.

Doctors who examined the 'corpse' stated that there was no sign of life. When the given time had elapsed, the adept came to life.

It is not an experiment fit for public view, the rigid body un-stiffens, the set lips relax, and from them issues a groan that none who have heard it can forget.

In February 1936 the *Sunday Times*, Madras, reported that a Yogi named Swami Vidyalankar, in the presence of several doctors, had reduced his heartbeat to unrecordable levels. 'He also showed several other feats, including that of remaining buried in a pit for 25 hours.'

In the same year, *The Madras Mail* reported:

BURIED ALIVE FOR THIRTY MINUTES
Yogi's feat witnessed by 15,000 people

Masulipatam, Dec. 15.

A remarkable feat of Yoga was exhibited by Yogi Sankara Marayanaswami of Mysore on Sunday evening in front of Sri Ramalingeswaraswami's Temple in the presence of a gathering of about 15,000 people. He was buried alive for about half an hour.

Lt.-Col. K. V. Ramana Rao, I.M.S., District Medical Officer, who acted as observer, took a letter from the Yogi before the ordeal, stating that he was performing the feat on his own responsibility.

The Yogi was seated in a box specially prepared for the purpose and let down into a pit, which was covered with earth. After about half an hour, the box was removed, when the Yogi was found sitting in a state of trance. The Yogi regained consciousness half an hour afterwards, when he was cheered by the people.

The most detailed description of the feat comes from the pen of a German doctor (130):

Runjeet Sing was told that a *saat*, or faqueer, living in the mountains, was able to keep himself in a state resembling death, and would allow himself to be even buried, without injuring or endangering his life, provided they would remove or release him from the grave after the expiration of a fixed time, he being in the possession of the means of resuscitating himself again. The maharajah thought it impossible. To convince himself of the truth of the assertion, he ordered the faqueer to be brought to court, and caused him to undergo the experiment, assuring him that no precaution should be omitted to discover whether it was a deception. In consequence, the faqueer, in the presence of the court, placed himself in a complete state of asphyxia, having all the appearance of death.

In that state he was wrapped in the linen on which he was sitting, the seal of Runjeet Sing was stamped thereon, and it was placed in a chest, on which the maharajah put a strong lock. The chest was buried in a garden, outside of the city, belonging to the minister, barley was sown on the ground, and the space enclosed with a wall and surrounded by sentinels. On the fortieth day, which was the time fixed for his exhumation, a great number of the authorities of the durbar, with General Ventura, and several Englishmen from the vicinity, one of them a medical man, went to the enclosure. The chest was brought up and opened, and the faqueer was found in the same position as they had left him, cold and stiff. A friend of mine told me, that had I been present when they endeavoured to bring him to life, by applying warmth to the head, injecting air into his ears and mouth, and rubbing the whole of his body to promote circulation, etc., I should certainly not have had the slightest doubt of the reality of the performance. The minister, Rajah Dhyan Sing, assured me, that he himself kept this faqueer (whose name was Haridas) four months under the ground, when he was at Jummoo in the mountains. On the day of his burial, he ordered his beard to be shaved, and at his exhumation his chin was as smooth as on the day of his interment; thus furnishing a complete proof of the powers of vitality having been suspended during that period. He likewise caused himself to be interred at Jesrota, in the mountains, and at Umritsir, and also by the English in Hindostan. In the *Calcutta Medical Journal* about 1835, there is a full description of the faqueer, and we are there informed that he preferred having the chest in which he was enclosed, suspended in the air, instead of its being buried beneath the earth, as he feared the possibility of his body being attacked by ants whilst in that middle state between life and death.

The German doctor was interested in Haridas's preparation for burial, which included some of the purification practices of Hatha Yoga.

Doubtless it is a difficult task, and not within the power of everyone, to acquire the skill necessary for the performance of this experiment, and those who do succeed must undergo a long and continual practice of preparatory measures. I was informed that such people have their *froenulum linguoe* cut and entirely loosened, and that they get their tongues prominent, drawing and lengthening them by means of rubbing with butter mixed with some pellitory of Spain, in order that they may be able to lay back the tongue at the time they are about to stop respiration, so as to cover the orifice of the hinder part of the *fosses nasales*, and thus (with other means for the same purpose, which I shall mention) keep the air shut up in the body and head. Novices, in trying the experiment, shut their eyes, and press them with their fingers, as also the cavities of the ears and nostrils, because the natural warmth of the body might cause such an expansion of the enclosed gas as otherwise to produce, by the violence of its pressure, a rupture of some of those delicate organs not yet accustomed by practice to endure it. This, I am told, is especially the case with the eyes and the tympan of the ear. For the better acquisition of this power, they are accustomed to practise the holding of the breath for a long period.

They swallow a small strip of linen, in order to cleanse the stomach, and by a tube draw a quantity of water through the anus into the intestines to rinse them. This is performed while sitting in a vessel filled with water to the height of the arm-pits. It is said that the faqueer in question, a few days previous to his experiments, took some kind of purgative, and subsisted for several days on a coarse milk regimen. On the day of his burial, instead of food, he slowly swallowed, in the presence of the assembly, a rag of three fingers in breadth and thirty yards in length, and afterwards extracted it, for the purpose of removing all foreign matters from the stomach. . . .

These preparations being made, the faqueer stopped all the natural openings in the body with plugs of aromatic wax, placed back his tongue in the manner I have before indicated, crossed his arms over his breast, and thus suffocated himself, in the presence of a multitude of spectators.

On his exhumation, one of the first operations is to draw his tongue into its natural position; after this, a warm aromatic paste, made from pulse meal, is placed on his head, and air is injected into his lungs and also through the ears, from which the plugs are withdrawn. By this operation, the pellets in the nostrils are driven out with considerable force and noise, and this is considered the first symptom of his resuscitation. Friction is then strenuously applied all over the body, and at length he begins to breathe naturally, opens his eyes, and is gradually restored to consciousness.

TUMO

Tumo is the technique of engendering body heat at will. Here again we have a control of importance to persons struggling for survival – this time in conditions of severe cold.

A detailed account of *tumo* is given by the French traveller and writer Mme Alexandra David-Neel, who visited remote parts of Asia. In her book *With Mystics and Magicians in Tibet* (113) she calls *tumo* 'the art of warming oneself without fire up in the snows'. This art enables hermit Yogins to spend the winter in snow-girt caves at altitudes between 11,000 and 18,000 feet, wearing only a single thin cotton garment, or even no clothing at all.

Tumo means 'heat' or 'warmth', but with various levels of meaning, from the gross bodily heat that can melt snow to 'fires' within the subtle body.

Tibetan adepts of the secret lore distinguish various kinds of *tumo*: exoteric *tumo*, which arises spontaneously in the course of peculiar raptures and, gradually, folds the mystic in the 'soft, warm mantle of the gods'; esoteric *tumo*, that keeps the hermits comfortable on the snowy hills; mystic *tumo*, which can only claim a distant and quite figurative connection with the term 'warmth', for it is the experience of 'paradisiac bliss' in this world.

In the secret teaching, *tumo* is also the subtle fire which warms the generative fluid and drives the energy in it, till it runs all over the body along the tiny channels of the *tsas*.

The *tsas* – the nerves, veins, or arteries of the subtle body – correspond to the *nadis* of Hindu Yoga, and the technique of kindling 'subtle fire' corresponds to the Hatha Yogin's awakening of serpent power (*kundalini*).

Mme David-Neel adds: 'However, only a few, even in mystic circles, are thoroughly acquainted with these several kinds of *tumo*, while the wonderful effects of the *tumo* that warms and keeps alive the hermits in the snowy wilds are known to every Tibetan.'

Initial cleansing breaths and later breath retentions are an essential part of the method, but these are combined with techniques of concentrative meditation, in which mystic syllables and fire are visualized vividly. In one method the sun is imagined in the palm of each hand, below the navel, and on the sole of each foot. The suns in the hands and in the feet are rubbed together, kindling the sun below the navel, which blazes up and fills the whole body with fire.

By combining advanced breath controls with intensive use of concentration and imagination, naked or skimpily-clad Yogins, sitting cross-legged and immobile, meditate for hours on exposed mountain slopes in sub-zero temperatures. Much as a Western Boy Scout is given some task whereby he gains an extra badge, so the Tibetan neophyte is given a test to prove his ability in engendering body heat. The test is to sit wrapped in a sheet that has been dipped in icy lake water. Dry three of these wet sheets in succession with your body heat, and you qualify for the title 'Respa', or Cotton-clad One. Qualified monks have been known to cheat and wear other clothing below their cotton shirt.

A 'little *tumo*' is within the capacities of most 'householder Yogins', and does not require the holding of the breath for several minutes or baroque visualization. With practice in concentrating the mind upon one part of the body, that part can be made to feel warm; and the technique can be extended eventually to the whole body. There are times in life when such adroit use of the powers of attention and imagination can prevent a chill or more serious illness, or simply hasten the onset of refreshing sleep.

LEVITATION

Under the headline 'Sitting in Air' the *Asiatic Monthly Journal* for March 1829 reported an event in Madras (104):

A Brahmin, old and slightly made, represented to be of high caste, contrives to poise himself in a most remarkable manner in the air. He performs this feat at any gentleman's house, not for money, but as an act of courtesy. The following is a description from an eye-witness, given in a Calcutta paper: 'The only apparatus seen is a piece of plank, which, with four pegs, he forms into a kind of long stool; upon this, in a little brass saucer or socket, he places, in a perpendicular position, a hollow bamboo, over which he puts a kind of crutch, like that of a walking crutch, covering that with a piece of common hide: these materials he carries with him in a little bag, which is shown to those who see the exhibition. The servants of the houses hold a blanket before him, and when it is withdrawn, he is discovered poised in the air, about four feet from the ground, in a sitting attitude, the outer edge of one hand merely touching the crutch, the fingers of that hand deliberately counting beads; the other hand and arm held up in an erect posture. The blanket was then held up before him, and they heard a gurgling noise like that occasioned by wind escaping from a bladder or tube, and when the screen was withdrawn he was again standing on terra firma. The same man has the power of staying under water for several hours. He declines to explain how he does it, merely saying he has been long accustomed to do so.' The length of time for which he can remain in his aerial station is considerable. The person who gave the above account says that he remained in the air for twelve minutes; but before the Governor of Madras he continued on his baseless seat for forty minutes.

This is fascinating: but it has all the elements – apparatus 'he carries with him', a blanket held before him – and atmosphere that one associates with a performance by a stage magician. The 'gurgling noise like that occasioned by wind escaping from a bladder or tube' is intriguing – had the old Brahmin, by some practice of *pranayama*, filled himself with air? Certainly this was a performance with which an exponent of the art could make a good living on the cabaret circuits today.

The evidence for levitation is based on only a handful of reports. With all respect to the author of a popular work on Yogic breathing who says that hundreds of Christian saints performed the feat, what evidence there is for levitation (though none of it was taken under conditions that would satisfy a scientific investigator) comes either from India or from Tibet. We will ignore the material of best-sellers that is clearly fiction. But Mme Alexandra David-Neel claims to have seen people levitating in Tibet, and Dr Alexander Cannon claims that he was taught to float through the air over a gorge in the Himalayas (111).

> He gave us instructions as to how we should cross this gulf by practising the levitation and transportation formula in which we had become ere this adept in its perfect manipulation.
>
> Within a few hours we made our bodily state fit to allow of this great miraculous transportation phenomenon taking place by pure mental effort, and in another moment of time landed safely on the other side.

Princess Choki of Sikkim, in her description of her uncle's daily levitation (quoted by Fosco Maraini in his *Secret Tibet*), makes the astonishing feat sound as homely as performing press-ups before breakfast. Her last sentence is priceless (149):

> He [my uncle] was the most extraordinary man I ever met. I remember that when I was a little girl he . . . did what you would call exercises in levitation. I used to take him a little rice. He would be motionless in mid-air. Every day he rose a little higher. In the end he rose so high that I found it difficult to hand the rice up to him. I was a little girl, and had to stand on tiptoe. . . . There are certain things you don't forget.

To these eye-witness accounts may be added a few lines by Professor Ernest Wood, though it is not clear whether he was actually among the spectators who made a close inspection of an old Yogin who was 'mystically inclined' (94):

> Levitation, or the rising of the body from the ground and its sus-pension a few feet up in the air above the seat or couch, is a universally accepted fact in India. I remember one occasion when an old yogi was levitated in a recumbent posture about six feet above the ground in an open field, for about half an hour, while the visitors were permitted to pass sticks to and fro in the space between.

Readers will form their own opinions on the basis of this evidence. Sceptics point out that no religion or ideology is without its mavericks, so it is surprising that not one exhibitionistic yogi has been found who is willing to levitate before scientists or to succumb to the temptation to demonstrate this most astounding of feats in the West or before film cameras – for fame and fortune surely await the first yogi to do so.

What does seem probable is that levitation is often confused with the floating feeling and the sensation of lightness which results from prolonged practice of *pranayama*, and which may be accompanied by hallucinations and the feeling of having become airborne. In his book *The Occult Training of the Hindus* (174), Ernest Wood writes: 'When I tried the long breathing, as a boy of fourteen or fifteen, for three quarters of an hour, I found when I stood up that I had lost my sense of touch and weight. I handled things without feeling them, and walked without any sense of touching the ground.' There are also bizarre accounts of yogins who, having swallowed huge quantities of air, bounce along the ground on their bottoms. The *Siva Samhita* describes it (91): 'Through the strength of constant practice, the Yogi obtains *Bhucharisiddhi* locomotory power , he moves as the frog jumps over the ground, when frightened away by the clapping of hands.' The Tibetan Yogins developed this Tantric technique to amazing lengths, according to the report by Mme David-Neel (113):

The student sits cross-legged on a large and thick cushion. He inhales slowly and for a long time, just as if he wanted to fill his body with air. Then holding his breath, he jumps up with legs crossed, without using his hands and falls back on his cushion, still remaining in the same position. He repeats that exercise a number of times during each period of practice. Some lamas succeed in jumping very high in that way. Some women train themselves in the same manner.

As one can easily believe, the object of this exercise is not acrobatic jumping. According to Tibetans, the body of those who drill themselves for years by that method become exceedingly light; nearly without weight. These men, they say, are able to sit on an ear of barley without bending its stalk or to stand on the top of a heap of grain without displacing any of it. In fact the aim is levitation.

A curious test has been devised. . . . A pit is dug in the ground, its depth being equal to the height of the candidate. Over the pit is built a kind of cupola whose height from the ground level to its highest point again equals that of the candidate. A small aperture is left at the top of the cupola. Now between the man seated cross-legged at the bottom of the pit and that opening, the distance is twice the height of his body. For instance, if the man's height is 5 feet 5 inches, the top hole will be at 10 feet 10 inches from the pit's bottom.

The test consists in jumping cross-legged, as during the training exercises which I have described, and coming out through the small opening at the top of the cupola.

Mme David-Neel says she did not witness this feat herself, but heard from Tibetans that it had been performed. The sitting jumps described above are part of the training of the Tibetan *lung-gom-pas* runners, who are said to run across mountainous country for several successive days and nights without stopping. 'Under the collective term of *lung-gom* Tibetans include a large number of practices which combine mental concentration with various breathing gymnastics and aim at different results either spiritual or physical,' says Mme David-Neel (113).

All the extraordinary feats described in this chapter are possible only, if at all, following years of very advanced breathing practices, well outside the furthest limits of our practical approach to the Yoga of Vitality. And this could be said too of the intensity of breath control taught in the Tantric texts to which we have frequently referred. This is how the *Hatha Yoga Pradipika* describes the stages of *pranayama* (77) : 'In the beginning there is perspiration, in the middle stage there is quivering, and in the last or third stage one obtains steadiness; and then the breath should be made steady or motionless. The perspiration exuding from exertion of practice should be rubbed into the body (and not wiped) i.e. by so doing the body becomes strong and light.'

Total dedication of this kind is intended for practitioners being taught *pranayama* by a *guru*. Readers should have a realistic picture of the determination he is likely to be called upon to sustain. 'I experienced the first stage at the very onset,' Dr Bernard (7) recorded.

After one or two rounds the perspiration began to flow freely. As I developed strength and power, it was slower in making its appearance and was not so extreme as when I was straining. It was several weeks before I observed the second stage, quivering, and this was at a time when I was perfecting *bhastrika*. First there appeared itching sensations. As I continued the practice, the sensations increased. Soon I began to feel as though bugs were crawling over my body. While I was working, my leg would suddenly shake. Later, other muscles unexpectedly contracted, and soon my whole body would shake beyond control. At this time I was told always to use the *padmasana* [Lotus] posture. This prevented the body from going into convulsions.

By adhering to my schedule, these manifestations all passed away. Another trying experience resulted from the agonizing pains that pierced the abdominal cavity. At first there were loud croaking noises as the intestines became filled with air. This was caused by swallowing the air as it tried to find its way out. The increased pressure was the source of this problem; but I was told that it would cease in time, and it did. At such periods, if one does not have an understanding of the principles upon which the practices are based, his faith is likely to forsake him. It is difficult to hold in mind the advice of the [*Siva Samhita*] text: 'Verily there are many hard and almost unsurmountable obstacles in Yoga, yet the Yogi should go on with his practice at all hazards; even were his life to come to the throat.'

To quote the *Siva Samhita* again (91): 'In the first stage of *pranayama*, the body of the Yogi begins to perspire. When it perspires he should rub it well, otherwise the body of the Yogi loses its *Dhatu* [humours]. In the second stage there takes place the trembling of the body; in the third, the jumping about like a frog; and when the practice becomes greater, the adept walks in the air.'

X Yoga and Sexual Health

YOGA AND SEXUAL FITNESS

The physiological factors which enhance sexual fitness are vitality, rich reserves of energy, good muscle tone, supple limbs and joints, and efficient functioning of the nervous system, circulation, and glands. On the psychological side, sexual well-being depends on freedom from tensions and anxieties, a relaxed openness of response, and total attention. Yoga practice promotes all of these factors.

That the disciplines of body and mind required for reaching the heights of contemplation and mystical illumination under the conditions of *ashram* schooling should demand chastity is understandable. There is no question here of repressing a force thought inimical to life, but rather of conservation of powerful life-currents and their transmutation into the finest vibrations of psychic energy. But celibacy (*brahmacharya*) is not asked of the 'householder Yogin' – the family man practising Yoga at home. Instead, it is expected of him that he will utilize sexual union to intensify and heighten his spiritual life. Coitus between loving partners can become an act of Yogic contemplation, taking on some of the qualities of the sacred rite that it becomes in Tantric Yoga. It is frequently reported that the sexual life of husband and wife takes on a fresh vitality and glow, and attains a heightened quality when one partner practises Yoga – better still if both do. The majority of readers of this manual will not wish to adopt chastity, unless for short periods, and will welcome enhancement of sexual health and experience within Yoga's harmonious life-style, based on the perfecting and balancing of physiological, psychological, and spiritual energies.

POSTURES AND SEXUAL VIGOUR

The *asanas* in general, by increasing vitality and lissomness, improve sexual fitness, but specific postures are held to act as restoratives of lost sexual vigour. Among these are the Thunderbolt Posture and the Supine Thunderbolt (in which one lies flat on the back after sitting on the heels in the basic pose), the Shoulderstand, the Plough, the Cobra, the Bow, the Locust, and the Spinal Twist. These, in their various ways, heighten libido, stimulate and tone the sex glands and reproductive organs, improve suppleness and pelvic and spinal mobility, and are beneficial for premature ejaculation, menstrual and menopausal disorders, enlarged prostate, frigidity, and impotence.

But it is certain *bandhas* and *mudras* of esoteric latent-power Yoga that act most directly upon the sexual muscles and organs.

BANDHAS AND *MUDRAS*

A *bandha* is a 'binding' or 'restraint', and a *mudra* is a 'seal' or 'lock'. Both are techniques for locking the breath and *prana* (or life-force) within the body, and the distinction between them is theoretical. These muscular locks and controls have on the whole been kept secret because of their links with the awakening of psychic powers and the harnessing of sexual energies, and they have been surrounded by unnecessary mumbo-jumbo. They have attracted people interested in occult and magical powers, and aroused prurient interest because they have been so persistently written about in guarded and abstruse language. Passages relating to them in the Tantric texts have been omitted in English translations or translated circumspectly into Latin, thus drawing attention to what the translators wished to conceal – like the old-fashioned bathing costumes.

THE TEN CHIEF *MUDRAS* AND *BANDHAS*

The *Hatha Yoga Pradipika* lists ten *mudras* and *bandhas* which 'should be kept secret by every means, as one keeps one's box of jewellery.' They are: *Maha Mudra, Maha Bandha, Maha Vedha,*

Khecari Mudra, Uddiyana Bandha, Mula Bandha, Jalandhara Bandha, Viparita Karani Bandha, Vajroli Mudra, and *Shakti Calana Mudra.* The *Siva Samhita* lists the same ten, but the *Gheranda Samhita* lists twenty-five.

Maha Mudra (Great Sealing)
The left leg is folded and the left heel brought in to press against the perineum (between anus and genitals). The right leg is fully extended, and you bend forward to grasp the toes of the right foot. The Chin Lock (*Jalandhara Bandha*) is applied, lowering the point of the chin into the jugular notch between the collar bones. The anus is contracted, repeatedly and strongly, and the abdomen is drawn back. Breathe deeply, filling the thoracic cavity, and press *prana* (life-force) down. Another life-current, called *upana*, which belongs to the abdominal region, is pushed up, and the two energy currents are united at the navel.

Reverse the roles of the legs frequently in practice. The big toe rather than all the toes may be grasped, or the hands may be locked around the ball of the foot. Beginners may grasp the ankle instead of the foot.

Maha Bandha (Great Binding)
This posture differs from the preceding *Maha Mudra* mainly in the placing of the legs. One heel is again drawn in against the perineum, but the other leg, instead of being stretched out straight, is folded and the foot is placed high up on top of the opposite thigh. Again, it is customary to retract the abdominal wall and repeatedly to contract the anus. And again, the esoteric aim is to unite upper and lower energy currents.

Maha Vedha (Great Piercing)
The sitting position for *Maha Bandha* may be adopted here, or any of the meditative cross-legged postures. A deep breath is taken and then held, the Chin Lock (*Jalandhara Bandha*) being applied. The palm of the right hand is placed on the ground beside the right buttock and the left palm on the ground beside the left buttock. The Yogi then presses down with his hands and bounces gently with his buttocks on the ground a few times. The anal sphincters and the lower abdomen are contracted as if in an attempt to bring anus and navel together. Hold the breath as long as is comfortable;

then release it slowly, at the same time relaxing the muscular contractions.

The *Gheranda Samhita* waxes lyrical (90): 'As the beauty and charms of women are in vain without men, so are *Mulabandha* and *Mahabandha* without *Mahavedha*. . . . The Yogin who daily practises *Mahabandha* and *Mulabandha*, accompanied with *Mahavedha*, is the best of Yogins. For him there is no fear of death, and decay does not approach. This *Vedha* should be kept carefully secret by the Yogins.'

Khecari Mudra

This is not recommended. Each day the frenum or membrane which joins the tongue to the lower part of the mouth is cut a little, until the tongue can be curled back into the gullet to block off the passage of air from the nostrils into the windpipe. In addition, the tongue is pulled out and lengthened by a milking action with the hands, until the tip of the tongue can touch the eyebrows. The intrepid Theos Bernard (7) gives a cut-by-cut account in his 'report of a personal experience'.

An ornate mythology surrounds the esoteric practice of this *mudra*, but it need not concern us here.

Uddiyana Bandha (Abdominal Retraction)

This is retraction of the relaxed abdominal wall on a full exhalation. It is considered to be one of the cleansing processes of Yoga hygiene, as well as a 'binding' in Yogic breath control. Its value as an exercise is what interests us most in our practical approach, and a whole chapter has been given to it and its accompanying muscle control, *Nauli*. Its practice is held by Yogins to improve sexual health.

Mula Bandha

For this exercise it is customary to sit in the Perfect Posture (*Siddhasana*), with one heel against the perineum and the other heel against the pubis. Sit in the Easy Posture if the Perfect Posture is too difficult. Dr Bernard (7) was instructed 'to take a position on elbows and knees'.

Mula means 'root'. The perineum, the soft part between anus and genitals, is contracted. At the same time the sphincters controlling the opening and closing of the anus are tightly squeezed, and so are the genital muscles. The lower abdomen, below the navel, is pulled back towards the spine. Try to pull anus and navel together. Hold the contraction for as many seconds as you can without discomfort. Contract the lower abdomen and whole pelvic area five times, relaxing for fifteen seconds each time between contractions.

Asvini Mudra
Tightening and holding shut the circular anal sphincters, as performed in *Mula Bandha* and other controls, is called *Asvini* or Horse *Mudra*. The contraction is named after the staling of a horse. This is an important muscle control in relation to sexual health and fitness, because the fibres of the anus join with those of the genital area.

Jalandhara Bandha (Chin Lock)
This is the Chin Lock employed to assist in suspension of breathing (*kumbhaka*) in advanced Yogic breath control. The chin is lowered into the jugular notch between the collar bones high up on the breastbone. During breath retention it is often combined with two other 'seals' – *Uddiyana Bandha* and *Mula Bandha*.

Viparita Karani Bandha (Inverted Body Binding)
Though a posture, this is listed in the classic texts among the *mudras*. Theos Bernard gives it as identical with the Headstand Posture (*Sirsasana*), but Ernest Wood describes the Shoulderstand Posture (*Sarvangasana*). The main Tantric texts appear to be describing the Headstand. 'Place the head on the ground and the feet up into the sky, for a second only the first day, and increase this time daily,' says the *Hatha Yoga Pradipika*. 'Place the head on the ground, with hands spread, raise the legs up, and thus remain steady,' is the instruction of the *Gheranda Samhita*. 'Putting the head on the ground, let him stretch out his legs upwards, moving them round and round,' says the *Siva Samhita*.

Vajroli Mudra
This *mudra* is often omitted from translations and discussions of Tantric texts, or is referred to in such guarded tones that disproportionate curiosity is aroused. It should be remembered that Tantrism is the Yoga of Sex, and contains a number of occult and magical concepts and practices. These are not the most appealing or practical of Yogic techniques, but the modern reader is entitled

to read the texts without resort to Latin. The *Hatha Yoga Pradipika* says (77):

> Even one who lives a wayward life without observing any rules of Yoga, but performs *Vajroli*, deserves success and is a Yogi. Two things are necessary for this, and these are difficult to get for the ordinary people – (1) milk and (2) a woman behaving, as desired. By practising to draw in the *Bindu* (semen) discharged during cohabitation, whether one be a man or a woman, one obtains success in the practice of *Vajroli*. By means of a pipe, one should blow air slowly into the passage in the male organ. By practice, the discharged *Bindu* is drawn up. One can draw back and preserve one's own discharged *Bindu*. The Yogi who can protect his *Bindu* thus, overcomes death; because death comes by discharging *Bindu*, and life is prolonged by its preservation. By preserving *Bindu*, the body of the Yogi emits a pleasing smell. There is no fear of death so long as the *Bindu* is well established in the body. The *Bindu* of men is under the control of the mind, and life is dependent on the *Bindu*. Hence, mind and *Bindu* should be protected by all means.

Here we perceive a concept which has received as yet no scientific backing, but which persists in folk-lore, and in occult, magical, and 'higher knowledge' cults: namely, that retaining semen is a way of conserving life-force. The association of semen with strength, potency, creative power, and the masculine principle in the universe is understandable. As the source of procreation, it was inevitable that it should be credited with magical and occult powers.

The sexual control (not recommended here) of absorbing the ejaculate seems incredible, but one recalls the technique of taking a cup of water into the bladder through the urethra, mentioned in the chapter on Yoga's cleansing processes. The same method is clearly involved here. It is unlikely to 'catch on' as a method of birth control – but what a puzzle for some theologians if it did!

The description of *Vajroli* given in the *Gheranda Samhita* bears no relation to the above sexual control, and is obviously a posture (90): 'Place the two palms on the ground, raise the legs in the air upward, the head not touching the earth. This awakens the *Sakti*, causes long life, and is called *Vajroli* by the sages.'

Shakti Calana Mudra

This is concerned with the arousal of latent psychic nerve-force in the body – symbolically a coiled serpent (*kundalini*) that sleeps between the rectum and the base of the spine. The symbolism of its arousal and ascent through the vital centres (*chakras*) to the crown of the head is colourful and complex, and belongs to the Yoga of Meditation. Shakti is the female power or principle in nature.

Sahajoli and *Amaroli Mudras*

Two more *mudras* may be briefly mentioned before moving on to the adaptation of some of the preceding muscle controls to enhancing sexual health. They are described along with *Vajroli* in the *Hatha Yoga Pradipika* (77): '*Sahajoli* and *Amaroli* are only the different kinds of *Vajroli*. Ashes from burnt up cow dung should be mixed with water. Being free from exercise of *Vajroli*, man and woman seated at ease, should both rub it on their bodies. This is called *Sahajoli* . . . the *Amaroli* is the drinking of the cool mid stream.'

YOGA AND SEX CONTROL

The prevalent problem of premature ejaculation (the Kinsey inquiry revealed that a majority of American males have an orgasm within two minutes of union) can be countered in several ways, one of which is breath control. Orgasm is triggered off by mounting physiological excitement – pulse rate, blood pressure, and breathing all accelerate during foreplay, eventually bringing about a climax and ejaculation in the male.

Yogins who have developed mind-body mastery to a high degree have control over all three excitatory responses, but for the majority of men it will be the last of the three named, breathing, which lends itself most readily to control. Respiratory regulation is at the centre of the practice of the Yoga of Vitality. Yoga makes use of the calming effect of slow smooth breathing on the total organism. The man who has a rushed orgasm within seconds of entry should learn to stay still and to breathe quietly. There are other supporting methods he can employ – choice of the least stimulating coital position, for example – but the second most important technique is another which Yoga practice induces: an ability to let go, relax the body muscles, and calm the mind's agitation. At the first sign of undue excitement heralding the onset of an orgasm, the man should let go with his body muscles, at the same time relaxing his mind – which may mean visualizing a pastoral scene, or some such act of imagination. Eastern couples sustain coitus longer than Western couples: Western attitudes of hurry, worry, and grab-what-pleasure-you-can-quickly are contributing factors.

For women, the problem is mostly one of not achieving orgasm at all. Here again, relaxation of breathing, musculature, and mind keeps away the kind of psycho-physical tension that militates against sexual fulfilment. Teachers of Hatha Yoga to women report that their pupils frequently report a happier and more relaxed sex life after a few months' regular Yoga practice.

Abdominal Retraction (Uddiyana Bandha)
This has been given a chapter to itself. Among the many benefits of this muscle control is its influence on sexual health and vitality. Besides massaging the abdominal viscera, it tones up the muscles of the pelvic floor, relieves congestion and activates circulation in that area.

Contraction of the Penile Muscles of Erection
The male sexual organ, in responding to sexual excitement, engorges with blood, lifts and rises to an angle above horizontal. The erector penis muscles responsible for the rise and the *transversus pevinei* and ejaculatory muscles contract to press on the root of the penis to 'bind' it and keep blood in the spongy tissues of the organ. Normally, the erection of the penis does not come under conscious control – but the penile muscles of erection can be contracted, toned, and strengthened, whether the penis is flaccid or erect. The result is a short quick 'jerk' that is more visible in an erect phallus. Make ten contractions without pause. Relax a few seconds; then repeat. Relax again for a short time, and repeat.

Contraction of the Penile Muscles of Ejaculation
The ejaculatory muscles can be exercised and brought under conscious control in the following way. When urinating, cut off the flow abruptly by conscious command, releasing the stream of urine again after a cessation lasting five seconds. This should be done several times until the bladder has been emptied.

Contraction of the Pelvic Floor
Both men and women can practise this *mudra*, which benefits sexual health. Hold each contraction strongly six seconds. Five successive

contractions is sufficient at any one time. As a result of contracting
the pelvic floor, an increased flow of blood circulates in the area, the
pelvic muscles are strengthened and toned, and neuromuscular
control is sharpened.

We are not born with this control, but we acquire it in training
to choose our own times for emptying bladder and bowels. The
contraction operates when an adult has to cope with a natural urge
to urinate or defecate at a time when circumstances force delay in
answering the call. It will be found that contraction of either set of
muscles means contraction of both. There is an anatomical reason
for this: the fibres of the two sets of muscles intermingle. It is
possible to develop control of each set of muscles separately, but
our concern here is to contract the whole area from pubis to rectum.
Squeeze and draw in the muscles as though you were trying to make
navel and anus meet. The more powerful of the two sets of muscles
are those of the anus (the anal sphincters). So by directing your
command to the stronger anal muscles you normally ensure effective
control of the whole area. Later, control of specific parts of the
pelvic floor may be acquired.

Contraction of the Vaginal Muscles
These muscles are contracted when a woman urgently wants to
empty her bladder but is forced to wait, and in the spasmodic
contractions of orgasm. The *bulbo-spongiosus*, which acts as a
vaginal sphincter, can be squeezed in, but the opening to the
vagina, unlike that to the rectum, is always slightly open, and the
muscles usually grip less strongly. A woman can also squeeze in the
levator muscle in the wider part of the vagina. Like the rectum, the
vagina has two main muscles controlling its action – a sphincter
muscle that grips or opens and a levator muscle that draws up. The
anal sphincter is trained to grip and open in childhood; the vaginal
sphincter tends to be neglected.

In contracting the pelvic floor, the vaginal muscles share in the
squeezing in and drawing up. If a woman concentrates her attention
upon the sensations experienced in this area, she can develop the
grip and pull, influencing sexual health and fitness and increasing
the enjoyment of coitus for both partners.

Each contraction should be strongly sustained for six seconds,
and ten contractions should be made, with brief relaxation between
them. Do not dissipate energy by contracting muscles other than

those in the pelvis. After one month's practice, an attempt should be made to contract the vagina separately from the anus. As there is an intermingling of the fibres of the two sets of muscles, separate control will not be one hundred per cent successful, but the relative strengths of the contractions felt in the two parts can be reversed, so that the vaginal squeezing in and drawing up becomes the stronger. At first the vaginal opening (sphincter) will noticeably be felt to contract, but later the sensations in the inner walls will also be experienced and recorded, to act as feedback information for full vaginal muscular control. The acme of this intimate female control is to contract the muscles of the deeper walls separately from those of the entrance. Some women can contract the clitoris separately.

The effects of applying this control during coitus are considerable. i. There are bunches of sensitive pleasure nerves concentrated at the vaginal orifice, which are stimulated by squeezing in the vaginal sphincter. ii. The clitoris, the most pleasurably sensitive of all the female sexual organs, is drawn down towards the phallus. iii. The male's pleasure is also enhanced – so much so, that for a man with the problem of hasty ejaculation it is prudent to leave his partner's 'milking' action until the final rush to climax. The Hindu love-manual, the *Ananga-Ranga*, says: 'To this end, i.e., to give pleasure to the husband, she [the wife] must ever strive to close and constrict the *Yoni* [vagina] until it holds the *Linga* [penis], as with a finger, opening and shutting at her pleasure, and finally acting as the hand of the Gopi-girl, who milks the cow.' iv. The penis can be held in the vagina following ejaculation and during detumescence, adding to the 'afterglow' for both partners, and also lessening the frustrating effects of premature ejaculation, should it occur. If the root of the penis is gripped firmly, blood will drain from the spongy tissues in a slow trickle. v. Where there are potency problems, full erection being difficult to maintain, this female art of vaginal control ensures that the penis is held in the vagina and squeezed repeatedly, assisting firmness. vi. By control of the vaginal sphincter, a woman can retain seminal fluid when she is seeking conception. vii. Lastly, the vaginal contractions tone muscles that may slacken through childbirth or age.

This intimate Yogic muscle control improves a woman's sexual health and well-being. She feels secure in her womanhood and in the knowledge that her sexual efficiency can be maintained late into life.

SEX AND MATURITY

For a fuller account of the use of exercises and muscle controls to improve and maintain sex fitness through the middle years and later, see the author's book *Techniques of Sex Fitness* (Universal, New York). The eminent British sexologist, Dr Robert Chartham, reviewing this work for *Forum*, called it 'one of the most important books on sex and health which has appeared in recent years'. Yogic postures, *bandhas* and *mudras*, provided the basic exercises described in *Techniques of Sex Fitness*, and more briefly in this chapter. It must be pointed out that the increased sexual health and sexual enjoyment that results from these controls will take its place easily and unobtrusively within Yoga's total life-style, which is one of moderation in all things and, when fully developed, of universal love. Of the type of person represented by the perfected Yogin, Alan Watts has written (172): 'for them an erotic relationship with the external world operates between that world and every single nerve ending. Their whole organism – physical, psychological and spiritual – is an erogenous zone. Their flow of love is not channelled as exclusively in the genital system as is most other people's.'

But even those of us who have just taken the first clumsy steps on the path to Yogic perfection will find that the *quality* of our sex life, as well as its vitality, is enhanced by Yogic exercises and controls. And the quality grows with the passing of the years. As I said in *Techniques of Sex Fitness* (129): 'Many men and women find supreme joys in lovemaking late in life when the opportunity presents itself for a kind of distilled sensuality, a blending of fleshly passion and spiritual love with subtle overtones and harmonies denied to clamorous youth. For many men and women the best, sexually, is yet to be.'

TANTRISM

A surviving Indian tradition, of ancient origin, aims at utilizing sexual energy to awaken higher consciousness. There are two contrasting approaches.

In the first approach, sexual energy is conserved through chastity. This is a matter of sublimation, not of viewing sex as sinful or inimical to the spiritual life. The sexual energies are precious and to be harnessed for self-realization. Yoga increases sexual energy, but also develops the ability to transmute this energy into creative mental activity if desired.

However, the student, unless studying with a *guru* under restricted conditions, is not expected to forego sex. On the contrary, he is encouraged to use yoga to improve the quality and depth of his love life. Not only are levels of sexual energy raised, but sexual efficiency is improved in the ways already indicated in this chapter. Teachers of Yoga in the West say that their pupils often report an enhancement of the sexual side of their marriages after a short period of yoga practice.

The second yogic approach to sex makes coitus a sacramental act of contemplation. The mystical end-goal of yoga is a union of positive and negative, male and female, *yang* and *yin* forces in the cosmos. The union of individual Self (*Atman*) and universal Over-self (*Brahman*) is symbolized in the physical coupling of man and woman. Much mystical language has sexual connotations – words like 'union', 'marriage', 'merge', 'dissolve', 'melt', 'bliss', and 'ecstasy'.

Ritual coitus may be actual or a vivid working of the imagination. Orgasm may be withheld, or permitted after prolonged union, perhaps for an hour or even two hours.

This second approach – coitus as sacrament – belongs to the Tantric tradition, which is the subject of my book *Yoga of Meditation*. Among the yogas, Tantrism is unique in character and tone. It views life as a dance, a play of universal energy, and sees in the physical union of man and woman a mystical 'way', a path to transcendental ecstasy.

XI Yogic Diet

CLASSIC GUIDELINES

The dietary instructions of the classic texts are more direct than those given for the postures and breath controls, but for the twentieth century occidental they provide guidelines rather than detailed advice on planning meals, since a high proportion of the foods listed are difficult to obtain outside of Asia. Nevertheless, it is worth looking at what the three main source-books have to say.

The *Hatha Yoga Pradipika* (77) lists:
Foods injurious to a Yogi; Bitter, sour, saltish, hot, green vegetables, fermented, oily, mixed with til seed, rape seed, intoxicating liquors, fish, meat, curds, *chhaasa* pulses, plums, oil cake, asafoetida [*hingu*], garlic, onion, etc. should not be eaten. Food heated again, dry, having too much salt, sour, minor grains, and vegetables that cause burning sensation, should not be eaten. . . .

Wheat, rice, barley, *sastika* [a kind of rice], good corns, milk, ghee, sugar, butter, sugar candy, honey, dried ginger, *Parwal* [a vegetable], the five vegetables, *moong*, pure water, these are very beneficial to those who practise Yoga. A Yogi should eat tonics [things giving strength], well sweetened, greasy [made with ghee], milk, butter, etc., which may increase humours of the body, according to his desires.

The *Gheranda Samhita* (90) tells us that:
He who practises Yoga without moderation of diet, incurs various diseases, and obtains no success. A Yogin should eat rice, barley [bread], or wheaten bread. He may eat Mudga beans [*Phaseolus mungo*], Masa beans [*Phaseolus radiatus*], gram, etc. These should be clean, white, and free from chaff. A Yogin may eat *patola* [a kind of cucumber], jack-fruit, *manakacu* [*Arum Colocasia*], *kakkola* [a kind of berry], the jujube, the bonduc nut [*Bonducella guilandine*], cucumber,

plantain, fig; the unripe plantain, the small plantain, the plantain stem and roots, *brinjal*, and medicinal roots and fruits (e.g. *rhhi*, etc.). He may eat ghee, fresh vegetables, black vegetables, the leaves of *patola*, and *Vastuka*, the *hima-locika*. These are the five *sakas* (vegetable leaves) praised as fit food for Yogins. Pure, sweet and cooling food should be eaten to fill half the stomach; eating thus sweet juices with pleasure, and leaving the other half of the stomach empty is called moderation in diet. Half the stomach should be filled with food, one quarter with water; and one quarter should be kept empty for practising *pranayama*.

And the *Siva Samhita* (91) says:

Now I will tell you the means by which success in Yoga is quickly obtained . . . The great Yogi should observe always the following observances: – He should use 1. clarified butter; 2. milk; 3. sweet food; and 4. betel without lime; 5. camphor; 6. kind words; 7. pleasant monastery or retired cell, having a small door; 8. hear discourses on truth; and 9. always discharge his household duties·with *Vairagya* (without attachment); 10. sing the name of Visnu; 11. and hear sweet music; 12. patience; 13. constancy; 14. forgiveness; 15. austerities; 16. purifications; 17. modesty; 18. devotion; and 19. service of the *Guru*.

From the above three quotations, the general principles of the Yogic approach to diet can be discerned. Note the association in the third quotation of diet and morality. Yogins have reverence for all life, and follow a lacto-vegetarian diet. Westerners who join Indian *ashrams* are expected to adhere to this principle, though Indian *gurus* teaching in the West recommend it but do not insist upon it. And Yogins hold that kinds of food influence consciousness itself.

FOODS AND HUMAN CONSCIOUSNESS

Traditionally, three kinds of food are held to influence human personality: *sattvic* or pure food, *rajasic* or stimulating food, and *tamasic* or impure food. Examples of *sattvic* food are milk, butter, fruit, vegetables, and grains. Examples of *rajasic* foods are spicy and strong-tasting foods, meat, fish, eggs, and alcohol – all of which stimulate the nervous system. *Tamasic* foods are putrefied, overripe, rotten, or impure in some way. Each of these three classes of food has a corresponding state of consciousness: gross, intermediate, and spiritual for *tamasic*, *rajasic*, and *sattvic* foods respectively.

A physician called Charok, attached to the Court of King Kanich Ka, composed a work about 200 AD called *Charaa Samita*, in which he advised on the right diet for health, strength, and longevity. He classified the foods into two main groups: heavy and light (by qualities not weight), corresponding to the above-mentioned *rajasic* and *sattvic* groupings. Heavy foods have the properties of earth and moon, and light foods those of air and heat. The light (or *sattvic*) foods should predominate in a healthful diet. Examples are vegetables, fruit, grains, milk, butter, and cheese.

Yogins say that a growing liking for pure, wholesome, nourishing food is part of a student's spiritual unfoldment, and that progress in Yoga and purity of diet go together.

ALKALINE-FORMING FOODS

Most of the *sattvic* foods are alkaline-forming. Health depends on a slightly alkaline pH for the bloodstream. Invading bacteria that could be harmful find themselves in an unfavourable medium. Professor E. V. McCollum, of Johns Hopkins University, says that the daily diet needs a considerable amount of alkaline-forming foods: salads, vegetables, fruits; and a moderate quantity of acid-forming foods: starches, sugars, meat, poultry, fish, eggs, and cheese. The majority of the inhabitants of Western countries eat too many acid-forming foods, causing acidosis, whose symptoms are lassitude, headaches, nausea, insomnia, and loss of appetite.

THE CASE FOR LACTO-VEGETARIANISM

Most Indian Yogins are lacto-vegetarians: that is, they do not eat flesh, but do include milk and milk products in their diet. (The phrase must be 'most Indian Yogins' because some Tantric Yogins eat meat.) They are vegetarians principally on ethical grounds – the association between the purity of the foods we eat and our spiritual development mentioned above, and the cruelty and crudity of killing for food. They also share, with vegetarians throughout the world, doubts about the long-term effects on health of eating meat and meat products.

For thousands of years vegetarianism has been practised by millions of people in the East, where Brahmanism, Buddhism, Jainism, and Zoroastrianism have long held all life to be sacred. Notable people in the West who have been vegetarians (the word was not coined until 1840) include Pythagoras, Plato, Socrates, Ovid, Hippocrates, Seneca, Plutarch, Tertullian, Clement of Alexandria, Leonardo da Vinci, Rousseau, Voltaire, Milton, Oliver Goldsmith, Sir Isaac Newton, Shelley, George Bernard Shaw, Albert Einstein, and Albert Schweitzer.

It is true that millions of people go without meat from circumstances rather than choice: a vegetarian does so on principle. Two groups of vegetarians may be distinguished:

i. Vegans, whose diet consists of fruit, vegetables, nuts, and grains, and who exclude all foods of animal origin, including milk and milk products, and even honey. Nor do they wear clothing obtained by animal slaughter. They follow, as best they can, the idea expressed in Pope's line: 'No murder clothes him, and no murder fed.'

ii. Lacto-vegetarians include milk and dairy products in the diet.

The austere Vegan diet needs very careful planning if it is to provide all essential mutrients, minerals, and vitamins. Advice is given by vegetarian societies found in many countries. The lacto-vegetarian diet has proved itself healthful for millions. Some winning Olympic athletes have been vegetarians.

Vegetarianism, as a chosen life-style, is marked by Yogi-like simplicity, moderation, and spirituality. It may be argued that idealistic and spiritual people choose vegetarianism, rather than that abstaining from flesh makes them the kind of persons they are – but the belief is strong among vegetarians that killing animals and eating them coarsens and harms the psyche, and that only a suspension of imagination prevents the majority of Westerners from giving up killing for food.

Vegetarians believe that, in addition to its being morally degrading, flesh-eating is harmful to health; that the vegetarian diet, if thoughtfully planned, is the healthier of the two. They point out that cancer, degenerative diseases of the heart, and other 'diseases of civilization' are most prevalent in flesh-eating communities; that the anatomy of man is that of a frugivore rather than a carnivore (long bowels, the ferment ptyalin in his saliva for predigesting starches, well-developed salivary glands, incisor teeth, and so on); that the muscle fibres of meat contain large concentrations of uric acid, which the meat-eater has to eliminate, putting a strain on the liver and kidneys; that meat quickly putrefies, releasing poisonous substances, whereas vegetables, fruit, and milk products decay or ferment.

There is a sense, deep down, biologically, in which we are all vegetarians. As David Le Vay (143) writes (the first italics are mine):

The essential chemical elements of protoplasm are carbon, hydrogen, nitrogen, sulphur, and phosphorus. Simple compounds of these, such as water and carbon dioxide, require an elaborate synthesis for their conversion into organic or living matter; this is effected by green plants under the influence of sunlight. Neither man nor animals can achieve this synthesis for themselves; they are dependent on the consumption of vegetable matter, either directly or indirectly, after it has been utilized by other animals lower in the food chain which serve as food in their turn. *Ultimately, we are all vegetarians, and all flesh is grass.* Thus, the energy transformations of living matter begin with light absorbed by plants and end with the heat waste of both plants and animals. In its passage this energy is subject to the laws of thermodynamics and can be utilized to do *work*.

MODERN YOGA DIET

Westerners are well established in their dietary ways, but the student of Yoga should aim to change his diet *gradually* in the ways that follow – if Yogic belief is correct, the more deeply the practitioner goes into Yoga the more he (or she) will be drawn effortlessly to do so.

i.   Cut down on meat and meat products. Too much protein is acid-forming. Textured vegetable protein (TVP) from soya and other pulses and grains is now available. Its flavour resembles that of meat and it costs much less. Nuts are a leading source of protein for vegetarians and a substitute for meat. They supply the important B-group vitamins and calcium, potassium, phosphorus, and magnesium. Eventually, some readers may find they wish to give up flesh-eating entirely.

ii.   Avoid, as far as is possible, denatured and chemicalized foods, such as white bread, white sugar, and white rice; artificially sweetened foods; heavily sugared drinks; highly spiced foods; and highly salted foods.

iii.   Eat a lot of alkaline-forming (*sattvic*) fruit and vegetables. Swami Vishnudevananda, an Indian teaching Hatha Yoga in America, says (92):

> the valuable organic mineral elements of iron, potassium, lime, soda, etc., which serve as eliminators, antiseptics, blood purifiers, and producers of electromagnetic energy are mostly found in the plant kingdom. The main supply of organic minerals comes from fruits and vegetables. Fruits and vegetables also aid in keeping an alkaline reserve in the blood. This is essential in maintaining its capacity for carrying carbon dioxide to the lungs for elimination.

He says also that 'fruits and raw vegetables contain antiscorbutic substances that prevent various diseases.'

iv.   Include milk and dairy products in your daily diet. They provide materials for growth and repair. Milk's lactic acid bacteria aid digestive processes. Cheese provides first-class protein, and is a rich source of calcium. To quote Swami Vishnudevananda again (92): 'Milk is a complete protein food. Thus, a diet containing milk and dairy products, fresh fruits, oranges, lemons, and pineapples, leafy vegetables (salads), and whole grains should be man's ideal vitamin-rich diet.' In short, a lacto-vegetarian diet.

v.   Make sure you eat some uncooked foods every day. The British Vegetarian Society recommends that fifty per cent of food eaten daily should be uncooked. The reason for this is that cooking destroys vitamins and enzymes, which play a leading role in all life processes. Temperatures well below boiling point – between fifty-six and eighty degrees centigrade – destroy many enzymes. Many processed and tinned foods are deficient in them. The more raw vegetables that are included in salads the better for health. Add flavour with herbs. Including more uncooked vegetables, fruits, and grains in your diet ensures an adequate supply of enzymes and healthy working of those already in the body.

vi.   Eat some wholewheat bread and uncooked wholewheat each day. The roughage of wholewheat bread encourages the movement of food in the intestines and colon, and the bread is rich in B-complex vitamins and in the minerals potassium, magnesium, phosphorus, calcium, and iron. There is great satisfaction, and great benefit to health, in baking wholewheat bread for oneself at home. Two recipes follow, one using yeast and the other without yeast.

A. 1 lb. wholemeal flour
    Just over ½ pint water (blood heat)
    1 teaspoonful salt
    1 teaspoonful sugar (or crude black molasses)
    ½ oz. fresh yeast

Warm the flour and mix in the salt. Mix the yeast and sugar with ¼ pt. hand hot water and leave ten minutes to froth up. Stir yeast mixture and remainder of water into flour and knead dough for ten minutes. Shape dough into a buttered or floured tin, cover with a cloth and leave in a warm place for about half an hour (until dough doubles, to just below top of tin). Bake 35-40 minutes in a moderate oven.

B. 1 lb. wholemeal flour
    ¾ pint buttermilk
    1 teaspoonful bicarbonate of soda
    1 teaspoonful cream of tartar

Mix a little of the buttermilk with the bicarbonate of soda and the cream of tartar to form a smooth paste. Mix all the ingredients together to form a moist dough. Line a tin with a sprinkling of flour and coat the dough with flour to prevent burning and sticking. Bake for one hour in a moderate oven.

Some readers will recognize this second recipe as the 'wheaten bread' much enjoyed in Ireland.

Baking the bread should be an act of mindfulness, of total attention, of Karma Yoga. Kahil Gibran put it beautifully in *The Prophet*: 'For if you bake bread with indifference, you bake bread that feeds but half man's hunger.'

Uncooked wheat is superior even to wholewheat bread for supplying enzymes and vitamin B which, because it benefits the nerves and digestion, is called 'the happiness vitamin'. It is also a rich source of vitamin E, which has associations with sexual health. Purchase organically-grown wheat grains from a healthfood store, and grind them, using an electric coffee-grinder. Either make a porridge with the freshly-ground wheat or mix it with water or milk and leave it covered overnight. In the morning add some of the following: raisins or chopped dates, nuts, apples, bananas, lemon juice, honey or maple syrup. This breakfast supplies energy for several hours and satisfies hunger.

vii.   Keep meals simple. This means having a few foods instead of many at one meal. Include a high proportion of natural fresh uncooked foods.

viii.   Eat moderately. The physician Charok said: 'One should take a proper measure of food.' This means leaving the table feeling one might have eaten a little more – so following the injunction of the classic text quoted earlier to leave a quarter of the stomach empty. As the aims of Yogic training are health, purification, and self-realization, the Yogin's diet should become a part of Yogic practice. This means simplicity and moderation – but never inadequacy. There are Hindu ascetics who seek to ingratiate themselves with the Divine Source by going without food until they are skin and bones. Hatha Yoga texts make it clear that this is not a true Yoga path. The founder of the Buddhist religion tried it and found it a hindrance rather than a help in finding man's essential nature.

ix.   Chew well. The first process of digestion takes place in the mouth, with the mixing of food and saliva. Strong chewing brings maximum flavour out of the food, as well as aiding digestion. Thorough mastication is yet another yoga exercise, and so to be performed with full attention.

CONCLUSION

If the reader has not been content merely to read through this book but has already put its techniques and exercises into practice, then he or she will probably have joined the many people who practise Yoga regularly and who have discovered that such practice improves the quality of living. It does this by improving health and by increasing vitality – and, integrated with the preceding two benefits, by inducing psycho-physical poise and relaxation. This writer first began to study and to experiment with Indian Yoga and Eastern systems of meditation twenty-five years ago at a time when he was writing his first book – on the subject of relaxation. He still feels that relaxation of a profound quality is the greatest benefit that Yoga offers to its European and American practitioners.

The pace and pressures of living in Western technological society destroy health and happiness through what are known as the 'stress diseases' and tensions within the psyche. Doctors estimate that over one million people in Britain suffer from tension headaches – a different problem from migraine, though often mistaken for it. The main cause of the headache is tension in the muscles at the back of the neck. Doctors know only one treatment – to prescribe tranquillizing drugs to dull the impact of stress and to reduce the pain. How much better to counter stress with the body's own defences! It is here primarily that Yoga has proved so effective and so valuable for Western men and women.

Posture Programmes For Life

The Yogic postures, by repeatedly stretching the trunk and limbs and because of their serene immobility, smooth away tension in those muscles where it most frequently lodges – in the lower back and in the neck.

The third chapter of this book should establish the reader in the practice of a sound and well-balanced programme of postures. However, after some months there is likely to develop a wish to extend the range of practice. In *Yoga of Posture* this writer has described more than four hundred postures, including limber-up exercises and Western adaptations and modifications of classic *asanas*. Books by the Indian masters, however valuable for the serious student, fail to allow for the lack of suppleness of the average European and American taking up Yoga. But this reference guide – the most complete ever published – meets the needs of students at every level of strength and suppleness, and there is guidance for planning programmes for beginners, intermediate, and advanced students.

Meditation For Physical Health and Psychological Well-being

Yoga of Meditation – the third volume in a trilogy on Yoga practice – covers a subject touched on only indirectly in the first two volumes. Consciousness is influenced to some extent by the breath controls and postures – but for the deepest changes, bringing serenity and inner freedom, you will need to practise Yoga meditation.

Persons interested in Eastern mysticism and metaphysics will not need any persuading to take an interest in the practice of Yoga meditation. But not all enthusiasts for the 'physical' type of Yoga are attracted by the mental disciplines. However, this indifference or aversion is mostly due to outdated notions of the nature and effects of meditation.

Yoga meditation is a technique, and not a religion. It was devised thousands of years ago to silence the 'monkey chatter' of thought and so reveal pure consciousness, which is held to be the ground of being. But the reasons for practising meditation today are no longer only those associated with mysticism or the occult. Recent studies at Western medical centres have shown clearly that meditation induces marked physiological and psychological changes associated with rest and relaxation of a transforming quality. Investigations into the physiology of meditation show that it reduces stress, reduces the breathing rate and the metabolic rate (oxygen consumption), lowers blood pressure in cases where the level is too high, and reduces the concentration of lactate in the blood. EEG equipment shows that deep meditation produces orderly brain patterns of beta and theta waves that are distinct from the patterns observed during drowsiness, sleep and hypnosis. These physiological effects are those that are associated with very deep rest and relaxation.

The psychological effects of meditation are also related to psychophysical poise and relaxation. Studies show that meditation reduces depression and neuroticism and also reduces the craving for drugs, cigarettes and alcohol. Furthermore, with repeated exposure to the deep thought-free awareness of meditation everyday living becomes more open, anxiety free, spontaneous, healthful, creative and rewarding in interpersonal relationships.

Traditionally, the Yoga taught in the present volume is viewed as a preparation for the Yoga of meditation. In the light of modern knowledge on the physiological and psychological effects of Eastern-style meditation this integral association of the two kinds of Yoga practice is justified more than ever. The Yoga of meditation intensifies and completes the transformation in the quality of living established by the Yoga of breath controls and posture.

Volume II
Yoga of Posture

I The Rewarding Practice of Yoga Posturing

A COMPLETE GUIDE FOR WESTERNERS

Many thousands of Westerners, men and women of widely varying ages, are finding in Yoga a way to greater energy, better health, a more youthful figure, and relaxed living. Daily their numbers are growing. This book offers for the first time a guide to the complete range of Yoga posturing, by which programmes can be planned to suit individual needs at every stage of progress. Drawing on the 418 postures described, beginner, intermediate, or advanced student can make a confident start and plan ahead for a lifetime of Yoga practice. For Yoga lasts for life, unlike most sports and physical-culture systems, which become too strenuous or disheartening once the strength, energy, and competitive enthusiasm of youth have passed.

Most people who take up Yoga continue with it – proof surely of its efficacy and value. The rewards of Yoga practice embrace both those areas which for conceptual and linguistic convenience we classify as 'body' and 'mind'. The aim of posture or *asana* (emphasis on the first 'a') is to attain steadiness of body and mind, a feeling of lightness, health, suppleness, and psycho-physical poise. There is a beneficial action upon the nerves, glands, and vital organs, as well as upon the musculature, and in perfecting the body, Yoga has ever in mind the harmony and health of the total organism. The mental disciplines of Yoga will be the subject of *Yoga and Meditation*. For the present it is enough to say that the postures evoke feelings of tranquillity, psychic strength, and lucidity of consciousness.

Manuals on the Yoga of Posture have tended to fall into two

categories. The first are specialist works for advanced students written mostly by eminent Indian teachers of Hatha (physical) Yoga. The second group are the popular text-books by Western writers. In the first group, for the numbers of *asanas* covered, three books are outstanding: Swami Vishnudevananda's *The Complete Illustrated Book of Yoga*, New York: Julian Press Inc., 1960; B. K. S. Iyengar's *Light on Yoga*, George Allen & Unwin Ltd, 1966; and Dhirendra Brahmachari's *Yogasana Vijnana*, Asia Publishing House, 1970. Of the three, Mr Iyengar's work is the most detailed textually and in the wealth of illustrations. Also worthy of mention is the American Dr Theos Bernard's *Hatha Yoga*, Rider & Co., 1950, a work of solid research into the traditional poses, based on the classic texts and on experiences in India. The illustrations show a degree of mastery of the most complicated poses unequalled by any Western expert himself illustrating a book on Yoga, but they are limited to thirty-six plates.

In the popular works written by occidental authors for Westerners, a new range of warm-up postures and adaptations and modifications of the traditional repertory becomes necessary. The average Westerner, especially if middle-aged, is lamentably out of touch with his muscles and joints, which have stiffened up and lost tone and elasticity. A great many of the poses of Yoga come more easily to an Indian than to an American or European. The most supple exponents of the complex poses are nearly all Indians. But such is the current enthusiasm for Yoga that the number of advanced performers in the West is increasing.

The term 'advanced' refers only to progression to more difficult postures, in terms of suppleness, of muscular strength (less often), and of balance and co-ordination. But it must be understood that if the rewards of Yoga practice were only for those who reach the equivalent of Judo's Black Belt standard, then there would be little point in most Westerners ever starting Yoga. Fortunately, this is not the case. Yoga is rewarding at any level; in one sense the beginner has more need of the postures than the very fit and supple person. And Yoga is not a sport: there are no opponents to defeat; the competitive attitudes inculcated in Western schoolchildren as virtues are alien to the spirit of Yoga.

The present work differs from the manuals of the first category mentioned above in that it incorporates the wealth of warm-up postures (essential for beginners); modern additions to the repertory of *asanas*; and simplifications and modifications of traditional poses, now widely taught in Yoga classes in Britain, Europe, and America, and described in manuals written for Western students of Yoga. These new postures grew out of the genuine need of Western students to free and limber muscles and joints more stiff in the main than those of the Indian, who is accustomed to sitting cross-legged on the ground throughout life and whose body tends to be more *svelte* than that of the American or European. Many Westerners are taking up Yoga after the age of thirty, forty, fifty, or sixty, by which time their ankle, knee, hip, wrist, elbow, and shoulder joints are stiff, their spines inflexible, their hamstrings shortened, their co-ordination, balance, and muscle tone poor. If such people immediately tackle the kind of poses found in Group B of this book, they are quickly discouraged and soon convinced that Yoga is for 'Indian rubber men', not for them. Painful joints and a stiff back are likely to reinforce the conviction.

This compendium therefore meets a real need for a comprehensive work that includes postures that are *practical* for every student, regardless of sex, age, or bodily condition. Full performances of the classic postures are not omitted, but neither are the stages whereby the average Western student can move towards standard and advanced technique, and probably a degree of suppleness beyond his expectations. For with regular practice, ideally *daily*, gradually the spine becomes more supple, the joints move freely, the hamstrings lengthen and loosen, the legs fold and the knees spread without discomfort.

THE NUMBER OF POSTURES

Three problems exist for the compiler of a comprehensive work on the Yogic *asanas*. The first arises from the seeming multiplicity of postures. The second is their naming, and the third is their classification. The classic Tantric texts are prone to inflated rhetoric, which fortunately need not be taken literally – for example the *Gheranda Samhita*'s statement: 'There are eighty-four hundreds of thousands of *asanas* described by Siva. The postures are as many in number as there are living creatures in this universe.' The book then goes on to say that 'eighty-four are the best,' and among these 'thirty-two have been found useful for mankind in this world.'

The postures described in this book have been gathered from both ancient and modern sources, from translations of key Sanskrit texts to the popular manuals of today. Examination of the brightly-coloured illustrations of an eighteenth-century album (the text of which was written in Braj-bhasa, a dialect of Hindi) provided a few *asanas* not recorded elsewhere – but in the main the album dealt with the standard postures, familiar now to thousands of Westerners: the Shoulderstand, the Plough, the Forward Bend, the Bow, and so on. British, European, and American housewives, businessmen, students, and others are today practising postures that were once the closely-guarded secret of Indian forest sages and seers. Ancient carvings reveal that some of these now widely-practised postures go back thousands of years.

NAMING OF POSTURES

In naming postures, either in English or in Sanskrit, one meets with some confusion both in classic texts and in those by modern authorities. A few *asanas* go under different names in the Tantric texts. On top of this, their descriptions are often difficult to follow. The teaching tradition in Yoga has been oral rather than written, esoteric rather than exoteric: and this explains why the classic texts are couched so ambiguously. The same thing is found in other esoteric systems: the priestly expert has to interpret for the student. The trouble is that different modern experts sometimes interpret a text in widely different ways. Thus the four authorities named earlier are on several occasions in conflict, both in naming and in interpreting. Mr Iyengar's *Virasana* or Hero's Posture is the other expert's *Vajrasana* or Thunderbolt Posture. The *Gheranda Samhita's* terse description of *Makarasana* or Crocodile Posture is given an effortful interpretation by Mr Iyengar, but to Mr Brahmachari it is a relaxation posture. Theos Bernard calls it the Dolphin Posture (see No 114 in this book). Mr Brahmachari's *Kurmasana* bears not the least resemblance to that of the other authorities, and there are at least six different views of what should be the main Hero's Posture. One could go on in this vein at some length. In this book we follow the most widely-accepted naming of poses and inter-pretations, but marked contradictions are indicated.

THE PROBLEM OF CLASSIFYING

Classifying the postures presents a third problem. Writers of manuals on Yoga adopt varying approaches to this task. Groupings may be determined by the part of the body principally used, such as the spine or legs; by the technical difficulty of the poses; or by what they are accomplishing. In this book we divide the postures into warm-ups, and A and B groupings based on the difficulty of the poses. The warm-ups are divided into standing, sitting, supine, prone, and slow-motion exercises. The Group A arrangement is as follows: standing, sitting and kneeling, relaxing and sleeping, supine, prone, inverted, and series postures, and muscular locks (*bandhas*). The advanced Group B postures are grouped: standing, sitting and kneeling, supine, prone, inverted, and balancing, with again the additional muscular locks. No method of classifying the *asanas* is fully satisfactory.

IS A TEACHER NECESSARY?

The answer to this question is that the *guru* (teacher) tradition, based on complete obedience, belongs to Eastern culture, but need not apply in the West where books are widely available and read. A teacher may still be necessary if one wishes to pursue certain esoteric aspects of Yoga, such as the arousal of serpent power (*kundalini*), but for improving the quality of everyday living with Yoga posturing a book such as this – of its kind the richest in content yet published – provides all the instruction you need. This does not mean that you should not join a class if one is available in your locality, and if you are the type of person who responds profitably to class atmosphere and the company of other students.

PROGRAMME PLANNING

Guidance for flexible compilation of individual schedules is given following each of the main sections: Warm-ups, Group A Postures (beginners and intermediate students), and Group B Postures (advanced). Posture to your *comfortable* capacity for maximum benefits.

CONTRA-INDICATIONS

Observe these where given. If in any doubt as to the suitability of a posture, either play safe and omit it or seek your doctor's advice.

THERAPY

Some of the *asanas* have a reputation for countering specific disorders. These have been tabulated at the end of this book. The postures are never a substitute for medical treatment, though they may well aid the correction of some disorders.

BREATHING

For maximum results in improving health and increasing energy, you should acquire the beneficial habit of breathing deeply, which means into the abdomen, as taught in No. 125, Figs 44 and 45. Yoga breathing exercises (*pranayama*), as much a part of Hatha Yoga as the *asanas*, can also be recommended for increasing vitality, clarity of consciousness, and peace of mind. This is outside the scope of *Yoga Postures*, but is dealt with fully in *Yoga and Vitality*.

The instructions 'breathe freely' or 'breathe normally', as given in this book, refer (unless otherwise indicated) to deep abdominal breathing through the nostrils, not the mouth. Usually the breathing should be slow and smooth, but occasionally the nature of a posture, in either stretching or compressing the diaphragm, necessitates rather fast and shallow breathing. This is generally indicated for the pose concerned.

PREPARING FOR PRACTICE

Before starting a Yoga programme, empty the bladder and evacuate the bowels if you can. Allow at least three hours to go by after a main meal, and one hour after a light meal. Rubbing the skin with a wet sponge or cloth imparts a feeling of freshness conducive to alert concentration. Clear both nostrils for easy breathing.

CONDITIONS FOR PRACTICE

Perform the postures on a level floor or ground. For comfort and safety, spread a folded rug or blanket. Beds and divans are too soft and yielding a surface for Yoga posturing. Not much space is required for Yoga practice, but furniture and other objects should be at a distance where they cannot cause knocks or injury should there be an overbalance or awkward lurch. The room should be well ventilated, the temperature free from extremes either of heat or cold, the air free from dust or other pollution. The surroundings should be as pleasant as possible for all the senses, and the session free from interruptions or distractions. Clothing should be loose-fitting and light: any clothing that might hinder movement or restrict breathing or circulation should be removed. Women who attend classes often wear leotards.

MANNER OF POSTURING

Finally an important matter: the manner in which postures are performed, the quality of attention brought to bear on each movement or stretch and during the poised immobility that is the peak of each pose, these are an essential part of Yoga. The spirit of Yoga is as much in the way it is performed as in the content of performance. The attitude is one of total whole-hearted attention – not a frowning, teeth-clenching concentration, such as is found in competitive sport or strenuous body-culture; rather a passive yet alert awareness, alive and wide-awake, but as psychologically balanced and poised as the muscular balance and poise of the postures themselves. Each movement and each holding of a pose should be accompanied by an attention that can almost be described as sacramental. Such an attitude not only contributes to the fullest physiological benefits from the postures of Yoga, but also makes their practice a form of meditation in the Eastern sense of 'mindfulness'.

II Warm-ups and Limber-ups

WARM-UPS AND LIMBER-UPS

These are usually missing from textbooks written by Eastern Yoga Masters, but appear in almost all manuals written by Western instructors. The reason is that whereas warm-ups are optional for the advanced practitioner, who has had years of daily practice and achieved a high level of lissomness, most Westerners are at the beginners' or intermediate stage of progress and their muscles and joints benefit from a few preliminary movements.

Warm-ups are valuable in two important ways. Firstly, the postures are more easily attained when the joints have been loosened and the muscles warmed by stretching and by the increased circulation of blood. Secondly, warm-ups reduce the risk of pulling a muscle or injuring a joint during the main programme of postures. They also reduce the likelihood of stiffness in the muscles and joints following a Yoga session.

Over several days the reader should work his (or her) way through the warm-up postures until all have been tried. Then he should devise a head-to-toe warm-up and limber-up programme on the lines suggested following the description of the postures.

STANDING EXERCISES

1. Palm Tree Posture I: *Palmyrasana*
In this posture, which has several variations, the body is held upright like the trunk of a tree, and the arm movements resemble the waving about of palm leaves.

Stand upright, back straight, head level, with legs and feet together, and the arms raised straight up alongside the ears, the backs of the hands facing each other. Inhaling, rise high on the toes, stretching the arms and body upwards as far as possible. Hold the stretched-up position for about five seconds. Then lower the heels to the floor, exhaling.

2. Palm Tree Posture II: *Palmyrasana*
Stand upright, feet together, arms raised as described for No. 1. The feet are kept flat on the floor this time (and in all variations of the Palm Tree Posture except No. I). Breathing out, slowly lower the arms to the sides, keeping them straight. Then raise the arms to the overhead position without bending them, breathing in as the arms sweep slowly up.

3. Palm Tree Posture III: *Palmyrasana*
Proceed as for No. 2, except that the arms are not brought down to the sides, but slightly in front of the body, so that the palms of the hands are pressed together in front of the lower abdomen. Again, exhale as the arms swing down, and inhale as they are taken up.

4. Palm Tree Posture IV: *Palmyrasana*
Proceed as for No. 2, except that only one arm is brought down to the side of the body. Bend over to that side and look up at the raised hand. The raised arm is kept perpendicular to the floor. Pause momentarily in the side-bending pose. Then slowly bring up the lowered arm, at the same time lowering the other arm, until the arm positions and the body bend have been reversed. Breathe in as the trunk straightens up, and breathe out as it bends over.

5. Palm Tree Posture V: *Palmyrasana*
Stand upright, with both arms straight up, feet together, as in No. 1. Keeping the arms unbent, bend first to one side, then to the other. Exhale as you bend the trunk sideways, and inhale as you straighten up.

6. Palm Tree Posture VI: *Palmyrasana*
Stand upright, feet together, one arm raised in the manner of the preceding exercises. Keeping the arm straight, slowly bring it down across the body, up again, then down, and so on. Circle first in a clockwise direction, and then anti-clockwise. Breathe out as the

arm comes down, and breathe in as it rises. Repeat with the other arm.

The Palm Tree series (Nos 1–6) improves posture, exercises the lungs, tones the arms, shoulders, back, thorax, and waistline, and dissolves muscular tension in the same body parts.

7. Standing Twist

Stand erect, feet together, arms extended in front of the chest, palms down and thumbs touching. Keeping your gaze on the backs of the hands, slowly swing the arms as far as possible to the left, without altering the position of the feet. Breathe out as you twist from the waist. Hold the twist to the left for a second. Then slowly return to facing forward, breathing in. Exhaling, twist to the right. You should be able to swing your arms round to a position at right angles to your forward-pointing feet. Inhaling, return to facing forward.

The Standing Twist develops spinal mobility and trims and tones the muscles that girdle the waist.

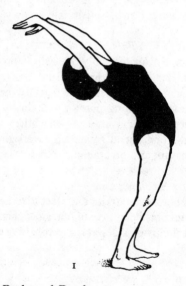

I

8. Standing Backward Bend

Stand upright, the arms raised straight overhead, palms forward, the feet a little apart. Breathe in. Bend backwards slowly from the waist, keeping the feet, legs, and pelvis steady. Tilt back the raised arms in line with the spine (Fig. 1). Take care not to jerk or to tilt backwards to the point of strain. Pause only momentarily before straightening up. Breathe out.

The Standing Backward Bend limbers the spine and strengthens the lower back.

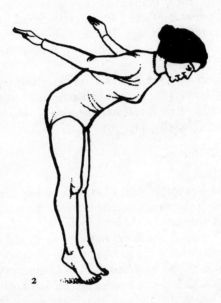

9.   Diver's Posture

Stand upright, legs together, arms by sides. Take a deep breath and rise high on the toes. Now lean forward about forty-five degrees and at the same time take the arms out and back. Legs, trunk, and arms are all kept straight (Fig. 2). Balance on the toes as though on the edge of a diving-board for ten seconds. Then, exhaling, stand up straight, bring the arms back to the sides, and lower the heels to the floor.

The Diver's Posture improves balance and co-ordination, and firms and tones the feet, ankles, legs, abdomen, back, arms, shoulders, neck, and jaw.

10.   Rag Doll Forward Bend

Stand erect with the feet one to two feet apart. Inhaling, stretch both arms as high as possible, palms forward. Exhaling slowly, fold forward from the waist, so that the arms, head, and torso hang down limply. The legs remain straight, though not tensely so. Let go fully with the upper body. Do not strive to touch the floor. The fingertips should either lightly brush the floor or swing just clear of it. If they rest firmly on the floor, bring your feet closer together. Swing the arms limply from side to side a few times, like a clock's pendulum. Then swing them a few times forwards and backwards between the spread-apart legs. The arms should dangle like empty coat-sleeves. The lungs are emptied by a long slow exhalation. Stand upright, inhaling.

The Rag Doll Forward Bend relaxes body and mind, exercises the lungs, and limbers the back and abdomen. It is at the same time preparatory training for *Padahastasana*, one of the classic postures of Hatha Yoga (No. 183, Fig. 79).

11. Chimp Bounce

Stand with the legs spread wide apart. Take a deep breath, and then squat down with the arms dangling between the spread-apart legs. Keep the back straight and the head in line with the spine. Rest the backs of the hands on the floor, and bounce up and down rapidly like a chimpanzee. Only the feet stay steady. It is important not to round the back. If you have that kind of humour, you might like to emit chimp sounds as you bounce up and down. At any rate, you should expel breath audibly with each bounce until the lungs have been emptied. Then stand upright, breathing in.

The Chimp Bounce provides an excellent warm-up and limber-up for the whole body.

12. Arm Rotation

Stand erect with the feet one foot apart and the arms fully extended in line with the shoulders, palms up. Slowly turn the arms forward and back, so that the palms of the hands face first the front, then the floor (Fig. 3), then behind, then upwards. Keep the body as upright as possible. Then reverse the rotation: palms back, down, front, and up, regaining the starting position. Breathe freely.

The Arm Rotation exercise improves the flexibility of the shoulder

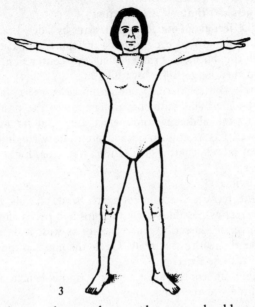

3

joints, and strengthens and tones the arms, shoulders and upper back.

13. Elbow Tap

Stand upright. Bend the arms so that the fingertips rest on top of the shoulder caps, the elbows out in line with the shoulders. From that position, bring the elbows together, tapping them together five times with short rapid movements. Meanwhile the fingers stay in position on the shoulders. Breathe freely.

The Elbow Tap exercise firms and tones the arms, shoulders, and upper back, and increases flexibility.

14. Standing Shoulder-blade Squeeze

Stand erect, feet together, hands on hips, elbows out wide to sides. Breathing in, draw the elbows slowly back and towards each other, squeezing the shoulder-blades together. As soon as the limit is reached, make two short rapid squeezes to a quick count of 'one-two'. Then slowly return the elbows to the sides, breathing out.

The Standing Shoulder-blade Squeeze strengthens, tones and releases tension in the shoulders and upper back.

15.   Abdomen and Buttocks Contracting

Stand upright, feet about one foot apart, arms by sides. Breathe out. Draw the abdominal wall back towards the spine, and at the same time clench the buttocks firmly. Hold the contraction for five seconds, and then let go fully, breathing in.

This muscle control develops mind-muscle *rapport*, firms and tones the abdomen and buttocks, and improves the posture and circulation to the abdomen and pelvis. The pulling in of the abdominal wall acts as a warm-up and preparatory conditioner for the important muscle control of *Uddiyana* (No. 162, Fig. 65).

16.   Hip Circling

Stand upright, feet about six inches apart, hands on hips. Keeping the back as erect as possible, circle the hips and pelvis slowly in a clockwise direction. Describe ten circles of as wide a diameter as you can make them. Breathe freely. Circle the hips ten times more in an anti-clockwise direction.

Hip Circling limbers the waist and hips, and is beneficial to the health and fitness of the pelvic area.

17.   Half Squat

Stand upright with the feet about eighteen inches apart, toes turned slightly out to the sides, and the arms extended straight out forwards from the shoulders. Take a deep breath. Keeping the back straight squat down until the thighs are parallel to the floor and right angles are formed between the upper and lower legs at the knees. Immediately rise to standing upright, and breathe out.

The Half Squat strengthens and firms the thighs and limbers the knee joints.

18.   Leg Raise in Front

Stand with the feet together and the hands on the hips. The legs remain locked at the knees throughout the exercise (this applies also in Nos 19 and 20). Breathing in, slowly raise the left leg forward as high as possible. Pause momentarily at the limit of the forward-and-upward movement, and then slowly lower the leg, breathing out. Repeat with the other leg. Maintain an upright posture.

This exercise firms and limbers the thighs and hips, strengthens the lower abdomen, and improves posture and balance.

19. Leg Raise to Side
Stand with feet together and hands on hips. Shift the weight of the
body on to the right leg, and slowly raise the left leg straight out to
the left side. Keep the spine as erect as possible. Breathe in as the
leg rises. Breathing out, slowly lower the leg. Repeat with the right
leg.
    This exercise firms and limbers the thighs and hips, and improves
posture and balance.

20. Leg Raise Behind
Again stand erect with feet together and hands on hips. Taking the
weight of the body on the right leg and keeping the back vertical,
slowly raise the left leg straight behind as far as is possible without
tilting the head and body forwards. Breathe in as the leg goes back.
Breathing out, slowly return the left foot to the floor. Repeat with
the right leg.
    This exercise strengthens the muscles of the lower back, firms
and limbers the thighs and hips, and improves posture and balance.

21. Shoulder Rotation
Stand with feet together and arms limply by sides. Concentrating
on the left shoulder-cap, circle it forwards, downwards, backwards,
upwards, forwards, and so on. Repeat with the right shoulder. Now
rotate the left shoulder in the opposite direction: backwards, downwards, forwards, upwards, and so on. Repeat with the right shoulder.
Complete the exercise by rotating the shoulders simultaneously,
first in one direction, and then the reverse. Breathe freely.
    Shoulder Rotation limbers and tones the shoulders and upper
back, bringing blood to nourish the nerves of the upper spine.

22. Head Roll
This exercise can be performed standing or sitting. Keep the back
upright, and the neck muscles as relaxed as possible. Roll the head
loosely in a clockwise direction, and then anti-clockwise. Be careful
to keep the rotation of the head slow and smooth. Breathe freely.
    The Head Roll removes stiffness from the neck muscles. See the
caution given for the next exercise.

23. Head Turning
Stand or sit with a straight back, head and neck in line with the

spine, chin level. Without tensing the neck muscles, turn the head slowly to the left until you are looking over the left shoulder. Stay three seconds in that position, and then slowly bring the face forward again. Repeat, turning the head to look over the right shoulder. Breathe in as the head turns towards the shoulder, and out as it returns to facing forwards. It is important to turn the head slowly and smoothly.

The neck is often the residence of muscular tension – other people can sometimes literally become 'a pain in the neck'. An unpleasant 'scrunch' or 'click' sould as the head turns is usually a sign that the joint needs freeing. Head Turning firms, tones, and relaxes the neck muscles, and has a beneficial effect on the top of the back where the neck joins the spine, a spot where an unsightly hump can develop. The exercise could be unsuitable for a person with a weak neck or neck injury: a doctor's opinion should be sought in such a case. The same caution applies to the preceding exercise, No. 22.

24.   Rag Doll Swing

Stand with the feet together and the arms hanging limply by the sides. This is a loosening-up exercise and a minimum of muscular contraction should be employed. Keeping the pelvis and legs as steady as possible, twist the upper body from side to side, swinging the arms loosely to right and left so that they wrap around the body like empty coat-sleeves. From the waist up you should have a rag-doll limpness; below the waist the knees can be slightly bent, and only enough muscular activity is employed to keep standing upright. Breathe out as the trunk twists, and breathe in as it faces forward.

This exercise loosens up and relaxes the upper body.

25.   Hand Inversion

Stand upright with the feet together. Bring the inner wrists together in front of the chest, with the palms of the hands spread apart as though supporting a bowl from below; the forearms and elbows are close together. Without altering the spread of the hands, invert the hands swiftly so that the fingers point down, raising the elbows high, and bringing the backs of the wrists into contact. Pause three seconds, and then return with a swift motion to the starting pose. Breathe in as you raise the elbows, and breathe out as you lower them. The raised elbows position has something of the look of a Spanish dancer.

This exercise increases flexibility in the shoulders and wrists, and limbers and tones the muscles of the hands, arms, shoulders, chest, and upper back.

26. Leg Pendulum
Stand upright, feet together, and hands on hips. Shift the weight of the body on to the right leg and swing the left leg forwards and backwards in a pendulum motion from the hip. The sole of the foot should just clear the floor at the lowest point of the swing. Stay as upright as possible, and allow the swinging leg to hang straight and relaxed. Breathe freely. Repeat with the right leg.

The Leg Pendulum exercise releases tensions, improves balance, and limbers the legs, hips, lower abdomen, and lower back.

27. Dog Shake Posture
Stand up straight with the feet about six inches apart and the arms hanging limply by the sides. Relax the body muscles from head to toe. The knees should bend just a little. Start shaking the arms, legs, and trunk from side to side rapidly like a dog shaking off water after a swim. Try to make your flesh as loose as possible on the skeletal frame. The hands should flap from the wrists as though they were empty gloves.

Muscle-shaking in this manner improves circulation and relaxation in all parts of the body.

SITTING EXERCISES

28. Sitting Alternate Toes Touch
Sit on floor, back erect, straight legs spread as far apart as is comfortable. Exhaling, lean forward and touch the left foot (toes if you can) with the right hand. Pause three seconds, and then sit up, inhaling. Exhaling, lean forward and touch the right foot with the left hand. Stay bent forward three seconds, and then sit up, inhaling.

This exercise stretches the back muscles, and strengthens and tones the legs and abdomen.

29. Sitting Walk

Sit on the floor with the legs extended together. Fold the arms across the chest. Keeping the spine erect, thrust forward first with one leg and hip, and then with the other leg and hip, so that you perform a sitting walk. Then reverse the action, thrusting backwards with alternate legs and hips. Breathe freely.

The Sitting Walk firms, limbers, and tones the legs, hips, and lower abdomen.

SUPINE EXERCISES

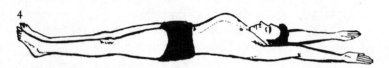

4

30. Recumbent Stretch

Lie flat on the back, legs extended together, arms by sides with the palms of the hands flat down. Breathing in deeply, slowly raise the arms to perpendicular to the body and the floor; then, exhaling, slowly lower the arms over head until the backs of the hands rest on the floor (Fig. 4). Keep the arms straight throughout the movement. Fully stretch for ten seconds. Inhaling, slowly raise the arms to perpendicular. Exhaling, slowly lower the arms to the floor by the sides. The breathing rule is to breathe in each time the arms are raised, and breathe out each time the arms are lowered. Try to keep the lower back in contact with the floor.

This exercise improves posture and circulation, tones and limbers many muscles, exercises the lungs and thorax, and dissolves stiffness and tension. It also provides preparatory training for the muscle controls of *Uddiyana* (No. 162, Fig. 65) and *Nauli* (No. 418, Fig. 191), because stretching the arms overhead on empty lungs hollows the abdominal wall, which draws back towards the spine.

31. Leg Raising and Spreading Apart

If you find this difficult lying flat on the back, sit up slightly, propped up on forearms and elbows. Keeping the legs straight, raise both legs together slowly to vertical (Fig. 5); slowly spread them far apart; and then lower the legs so that the heels are just an

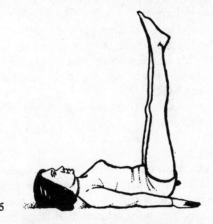

5

inch or so from the floor. Bring the legs together, raise them, and repeat the movements. Perform five times. Breathe in as the legs are raised and spread apart, and breathe out as they are lowered and brought together.

This exercise strengthens, limbers, and tones the legs, hips, and abdomen.

32.   Leg Raising and Sit up

Inhaling, raise the legs together, locked at the knees, and simultaneously sit up, forming a V with trunk and legs. Balance on the buttocks for five to ten seconds. Then, exhaling, lower the legs and back slowly to the floor. The posture can be made more difficult by clasping the hands behind the head or by folding the arms across the chest.

The legs, hips, and abdomen are limbered, firmed, and toned by this exercise.

33.   Side to Side Rolling I

Lie flat on the back, the legs fully extended together, the arms folded across the chest. Keeping the whole body in a straight line and the muscles tautened, roll over on to the right side; then on to the left side; right side; left side; and so on. Breathe freely. The rolling movement may be brisk.

Side to Side Rolling massages the hips and is a general conditioner.

34.   Side to Side Rolling II

Lie flat on the back. Draw the knees up and back and, clasping the hands around the knees, press the thighs against the abdomen and chest. Roll over to the floor on the right; on to the back again; then over to the left. Breathe out as you roll to the side, and breathe in as you roll on to the back.

This exercise tones and limbers the hips, thighs, and spine, and dissolves bodily tensions.

35.   Knees Swing I

Lie flat on the back, arms out to sides, and draw knees up together with the soles of the feet flat on the floor. Keeping the knees together and the back flat on the floor, lower the knees to the floor, first to one side, and then to the other side, twisting the head to the side opposite to the lowering legs. Continue at a moderate speed, breathing out as the knees swing down, and breathing in as they swing up.

Keeping the lower back flat on the floor presents a difficulty, but the attempt is an aid to good posture. Legs, hips, and waistline are limbered.

36.   Knees Swing II

Begin as for No. 35, but with the feet apart so that the left knee touches the right foot on lowering to the right, and vice versa.

The benefits are as for No. 35, but the different action on the leg, hip, and abdominal muscles will be discernible to the practitioner.

37.   Cradle Rock

Lie flat on the back. Cross the ankles, draw the knees up and back to the chest, and clasp the arms around the knees (Fig. 46). Round the spine, bringing the forehead up near the knees. Rock gently from side to side, breathing freely. If you should rock too far and go over to one side, a thrust from the elbow on that side should restore balance.

This exercise provides a spinal massage and quietens the nervous system, which explains why it is said to overcome insomnia. It can be inserted into Yoga programmes immediately following such back-bending *asanas* as the Locust and the Bow.

38.   Spinal Rock I, also called Rocking-chair Posture, Limbering-

up Rock, and Rock 'n' Roll

Lie flat on the back and press the knees against the chest as described in No. 37, but this time keep the feet together without crossing the ankles, and clasp the hands *behind* the knees. In No. 37 you rolled from side to side. In the Spinal Rock you rock gently backwards and forwards on the rounded back. Keep the forehead close to the knees. Roll backward on to the upper back, and forward until the soles of the feet almost touch the floor. Breathe out as you rock backward, and in as you rock forward.

This is probably the warm-up most widely recommended by Yoga teachers. It massages the spine and abdomen and releases stiffness from the spinal column. It is a fine exercise in its own right, apart from its use as a warm-up, for it has a beneficial effect on the liver and spleen, aids digestion and elimination, and quietens the nervous system. No limber-up, even when time is limited, should exclude it.

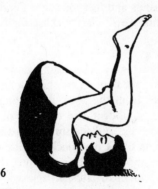

6

39. Spinal Rock II

Lie as for No. 38, but this time rock further back on to the shoulders, so that the knees are together above the face and the lower legs vertical, forming a right angle with the thighs (Fig. 6). Breathe out as you rock backward, and breathe in as you rock forward.

This is a more difficult version of No. 38, with intensified benefits.

40. Spinal Rock III

Only after you can comfortably perform Nos 38 and 39 should you include this advanced variation in your warm-up programme. Continue the backward swing, extending the legs so that the toes

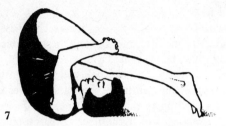

7

touch the floor beyond the head (Fig. 7). Breathe out as you rock backward, and in as you come forward.

This intensified version of the Spinal Rock stretches and limbers the body very strongly.

41.   Spinal Rock IV
In this advanced variation the ankles are crossed. Grasp the right toes with the left hand and the left toes with the right hand, and roll back until the hands and feet touch the floor.

The bodily benefits are similar to those for No. 40.

42.   Hammock Swing
Lie flat on the back, arms by sides, palms down, knees drawn up, soles of the feet flat on the floor about one foot apart. Raise the hips to about three inches from the floor, supporting the body on the back of the head, the shoulders, and the soles of the feet. Keeping the head, shoulders, arms, and feet firmly on the floor, swing the body from side to side like a hammock. Breathe freely.

The Hammock Swing strengthens and tones the legs, hips, and back muscles. The abdominal wall stays relaxed, but the abdominal contents receive a deep rolling massage, providing a corrective for constipation and an aid to intestinal fitness.

PRONE EXERCISES

43.   Alternate Leg Raising, Lying Face Downwards
Lie face downwards on the floor, the legs fully extended together, the arms along the sides, palms up. Breathe in. Slowly raise one leg as high as possible without bending it. Slowly lower it to the floor, and breathe out. Inhale and raise the other leg. Perform with alternate legs, establishing a smooth rhythm (No. 334, Fig. 156).

This exercise strengthens the muscles of the lower back, and tones and limbers the spine, hips, and legs. It provides preparatory training for the Locust Postures (Nos 335-7, Figs 157-8).

44. Shoulder-blade Squeeze, Lying Face Downwards
Lie face downwards, hands clasped behind the lower back. Breathing in, raise the head, shoulders, and upper body, and draw the shoulders and the elbows back and towards each other, squeezing the shoulder blades together. Hold the squeeze for five seconds; then slowly return to the starting position.

The Shoulder-blade Squeeze strengthens, tones, and releases tension in the neck, the shoulders, and the upper and lower back.

SLOW-MOTION EXERCISES

Indian slow-motion (*dhandal* and *bhasky*) exercises appear to be an imitative system entirely, in which working and sporting movements are performed very slowly and with maximum concentration. Pour into each movement all your psychic force (*prana*). Correctly performed, the exercises take on the appearance of a graceful and stylized dance or mime. Only a few motions are suggested here: the possibilities are legion, and depend on the knowledge and experience of each individual and his ability to mimic. A great variety of muscular movement is possible, and it is not difficult to ensure that all the major muscles of the body are brought into play. Slow-motion exercises firm, tone, and shape the body – they also strengthen concentration and calm and develop the mind.

45. Standing Breast Stroke
Stand up straight. Bring the palms of the hands together in front of the chest, wrists against chest, fingers pointing straight out. Exhaling, slowly extend the arms together to their full length. Twist the hands so that their backs are in contact instead of the palms. Then, breathing in, slowly sweep the straight arms back until they are in line with the shoulders. Here the action has been borrowed from swimming, and the arms, chest, and lungs all benefit. The Crawl, Butterfly, and other swimming strokes could also be copied.

46. Bow and Arrow
Very slowly draw the bow and release the arrow. Sustain the tension of the powerful bow all the way, breathing in. Exhale as you release the arrow.

47. Throwing
Here the field events of athletics provide a number of slow movements: throwing the javelin, throwing the discus, throwing the hammer, putting the shot (though this is a heave rather than a throw). Throwing a ball also comes to mind.

48. Pulling
Have a tug-of-war with an imaginary opponent: man, horse, or elephant, according to imaginative zest. Pull yourself up a gymnasium rope, or toll a great bell. Pull a boat from the water on to the land.

49. Lifting
Weight-lifting and weight-training provide numerous movements. The first-named is a competitive sport, and the last-named a system of body-building with exercises for every part of the body. Weight-training exercises with dumb-bells and bar-bells (one-handed and two-handed weights) thus provide a neck-to-calves body-culture programme that can be simulated in slow motion. Your local library should have illustrated books on the subject.

A typical weight-training excercise is to hold the bar-bell across the top of the chest, gripping the bar at shoulders' width, and 'press' it slowly aloft ten times, breathing in as you extend the arms, and breathing out as you lower the bar-bell back to the chest.

50. Hammering
A blacksmith hammering on an anvil comes first to mind. Hammer first of all with the right hand, and then with the left hand.

51. Expander
Hold a body-building expander in front of the chest and, breathing in deeply, slowly straighten the arms to the sides. Exhaling, slowly bend the arms to the starting position.

52. Digging
Turn over the soil in an imaginary garden, or dig a large hole. Dig for treasure if you need an incentive.

53. Kicking
Football provides yet another opportunity for slow-motion muscular movement, this time for the legs.

54. Punching
Have a slow-motion work-out with an imaginary punching-bag or sparring partner.

55. Tennis
Serve, volley, lob, smash – all the strokes of the game can be made in slow-motion.

The above examples of slow-motion exercise will suffice. It requires only a modicum of imagination to construct a rich and varied programme.

III Warm-ups:
Programme Planning

The most important aspect of programme planning is to ensure
that all body parts are contracted and stretched, toned up, limbered
up, and warmed up. A sound and thorough programme that meets
these conditions would be on these lines:

Nos 1–8; 9 or 10; 12 or 13; 15; 16; 11 or 17; 18; 19; 20; 14 or
21; 22 or 23; 24, 25, 26, or 27; 28 or 29; 30; 31 or 32; 33, 34, 35,
36 or 42; 37, 38, 39, 40, or 41; 43; 44.

The Slow-motion Exercises (Nos 45–55) may occasionally be
substituted for the preceding warm-up programme, but can also
be performed as a separate series at another time of the day. Warm-
ups are optional for advanced students, but they may use them as a
greet-the day limber-up on first rising in the morning.

For the greatest effect from only a few exercises, combine the Palm
Tree series (Nos 1–6) or Recumbent Stretch (No. 30) with any one
of the Spinal Rock series (Nos 38–41).

IV Group A Postures

These are for beginners and intermediate students. They include, however, some basic Yoga poses, including such classic *asanas* as the Cobra and the Shoulderstand. There are also many postures that are simplifications and modifications of the full performance of basic poses which prove too difficult in full performance for all but the advanced practitioner. In addition there are a number of Western insertions into the Yoga repertory of postures which are now widely taught in classes in Europe and America. As they have been specifically introduced for the novice or intermediate student, and also to meet occidental physiological and psychological requirements, they play an important part in Group A posturing. When perfect performance of Group A, with total comfort and ease, is assured, the student can investigate whether his or her joints and limbs will permit an advance to Group B performance. The posture numbers given in the index provide a guide to the development of individual postures.

It is impossible to attempt to predict how long it might take the average beginner to master Group A posturing and to progress to Group B posturing. So many factors are involved: age, suppleness, strength, co-ordination, bodily proportions, health. It can take months or years, and some people will never reach the advanced level. This need not cause dismay. Bear in mind that the postures suitable for your present level of suppleness and strength are those that will enable you to garner the valuable benefits of Yoga. This applies in all stages, from beginner to advanced.

Guidance in planning Group A programmes is given following the description of the postures.

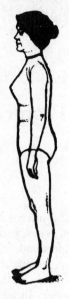

8

STANDING POSTURES

56.   Standing Upright Posture: *Samasthiti*

Sama means 'upright' or 'erect', and *sthiti* means 'steadiness'. This is the basic standing pose in Hatha Yoga, and the starting position for most of the standing postures.

In this posture you stand erect and steady, feet together, arms by sides, head, neck, spine, pelvis, legs, and feet forming a straight, but poised rather than rigid, vertical. By standing sideways to a full-length mirror and swivelling your eyes, you can observe how far your posture matches that depicted in our illustration (Fig. 8). (A frank observer is even better; or be photographed front, back, and side views.) There are two fundamental deviations from the poised standing posture. Slouching, round-shouldered, flat-chested, with protruding and sagging stomach, is one common fault. Equally harmful is a stiff, exaggeratedly-erect stance, pigeon-chested, back arched, head pulled back; this compresses the spine and damages health with its rigidities. One may have these faults in a minor or major degree. Adopt each of these two erroneous postures in an exaggerated way, and note that each has a characteristic psychological as well as physical tone. Poised posture is the only posture that imparts a psycho-physical feeling tone that is in accord with Yoga: one of alertness, balance, integrated energies, and wholeness. It is the life-feeling itself, firmly rooted in Nature, which the Chinese call the Tao.

In the poised posture the chin is held level and the head balances easily on the neck; the spine is straight, with no hump where it joins the neck; the thorax is naturally lifted (not deliberately thrust out) and deep; the pelvis feels centred and firm; and the legs firmly support the body, whose weight is evenly distributed over both feet and the full length of each foot. There is a sense of uplift and 'thinking high'. The abdomen is gently braced, feels firm yet pliant, and gives sound support to the abdominal viscera, which are free from downward pressures. The total feeling is of an unforced natural firmness and poise.

Yoga posture should be carried into walking, and its principles (straight back, even distribution of weight, and so on) applied to lifting, pushing, pulling, and all the multifarious bodily activities of daily work and play.

57.   Tree Posture I: *Vrksasana*

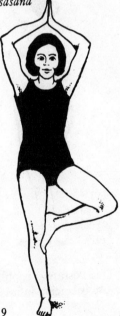

9

Vrksa is Sanskrit for 'a tree'. Stand upright, feet together. Bend the left leg and place the sole of the left foot against the inside of the right knee. Keeping the body upright, bring the palms of the hands together overhead, with the arms slightly bent and the elbows pulled out wide. Balance steadily on the right leg for at least ten seconds (Fig. 9). It helps balance to fix your gaze on a precise point on the wall straight ahead, level with the eyes. Breathe freely. Repeat, standing on the left foot. Later you should be able to place the sole of the foot higher up the inside of the thigh or rest the instep high up on the front of the thigh (see No. 163, Fig. 66).

The Tree Posture improves balance, posture, and concentration, limbers the hips, deepens the thorax, strengthens the ankles, and firms and tones the muscles of the legs, back, and chest.

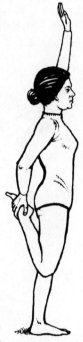

10

58.   Tree Posture II: *Vrksasana*
This variation of the Tree Posture is popular with Western students of Yoga, perhaps because balancing in it is less difficult than in the orthodox No. 57.

Stand up straight and, shifting your weight on to the left foot, fold the right leg so that the heel goes backwards and up towards the right buttock. Grasp the right foot with the right hand and pull the foot up close to the buttock; the two thighs stay in contact. Breathing in, lift the left arm to perpendicular, the upper arm against your ear, the palm of the hand forward and the fingers pointing straight up. Keeping as erect and steady as possible, stretch the left hand high (Fig. 10). Hold this position of stretch and balance for six seconds; then return smoothly to the starting position, breathing out. Repeat, balancing on the right leg and raising the right arm. If you hold the pose longer than six seconds, breathe freely.

The benefits of this variation of the Tree Posture are similar to those of No. 57, except that the limbering of the hips is less marked.

59. Doorway Posture

Stand erect with the feet spread slightly apart. Cup the elbows with the palms of the hands and raise the arms to shoulder height. Maintaining this grip, raise the forearms to above (and almost touching) the head, breathing in. Hold the pose for six seconds; then lower the arms, breathing out. If you hold the pose for longer than six seconds, breathe freely.

This posture expands the chest, exercises the lungs, improves posture, and limbers the arms, shoulders, chest, and upper back.

60. Tall Person Posture

Stand upright, feet together, arms by sides. Without raising the shoulders and keeping the feet firmly on the ground, become as tall as possible by slowly stretching the spine and the rest of the body upwards. Sustain the upwards stretch for ten seconds, breathing normally.

There is nothing dramatic about the appearance of this posture, but the spine and body muscles are subtly stretched and posture is improved.

61. Forward Tilt Posture

Perhaps this should be called the Leaning Tower of Pisa Posture. Stand erect, feet together, arms by sides. Imagining your feet to be weighted down, lean very slowly forward without losing the straight line of head, neck, spine, pelvis, and legs. You will only be able to tilt forward a little without losing your balance – learn to recognize the furthest point you can reach. Hold that forward-tilting limit for six seconds; then slowly return to standing upright. Breathe freely.

The Forward Tilt Posture improves posture, balance, and circulation, and strengthens and firms the feet, ankles, legs, buttocks, and back muscles.

62. Arm Stretch

Stand erect with the feet spread one foot apart and the arms straight out to the sides at shoulders' height, the palms of the hands facing downwards. Inhaling, stretch the arms outwards as far as you can and hold the stretch for six seconds (No. 12, Fig. 3). Exhaling, slowly lower the arms to the sides.

The Arm Stretch firms the undersides of the arms, improves posture and circulation, expands the chest, and tones the muscles of the shoulders and upper back.

63. Swaying Palm Tree Posture: *Palmyrasana*

This is another of the *Palmyrasana* series, used to open our warm-up programme.

Stand upright with the feet about two feet apart and the arms extended in the crucifix position (upwards and to sides forty-five degrees), the palms of the hands facing each other. Rise on the toes of the right foot and reach higher with the right hand. Keeping the left foot flat on the floor, swing the right arm gracefully across to the left and bring the right palm down on to the left palm. The left arm should not have moved. Follow the 'flight' of the right hand with the eyes. Hold the palms together for six seconds; then slowly return to the starting position, again following the movement of the right hand with the eyes. Repeat to the other side, rising on the toes of the left foot and taking the left hand across to the right. Exhale as one arm moves towards the other, and inhale as they separate.

The Swaying Palm Tree Posture improves posture, balance, and circulation, stretches the whole body in a graceful, flowing action, limbers the spine, and firms and trims the waistline.

64. Up-stretched Arms Posture I: *Urdhva Hastottanansana*

Stand upright with the feet together. Stretch the arms overhead

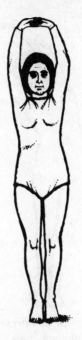

11

and interlock the fingers, turning the palms upwards with a twist of
the wrists. If, due to weak wrists, you find this hand position painful, interlace the fingers with the palms pointing downwards.
Breathing in, stretch up, standing high on tiptoe for six seconds
(Fig. 11). Lower the heels to the floor, exhaling.

This pose improves posture and balance, increases physical and
mental poise, exercises the lungs, strengthens the wrists, calves, and
feet, and firms and tones the muscles of the arms, shoulders, chest,
back, abdomen, hips, and legs.

65.   Up-stretched Arms Posture II: *Urdhva-Hastottanasana*
Stand upright in the overhead-stretch pose described at the start of
No. 64, fingers interlocked. Breathing in, stretch the hands high,
but keep the feet flat on the floor. Breathing out, slowly bend to
the right. Pause for three seconds at the limit of the bend; then
straighten up slowly, breathing in. Stand erect for three seconds;
then bend slowly to the left, breathing out (Fig. 12). Pause three
seconds; then straighten up slowly, inhaling. Repeat twice more.

This exercise improves posture and circulation, limbers the spine,

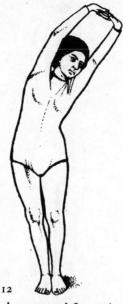

12

trims the waistline, and tones and firms the muscles of the arms, shoulders, chest, back, abdomen, hips, and legs.

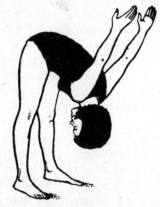

13

66. Flying Bird Forward Bend: *Padahastasana*

Stand erect with the feet spread about two feet apart, arms by sides. Keeping the legs locked at the knees, breathe out and bend forward from the waist so that you are gazing between your legs, and at the same time swing the straight arms backwards and upwards (Fig. 13). Stay bent forwards for six seconds; then slowly raise the upper body, breathing in.

This posture is excellent for loosening the shoulders and upper back, limbering the spine, and toning and firming the arms, hips, and legs. It also feeds the facial tissues and scalp with blood, and improves circulation. It corrects round shoulders and poor posture.

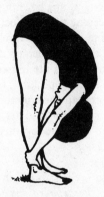

14

67. Standing Forward Bend for Beginners: *Padahastasana*

Stand upright, feet together. Breathing in deeply, raise the hands high overhead, palms forward, the upper arms covering the ears. Exhaling and keeping the legs locked at the knees, bend forward from the waist and grasp, according to suppleness, either the ankles or the legs above the ankles. Press the forehead towards the knees (Fig. 14). Stay in the folded-over position for six seconds; then slowly return to upright, breathing in.

Regular practice brings increasing suppleness. The nervous system is toned, the spine stretched and limbered, the abdominal organs are massaged, the legs firmed and toned, and the hamstrings at the backs of the thighs loosened. The facial tissues and scalp are nourished with an additional supply of blood.

68. Elbow to Knee Forward Bend: *Padahastasana*

Stand upright, feet spread about two feet apart, palms cupping elbows and the arms held out in front at chest height, as at the start of the Doorway Posture, No. 59. Inhale; then exhale and bend forward, keeping the legs straight, and rest the right elbow on the left knee. Stay bent forward for six seconds; then rise to the starting position, breathing in. Inhale; then exhale and bend forward again, this time placing the left elbow on the right knee, keeping both legs locked. Stay down six seconds before coming up slowly, inhaling.

Benefits are as for No. 67, but reduced in intensity.

69.   Beginner's Head to Knee Forward Bend: *Padahastasana*

Stand erect with the feet spread about two feet apart. Breathing in deeply, raise the arms straight up, covering the ears, palms forward. Breathing out and keeping the legs locked at the knees, bend forward from the waist and lower the forehead towards the left knee, grasping the left ankle (or higher up the leg if you are less supple). Press the forehead towards the left kneecap for six seconds before rising slowly to the starting position, inhaling. Repeat to the other side, lowering the forehead towards the right kneecap.

The effect of this exercise on the body is much the same as for No. 67, in which the feet are kept together and the forehead is lowered towards both knees.

70.   Arrow Posture, also called Bird in Flight Posture, or Virabhadra's Posture: *Virabhadrasana*

Stand upright. Shift the weight on to the left leg and slowly bend forward, at the same time raising the right leg slowly behind you until the trunk and raised leg are in line and parallel to the floor. The arms are spread wide, level with the shoulders, like a bird in flight. All three movements – forward bending, raising the leg backwards, and spreading the arms wide – are performed simultaneously, slowly and smoothly. In the final position, raise the head and look straight forward, balancing steadily for at least six seconds. Breathe freely. It will aid balancing if you fix the eyes on a point or object straight ahead and level with the eyes. Repeat, balancing on the right leg.

This graceful pose increases physical and mental poise, improves concentration, tones the nervous system, and strengthens, firms, and tones the legs and lower back. See No. 177, Fig. 76 for a more advanced form of this pose.

71.   Flying Bird Backward Bend

Stand upright with the feet a little apart. Stretch the arms straight out to the sides at shoulder level. Inhaling, bend back from the

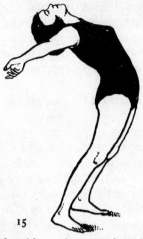

15

waist as far as is comfortable, at the same time throwing the arms out
and back (Fig. 15). In the final position you should be looking
straight up at the ceiling or sky. Hold the pose for six seconds.
Straighten up, breathing out.

The spine is here arched, in contrast to the forward bending of
earlier poses. The spine is strengthened and limbered, the front of
the body stretched, and the circulation stimulated.

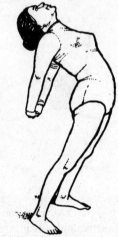

16

72. Standing Backward Bend
Stand upright, the feet about one foot apart, and the hands clasped

with interlaced fingers behind the back. Inhaling, bend back, without moving the legs, until you are looking up at the ceiling or sky. Push the hands and arms strongly out from the body, contracting the back muscles (Fig. 16). Stay in the immobile pose for six seconds; then slowly straighten up, breathing out. Perform a second time.

The effects are as described for No. 71, but intensified.

73. Red Indian Twisting
Stand up straight, feet together, arms folded and held out before the chest as we have seen the proud Red Indians do in films. Exhaling, twist slowly to the right, keeping the legs and pelvis steady. Stay six seconds at the limit of the twist; then slowly return to facing forward, inhaling as you do so. Then twist to the left, exhaling. Again a pause of six seconds before you return slowly to the starting position, inhaling.

Red Indian Twisting limbers the spine, and trims and tones the muscles that girdle the waistline.

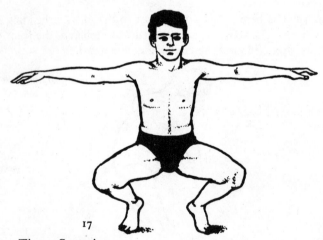

17

74. Tiptoe Squatting
Stand upright, the feet about one foot apart. Take a deep breath, and rise up on the toes, at the same time extending the arms straight out to the sides at shoulder height. Balancing on the toes, squat right down, exhaling and keeping the spine vertical (Fig. 17). Stay in the squat for six seconds; then stand up straight, inhaling,

and lower the arms to the sides and the heels to the floor. Perform once more, this time holding the arms straight out in front parallel to the floor, instead of to the sides.

Tiptoe Squatting improves balance and posture, and limbers and strengthens the feet, knees, and thighs.

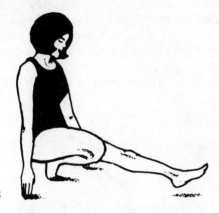

18

75. Single-foot Balancing Squat I

Stand upright, feet together, arms by sides. Inhale deeply, rising on the toes. Exhale, at the same time squatting right down, keeping the spine straight. Steady the balance by pressing the fingertips on the floor. Keeping the trunk upright, stretch out and straighten the left leg in front with the heel clear of the floor (Fig. 18). Hold this position of balance for at least six seconds; then retract the left leg and rise to the starting standing position, inhaling. Repeat the squat and balance on the left foot, extending the right leg.

The Single-foot Balancing Squat improves physical and mental balance, poise, and concentration, limbers the knee and ankle joints, and strengthens, firms, and tones the feet, legs, pelvis, and abdomen.

76. Single-foot Balancing Squat II

Once you have achieved steady balance and ease in the preceding posture, you can raise the fingers from the floor and extend both arms straight in front parallel to the floor. Performance is otherwise as described for No. 75.

Benefits are as for No. 75, with developed balance.

77.   Squatting Knee Squeeze

The first stages are as for No. 75. Stand upright, feet together, arms by sides. Breathe in deeply and rise on the toes. Exhaling, squat, and steady the balance by pressing the fingertips on the floor. Once balance is secured, fold the arms just below the knees, hands gripping the elbows, and press the body against the knees and thighs, taking care not to overbalance. Hug the knees firmly for six seconds at least; then rise to the starting standing position, inhaling. If you stay down longer than six seconds, breathe freely during the knee-hug.

Benefits are as for No. 75, with massage of the abdomen. Corrects constipation.

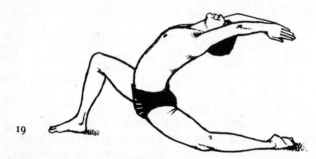

19

78.   Homage to the Sun Posture: *Surya Namaskar*

Stand up straight, feet together, arms by sides. Take a long step forward with the right leg and drop down on to the left knee, so that the body is supported on the forward right foot and on the left knee, and the fronts of the lower left leg and left foot. The lower right leg should be vertical, and at this stage the spine also. The arms are still by the sides. Now stretch both arms up high, palms forward, and tilt the spine and the arms backwards as far as you can (Fig. 19). Hold this pose for at least six seconds. Steady balance is achieved with practice. Breathe freely. Repeat, reversing the roles of the legs.

I have named this pose Homage to the Sun because of its similarity to some of the stages of the Sun Salutation series (*Surya Namaskars*), Nos 158 to 161. It is in fact inserted into this series by one eminent teacher of Hatha Yoga, Dhirendra Brahmachari.

This posture inproves posture and balance, stretches the front of the body, and limbers and strengthens the spine, hips, and legs.

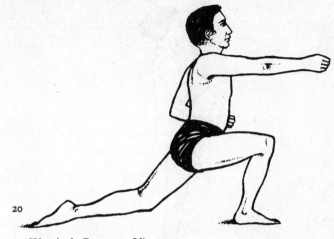

20

79. Warrior's Posture: *Virasana*

Virasana or Warrior's Posture is one of the 'thirty-two *asanas* considered auspicious' by the classic text, the *Gheranda Samhita*. The most common version of it is that described later, (No. 213, Fig. 92). Dhirendra Brahmachari gives a version in which the leg positions are similar to those we have just described for Homage to the Sun, No. 78.

Again we have the long forward step and the drop on to one knee. In No. 78 both arms were raised up and back. Here, when the right foot is forward, the straight right arm is thrust strongly out in front at shoulder height, the right hand clenched with its back facing to the right and the thumb tucked inside. The left arm is half bent and brought in against the left side, and the clenched left hand is pressed against the diaphragm, just above the navel. You stare fiercely ahead for six seconds at least (Fig. 20). Breathe out as you step forward and go down on one knee; breathe in as you thrust your arm forward. Breathe freely in the final pose if you hold it longer than six seconds. Repeat, stepping forward with the left foot, dropping down on to the right knee, and extending the left arm.

This posture strengthens and limbers the legs and hips, firms the muscles of the back, chest, and arms, and tones the nervous system. Brahmachari says of it: 'The practice of this *asana* generates unprecedented strength, vigour, courage, fortitude and power. It also removes lethargy.'

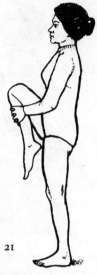

21

80.   Standing Knee Squeeze

Stand upright, feet together, arms by sides. Shift the weight on to
the left leg and raise the right knee as high as possible without losing
balance. Keeping the spine straight, clasp the right leg just below
the knee, interlocking the fingers. Stretch the spine upwards, pull
the knee firmly against the body, and look at a point ahead level
with the eyes (Fig. 21). Hold the pose for at least six seconds.
Breathe freely. Repeat, standing on the right leg and raising the
left knee.

The Standing Knee Squeeze improves posture, balance, and
concentration, limbers the legs and hips, and strengthens the spine.

SITTING AND KNEELING POSTURES

The popular image of a Yogi is of an Indian sitting on the ground
with his legs crossed and his feet upturned on his thighs – the pose
of the serene meditating Buddha, the Lotus Posture of Yoga.
Occidentals on first taking up Yoga despair of accomplishing this
pose. Many never do, it is true; but many achieve it in a matter of
months or years. But there are sitting *asanas* other than the Lotus,

most of them simpler. The simplest (and ideal for beginners) is the Easy Posture (*Sukhasana*).

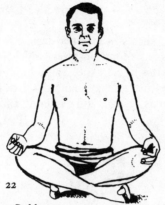

22

81. Easy Posture: *Sukhasana*

Sit on the floor with the legs crossed (tailor's fashion) at the ankles. Head, neck, and spine should be held poised in a vertical straight line. The knees and outer edges of the legs should be kept as low as is comfortable; if the knees are raised very high the pose will not be as firm as it should be, and the spine will not be kept erect easily – an essential feature of the sitting postures of Yoga. Nor can the body's weight be taken solidly on the seat. Rest the left and right hand limply on the left and right knee respectively (Fig. 22). Breathe freely. Gradually, with practice, the knees will lower: when they comfortably rest on the floor you can move on to one of the more advanced sitting postures.

Sitting cross-legged on the ground is common practice among Indians, for whom it is the most comfortable way of sitting. Occidentals, used to sitting mostly on chairs once childhood has passed, need a period of limbering the legs and hips before comfortably being able to stay for minutes on end in the sitting *asanas*. However, the Easy Posture can be taken up immediately by most Westerners, who should use it several times a day for short periods of reading, listening to the radio or records, watching television, and so on. Thus the knees can be spread further apart, and the legs and hips are limbered in preparation for more advanced postures.

Elderly persons and others who have difficulty in sustaining this posture for several minutes can experiment with tying a belt around the knees and lower back, to bring increased stability and comfort. But this should rarely be necessary.

Vary the crossing of the ankles – a few minutes with right ankle crossed over left; then a few minutes with left ankle crossed over right.

The Easy Posture shares in modified form the benefits accruing from Yoga's traditional sitting postures, which include limbering and strengthening the ankle, knee, and hip joints, countering rheumatism and arthritis, strengthening the back muscles, calming and toning the nervous system, and gathering and conserving vital energies.

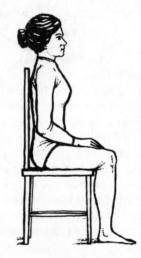

23

82.   Egyptian Posture

This is an even simpler posture than *Sukhasana*, No. 81. When, due to infirmity or any other cause, even the Easy Posture proves uncomfortable for Yoga breathing exercises or meditation, the Egyptian Posture may be used, sitting on a straight-backed chair. One sits firmly, feet and knees together, soles of the feet flat on the floor, the back perfectly straight, head poised on the vertical neck, chin level. The palms of the hands rest flat on the thighs, just above the knees, right hand on right thigh, left hand on left thigh. Breathe freely. One sits tall, yet without rigidity (Fig. 23).

The statues of ancient Egypt depict royal figures sitting with the poised dignity we have described. The posture was given the name

'Egyptian' by Sir Paul Dukes, an English authority on Hatha Yoga.

This sitting pose misses out on the limbering and strengthening of the ankle, knee, and hip joints obtained from the cross-legged postures, but does share some of their calming and toning influence on the nervous system and the sense of gathering and conserving vital energies.

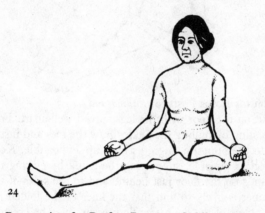

24

83.   Preparation for Perfect Posture: *Siddhasana*

A *Siddha* is a sage, seer, or perfected person. The extraordinary psychical faculties he has developed are called *siddhis*. The sitting posture named after the *Siddha*, in which he is wont to sit still and meditate, is described as No. 195 and illustrated (Fig. 83). Here we go in for some preparatory leg and hip limbering.

Sit on the floor with the legs spread well apart. Fold one leg fully and pull the ankle so that the heel is brought up against the crotch and the sole of the foot rests against the inside of the upper thigh of the extended leg. The outer edges of the folded leg and foot lie flat on the floor. The other leg remains fully extended. Sit up straight and rest the backs of the hands limply on the knees, right hand on right knee, left hand on left knee (Fig. 24). Breathe freely. Stay half a minute or longer in the pose; then repeat, reversing the roles of the legs.

This pose limbers the hips and legs, strengthens the back muscles, and calms and tones the nervous system. It conditions the legs, hips, and back for performance later of the full version of the posture, No. 195.

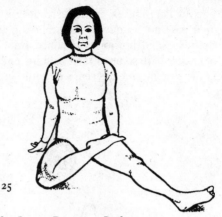

25

84. Preparation for Lotus Posture: *Padmasana*

As in No. 83, sit on the floor with the legs spread well apart. Fold
one leg, and assisting by pulling the ankle, draw the toes and instep
of the foot on to the opposite thigh, as high up as possible. Keep
the spine as erect as possible, supporting the trunk by placing the
palms of the hands on the floor just behind and to the sides of the
hips. The beginner is likely to find that the knee of the folded leg
stays obstinately clear of the floor. Gentle pressure may be exerted,
pressing it down for a few seconds with one hand. Breathe freely.
Stay half a minute or longer in the posture; then repeat by reversing
the roles of the legs. Try to keep the thigh and knee of the folded
leg on the floor (Fig. 25).

This simplified Half-lotus conditions the legs, hips, and back for
performance later of the full Lotus Posture (No. 199, Fig. 87), the
best-known sitting posture in Yoga. It is also a valuable exercise in
its own right, limbering the hips and legs, and strengthening the
back muscles.

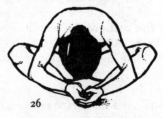

26

85. Star Posture

Sit on the floor with the knees spread very wide, the soles of the feet pressed together, and the feet clasped by the hands. Take a deep breath. Exhaling, slowly bring the forehead down as near to the feet as you can comfortably manage, at the same time lowering the elbows outside the shins. Draw in the stomach as you bend forward (Fig. 26). Bend forward for six seconds; then raise the head and trunk slowly, inhaling. Repeat once more. Advanced performers can bring their heads on to the feet, resting the forearms and elbows on the floor. Do not strain; just drop the head as far as you can without discomfort.

The Star Posture limbers the spine, the hip joints, and the legs, strengthens the legs and lower back, improves digestion, corrects constipation, and makes childbirth easier. It is contra-indicated in cases of high blood pressure or spinal weakness.

86. Knee Stretch, or Preparation for Gentle or Auspicious
     Posture: *Bhadrasana*
This is like No. 85, except that one concentrates on the spread of the knees and does not bend forward.

Sit on the floor with the knees spread as wide as possible and with the soles of the feet pressed together. Clasp the feet with the hands, without rounding the back. Pull the feet as far back as you can. Lift the hands from the feet and press the knees down towards the floor. Hold the pose for at least six seconds. Breathe freely.

The Knee Stretch adds rapidly to the flexibility of the knee and hip joints. Useful for women who wish to make childbirth easier.

87. Diamond Posture
Sit on the floor with the knees spread as wide as possible and the soles of the feet pressed together, forming a diamond shape with the legs. Grasping the ankles, draw the heels back towards the crotch as far as you can. Inhale. Exhale and straighten the right leg, without letting go of the ankle; bend forward as the leg straightens. Hold the pose for six seconds. Then draw back the right foot and press the soles of the feet together again, inhaling as you do so. Exhaling, repeat by extending the left leg. Perform a second time with each leg.

The Diamond Posture strengthens and limbers the legs and the hip joints, limbers and stretches the spine, improves digestion, and corrects constipation.

88.   Sitting Knee Squeeze Posture I, Also Called Wind-relieving
      Posture: *Pavanmuktasana*

Sit on the floor, legs extended, feet together. Exhaling, draw the
knees back and up to the chest, keeping the back straight and the
soles of the feet flat on the floor. Wrap the arms around the knees.
Inhaling, press the knees firmly against the chest for six seconds.

The abdominal viscera are massaged by the Knee Squeeze.
Intestinal gases may be released. Spine and legs are limbered.

89.   Sitting Knee Squeeze Posture II, also called Wind-relieving
      Posture: *Pavanmuktasana*

In this version each knee is squeezed against the chest separately.
One leg is folded so that, in the case of the right leg, the heel of
the right foot is under the left buttock and the right knee and outer
leg is pressed down on the floor. The left knee is drawn up close
to the body and pressed against the chest with both arms. Duration
and breathing are as for No. 88, and the effects are the same.

90.   Resting Warrior's Posture, sometimes called Hero's Posture:
      Virasana

This sitting position just described, No. 89, was that often used for
resting by Asian soldiers. In No. 89 we gave it as a knee squeeze,
but the resting warrior merely rested both hands on the drawn-up
knee o rested a hand on each knee. The pose was the same but
was put to a very different use. It was used when the warrior wished
to rest without being caught off guard.

91.   Little Twist Posture, or Preparation for Spinal Twist Posture,
      also called Matsyendra's Posture: *Matsyendrasana*

Sit with the left leg extended straight in front. Step over it with the
right leg and place the sole of the foot outside the left knee. Twist
the upper body as far as you can to the left and place the palms of
the hands on the floor to your left. Keep both the right knee and
the left foot steady and upright. Breathe freely. Stay in the twisted
pose at least ten seconds, breathing freely. Repeat, twisting to the
right-hand side.

The Little Twist Posture offers in milder form the benefits of
the full Spinal Twist Posture (No. 251, Fig. 115). It makes the
spine supple, squeezes and tones the adrenal glands, and tones and
calms the nervous system.

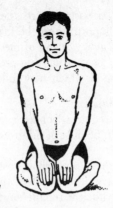

27

92.   Thunderbolt Posture: *Vajrasana*

This is also called the Adamantine, Diamond, and Adamant Posture. B. K. S. Iyengar goes against the general run by making it *Virasana*, the Hero's or Warrior's Posture, of which there are at least six different descriptions.

A number of the most valuable postures of Hatha Yoga have their starting-point in this position of sitting between the heels. The Thunderbolt Posture (*Vajrasana*) is the basic pose. *Vajra* means 'thunderbolt'. As with the cross-legged Easy Posture, No. 81, one should practise regularly until it is fully comfortable, which it is for the Japanese and some other races.

Kneel with the knees together and sit on the inner edges of the upturned feet. The fronts of the feet rest on the floor, the toes flat and not bent forward. Though the knees are together and the toes may touch, the heels are spread apart so that their inner edges support the outer edges of the buttocks. In advanced performance, Yogins sit on the floor between the feet. The left hand is placed, palm down, on the left knee, and the right hand is placed, palm down, on the right knee. Sit erect, with easy poise, keeping the head and back in a vertical straight line (Fig. 27). Breathe freely and sit perfectly still for at least a minute.

Beginners can expect to experience some protest from the knee-joints, but this should fade away with regular practice. One can speed up the loosening of the synovial ligaments by sitting and *gently* bouncing up and down a few times at each Yoga session.

Sitting still in the Thunderbolt Posture calms the mind and quietens the nervous system, improves posture, firms the legs, and limbers the knee-joints. As with the cross-legged sitting postures, this basic sitting-on-heels posture can be used for the practice of Yogic breath control (*pranayama*) and of meditation. *Vajrasana*, as was mentioned earlier, is also the starting position for a number of important postures, some of which now follow.

93. Lion Posture: *Simhasana*

Simha means 'lion'. It requires leonine courage to perform this pose other than by oneself, because of the grotesque facial expression that is produced.

Sit with back erect in the Thunderbolt Posture (No. 92, Fig. 27). Exhale until the lungs have been emptied; then open the eyes and the mouth wide and protrude the tongue down as far as is possible, at the same time straightening the arms and tensing the whole body. Hold this static contraction for six seconds; then relax for a short time, breathing normally, before repeating the posture once.

The Lion Posture is an early example of a static or isometric contraction exercise. Isometrics – a form of strengthening and firming the body without moving the muscles – entered the physical fitness scene in America with a bang in the 1960s. The Lion Posture stimulates the circulation of blood throughout the body and directs a flow to the throat and the larynx, which rarely receives such additional nourishing. The pose is said to improve the quality of the voice and to prevent or cure sore throats. By pushing the tongue out to its limit of extension, the muscles of the throat and face are strengthened and toned – a form of rejuvenation. It is a bizarre posture, but held in high regard in Yoga.

94. Cowface Posture: *Gomukhasana*

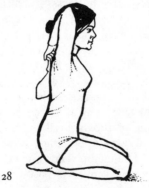

28

Sit on the floor in the Thunderbolt Posture (No. 92, Fig. 27). This means that the back is erect, the knees are together, and the buttocks are against the inner edges of the heels and the soles of the feet. Bend the right arm, raise the elbow high, and stretch the hand over the right shoulder and down the middle line of the back as far as it will reach without disturbing the spine's vertical poise. At the same time bend the left arm and bring the left hand up the centre of the back from below until the fingers of the two hands meet. Clasp them firmly by curling the fingers of both hands and hooking them together. The palm of the right hand faces the back and the palm of the left hand faces outwards (Fig. 28). Breathing freely, stay in the pose for at least six seconds. Then repeat, reversing the arm positions.

Beginners who find they cannot interlock the hands should grip a handkerchief, towel, or belt with the hands, shortening its length as suppleness increases. If the kneeling position proves too painful, you should sit in the Egyptian Posture (No. 82, Fig. 23) or stand upright.

The pose, viewed from the back, is said to resemble the face of a cow. Not everyone can see this. *Go* in Sanskrit means 'cow' and *mukha* means 'face'. The pose improves posture, limbers the shoulder joints, strengthens and tones the muscles of the shoulders, upper back (trapezius, latissimus dorsi), and rear upper arm (triceps), and gives a stronger grip. It helps prevent bursitis.

95. Expansive Posture

Sit on the floor in the Thunderbolt Posture (No. 92, Fig. 27). Raise the arms straight out at chest height and hold the palms of the hands together. Exhale. Inhaling, take the straight arms slowly out wide until they are in line with the shoulders. Pause for six seconds; then slowly bring the palms of the hands together again, exhaling. Repeat once.

The Expansive Posture expands the chest, exercises the lungs, improves posture, strengthens the back, limbers the legs, and calms the nervous system. Each posture of Yoga has its concomitant psychological tone. This one has expansive, reverential overtones – an unconscious matter that should not be consciously looked for or dissected.

96. Hugging Posture

It looks narcissistic – but the idea is not to love yourself but to draw

upon universal energy, which the Yogins call *prana*. Sit in the
Thunderbolt Posture (No. 92, Fig. 27). In slow motion stretch the
arms diagonally up to the front as though in a gesture of overjoyed
welcome. Exhale as the arms are raised. Inhaling slowly, and again
in slow motion, bring the arms down towards the chest. As the
arms start to cross in front of the chest, bend them and curl the
hands slowly. Cross the arms and wrap them around the upper
torso, the fingers placed just under the shoulder-blades – the
fingers of the right hand under the left shoulder-blade and the
fingers of the left hand under the right shoulder-blade. So much
for the physical action: the imaginative part of the exercise has
still to be described. As you inhale and bring the arms down very
slowly, think of drawing *prana* or life-force from the air and
appropriating the gathered armful as you squeeze your body, for
six seconds or more, exhaling. Repeat the exercise once.

The posture has added worth if performed out of doors. It
imparts the benefits described for the Expansive Posture (No. 95),
with an additional discernible but unmeasurable factor according
to how successfully you free your imagination to flood the body with
energy.

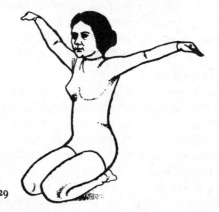

29

97. Flying Swan Posture

Again sit in the Thunderbolt Posture (No. 92, Fig. 27). Keep the
back straight throughout the exercise. Extend the arms to the sides
in line with the shoulders. Commence slow up-and-down undulat-
ing sweeps of the arms, in unison, as though they were great
wings. Imagine feathered extensions beyond the hands. Each hand

moves gracefully from the wrist, fingers drooping on the upstroke, flattening out and lifting on the downstroke. The arm action should have something of the power and beauty of the slow wing-movements of the flying swan. Breathe in on each upstroke, and breathe out on each downstroke. Take the arms high; then take them down to the sides. On each downward sweep of the arms imagine that you are pumping energy (*prana*) into the body (Fig. 29). Perform at least ten up-and-down sweeps of the arms. Only the arms should move; keep the rest of the body steady.

The Flying Swan Posture improves posture, tones the nervous system, energizes, limbers the ankles, knees, shoulders, and wrists, and firms the muscles of the upper back.

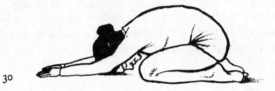

30

98. Salaam Posture

Yet again the starting position is the Thunderbolt Posture (No. 92, Fig. 27). Sitting with the back straight, inhale and raise the arms straight up, palms forward. Exhaling, lower the straight arms slowly forwards, at the same time lowering the head, shoulders, and torso towards the floor. Place the palms of the hands flat on the floor and lower the forehead also to the floor. Keep the buttocks down between the heels (Fig. 30). Stay down for six to ten seconds; then, inhaling, raise the arms and upper body slowly upright. Remain a few seconds with arms raised and the back straight; then bring the arms down on to the knees, exhaling. You have returned to the Thunderbolt Posture again. Repeat once.

The Salaam Posture limbers the spine, shoulders, and legs, stretches the neck, back muscles, and arms, and calms and tones the nervous system. Circulation is improved and a nourishing flow of blood is brought to the facial tissues and scalp. The pressure on the abdomen provides an internal massage, aiding digestion and correcting constipation. The psychological overtones are those associated with making an obeisance.

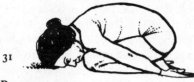

31

99. Child Posture

Sit in the Thunderbolt Posture (No. 92, Fig. 27). Hang the arms limply by the sides with the backs of the fingers touching the floor beside the feet. Inhale. Exhale, lowering the forehead and rounding the back until the forehead rests on the floor in front of the knees. The pose is similar to the Salaam Posture, except that here the arms stretch backwards, not forwards, with the backs of the hands flat on the floor alongside the feet (Fig. 31). Keep the head down and stay still for six to ten seconds. Then, inhaling, slowly come up into the sitting position with a straight back. Exhale. Repeat once.

The effects on the body and nervous system are as for the Salaam Posture (No. 98), except for those on the shoulders and arms, which do not apply in this milder pose.

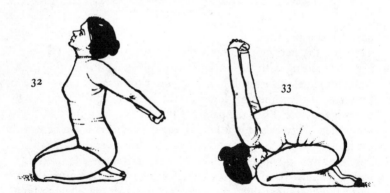

32

33

100. Anchor Posture, or Preparation for Yoga Posture: *Yogasana*

Sit in the Thunderbolt Posture (No. 92, Fig. 27), but with the hands clasped behind the back, fingers interlocked, palms up. This posture has two parts. In the first you inhale and stretch the arms backwards as far as you can, contracting the back muscles, for six seconds (Fig. 32). In the second part, breathing out, bend forwards, rounding the back and lowering the forehead until it rests on the floor in front of the knees. Keep the buttocks down against the inner edges of the heels, and stretch the arms and the clasped hands high and perpendicular (Fig. 33). Stay bent forward for six to ten seconds; then slowly sit up, inhaling. Repeat once.

This is the most vigorous of the series of forward bends from the Thunderbolt Posture. The upward swing from the straight arms strongly contracts the muscles of the upper back and the shoulders and presses the shoulders and head firmly down. The shoulders, spine, and legs are limbered and the circulation is stimulated, with a nourishing flow of blood to the spine, neck, face, and scalp. The abdominal pressures and massage aid digestion and correct constipation. The ankles and feet are strengthened. The body is conditioned for the more advanced Yoga Posture (*Yogasana*), No. 216, Fig. 95.

101. Champion's Posture: *Vajrasana* or *Virasana*

Sit in the Thunderbolt Posture (No. 92, Fig. 27). Clasp the hands so that the fingers interlace and interlock, and stretch the arms straight up as high as you can without lifting the buttocks, twisting the hands from the wrists so that the palms are turned upwards. Take a deep breath as you raise the arms. Look straight ahead. Hold the stretch for six to ten seconds; then lower the arms, exhaling. Repeat once.

This posture gives a powerful stretch to the whole body from the pelvis upwards – waist, spine, back, shoulders, neck, and arms all benefit. The hands and wrists are strengthened. The lungs are exercised and posture is improved. The muscles of the upper body and the nervous system are toned. Circulation in the upper body is stimulated.

102. Tortoise Posture: *Kurmasana*

The advanced exercise usually designated as the Tortoise Posture (*Kurmasana*) is shown in Fig. 98 (No. 225). It bears little resemblance to this much simpler and somewhat strange pose, described and illustrated by Dhirendra Brahmachari in his *Yogasana Vijnana*; his source is the classic text, the *Gheranda Samhita*.

Again one begins by sitting in the Thunderbolt Posture (No. 92, Fig. 27). The elbows, forearms, and hands are brought together. The hands (palms up) are squeezed into tight fists, and the elbows are pressed against the navel. Holding the fists between the knees, bend forward and stretch out the upper body as far as possible.

Breathe freely. Stretch for at least six seconds. You do not rise from the sitting position.

The upper body is stretched by this pose, and the abdomen and its contents receive a massage from the pressure of the elbows. The digestive fires are said to be stoked.

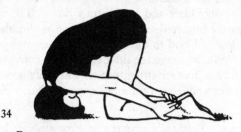

34

103. Hare Posture

Kneel on the floor, the back and thighs in a straight vertical line, thighs and lower legs forming a right angle. Inhale. Exhaling, round the back and lower the top of the head (not the forehead, as in several preceding postures) to the floor. Carry the arms back so that the palms of the hands grasp the legs just above the ankles (Fig. 34). Stay down for six to ten seconds; then come up slowly to the kneeling position, inhaling. Repeat once. In the head-down position, the thighs should still be upright and forming a right angle with the lower legs.

The Hare Posture limbers the feet, legs, and spine, and tones the legs, back, shoulders, and neck. The brain and the glands of the head and neck are nourished with blood – so are the scalp and facial tissues. The body is conditioned for the inverted poses of Yoga.

Do not rise abruptly at the conclusion of this posture – this could cause giddiness. The Hare Posture should not be practised by persons with high blood pressure or heart trouble.

104. Embarrassed Child's Posture

Kneel on the floor as at the start of the Hare Posture (No. 103). Interlace and interlock the fingers and cup the back of the head with the palms of hands. Exhaling, bend forwards and place the top of the head on the floor. The inner edges of the hands should rest on the floor; so should the forearms and the elbows, the latter spread not wider than the shoulders. (See No. 345, Fig. 162 for hand and

arm positions.) The thighs are upright, forming a right angle with
the lower legs. The pose could in fact be the Hare Posture, except
for the different position of the arms and hands. Stay bent forwards
for six to ten seconds; then rise slowly to the kneeling position,
inhaling. Repeat once.

The benefits, and the contra-indications, are as for the Hare
Posture (No. 103).

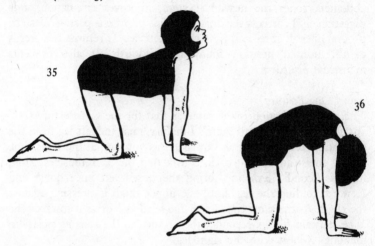

105.   Cat Posture

There can be no disputing the aptness of the naming of this posture,
which by copying movements characteristic of the cat – both
arching and bending the spine along its full length – helps us gain
some cat-like suppleness.

The starting position is 'on all fours', the body supported on the
floor by the palms of the hands, knees, fronts of the lower legs, and
and fronts of the feet, toes flat. The hands are placed at shoulders'
width, fingers forward. The arms are locked at the elbows and
vertical. The thighs too are vertical, and form a right angle with
the lower legs. The knees are kept together. The back is parallel
to the floor, and the neck and head are in line with the back, so
that you look down at the floor.

The Cat Posture has two parts. In the first part you breathe in
and lower the back, lifting the head up and back. The body between
shoulders and hips is lowered as far as posssible, without bending
the arms (Fig. 35). Hold this for six to ten seconds; then move

smoothly into the second part of the posture. Breathe out slowly and at the same time hump the spine upwards as high as you can and bring the head down between the arms, which (as in the first part) stay immobile. The exhalation will make it possible for you to pull the abdomen well in towards the spine (Fig. 36). Hold for six to ten seconds. Repeat once or twice.

The Cat Posture makes the spine more supple, reduces fat on the abdomen, tones the nervous system, improves circulation, aids digestion, and corrects constipation. This posture is part of Western programmes of ante- and post-natal exercises. It returns the uterus to the normal position following childbirth. It also prevents menstrual disorders.

106. Dog Posture

The starting position is the same as that for the Cat Posture (No. 105, Figs 35–6) – 'on all fours'. Inhaling, raise the left leg from the floor and stretch it back and up as far as you can, at the same time raising the head up and back, contracting the back muscles. Hold for six seconds. Exhaling, bring the raised left knee down and forward, folding the leg, until the upper thigh is pressing against the chest. At the same time lower the head and press it towards the knee. Sustain for six seconds; then return to the starting position, inhaling. Repeat with the right leg.

The Dog Posture strengthens, firms, and tones the back, neck, abdomen, hips, and legs. It massages the abdomen and its contents. It aids digestion and corrects constipation. It stimulates the circulation and brings blood to the brain, scalp, and face. It tones the reproductive organs.

107. Wheelbarrow Posture I

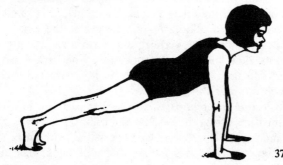

37

Lie face down full length on the floor, the legs together, the toes bent up ready to provide support. The palms of the hands are placed flat on the floor beside the shoulders, fingers pointing forwards. Take a deep breath and push up until the arms are straight and the body is supported only by the palms of the hands and the toes. Head, spine, and legs should be in a straight line (Fig. 37). Hold for six to ten seconds; then bend the arms and lower the body slowly to the floor, exhaling. Repeat once. If staying in the posture longer than ten seconds, breathe freely after the first ten seconds.

The Wheelbarrow Posture is of course the completed press-up of Western keep-fit enthusiasts. In Yoga the important feature is not the pressing up, or the number of press-ups you can do, but the sustaining of the final pose with good form and immobility. The pose stimulates circulation, improves posture, and strengthens and firms the arms, shoulders, back, legs, and feet. It provides the starting position for the more difficult version of the Wheelbarrow Posture that follows.

108. Wheelbarrow Posture II

Place yourself in Wheelbarrow Posture I (No. 107, Fig. 37), though not necessarily by means of a press-up. Head, back, and legs should form a straight line slanting down to the supporting toes. This posture has several parts, as follows.:

i.   Having breathed in as you moved into the Wheelbarrow Posture position, exhale smoothly, establishing a steady pose. Then inhale and raise the right leg as high as possible without bending it. Keep the leg up for six seconds; then lower it so that the toes rest on the floor, exhaling.

ii.   Inhaling, raise the left leg without bending it. Hold it up for six seconds. Lower it, exhaling.

iii.   Inhaling raise the right arm straight up in front. Hold it up for six seconds. Try to avoid wobbling. Exhaling, lower the arm until the palm rests on the floor again.

iv.   Inhaling, raise the left arm straight up in front. Hold it up for six seconds. Exhaling, lower the arm.

Conclude by bending the arms and lowering the body to the floor.

Some strengthening of the muscles by Wheelbarrow Posture I, (No. 107, Fig. 37) may be necessary before this more difficult version can be performed smoothly and without strain. Wheelbarrow Posture II strengthens the neck, shoulders, arms, back, legs, and feet, speeds up the circulation, and limbers the legs and hips.

109.   Camel Posture: *Ustrasana*

In the full version of this posture one kneels, and then throws back the head and bends back the spine, grasping the ankles with a thumb to the outside of each ankle (No. 258, Fig. 119). Here, for a simpler Group A version, we are content to rest the hands (or the fingers) on the heels. Having the knees and feet apart makes it easier; draw them closer together as suppleness increases. Keep the arms stiff, raise the pelvis and abdomen forward and up, and let the head fall back loosely. Breathe in and out freely as you hold the pose for at least six seconds.

The Camel Posture limbers and strengthens the spine, firms the neck, waist, abdomen, and legs, and benefits the thyroid gland and the reproductive organs. It corrects round shoulders.

110.   Camel Posture, Using a Chair: *Ustrasana*

If the version of the Camel Posture given in No. 109 proves difficult, a simple version should be possible using a dining-chair. Sit well forward on the chair, keeping the back erect and the feet flat on the floor about six inches apart. Place the heel and palm of each hand firmly on the chair seat just behind the hip, with the fingers gripping the edge of the chair seat. Now raise the pelvis forwards and upwards, arch the back and let the head hang back loosely. Breathe freely. Hold the pose for at least six seconds.

The effects of the beginner's Camel Posture using a chair are similar to those given for No. 109, but of reduced strength.

111.   Hunkering Posture: *Utkatasana*

This is also called Squatting, Difficult, Hazardous, Raised, Eager, Powerful, Fierce, or Uneven Posture. *Utkatasana* is one of the thirty-two *asanas* listed as being the most important in Hatha Yoga by the *Gheranda Samhita*. As described by Dhirendra Brahmachari – the version given here in Group A – it is not particularly difficult, hazardous, eager, powerful, fierce, or uneven. The version given by B. K. S. Iyengar – our No. 192 – is another matter, and would justify most of these appelations.

In the simpler form you stand upright, rise on the toes, and then hunker down, sitting on the heels, which are raised. The feet are

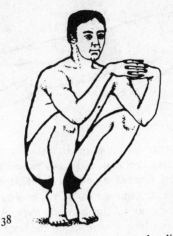

38

together, or nearly so, the knees are spread a little apart, and the elbows rest on the knees with the arms bent and the hands clasped with the fingers lightly interlaced (Fig. 38). Stay down at least fifteen seconds, breathing freely, and then return to standing upright.

This kind of tiptoe squatting is used for some of the intimate cleansing processes of traditional Hatha Yoga. The pose is also used for some of the Tantric exercises connected with control of the sexual energies – see *Yoga of Breathing*.

RELAXING AND SLEEPING POSTURES

Yoga in all its aspects – postures, breath controls, contemplation, and so on – effectively overcomes and wards off stress, soothes taut nerves, replenishes energy, and cultivates poise, harmony, and tranquillity. But among the postures are some which aim specifically at psycho-physical relaxation and sleep of the highest quality. Their origins go back many centuries, but they have the utmost value today, when the pace and stresses of living make letting go so difficult and when the 'stress diseases' are on the increase. Many people who take up Yoga find relaxation to be its most marked and most welcomed benefit.

It is customary to conclude a session of Yoga *asanas* with a few minutes' recumbent relaxation, usually in the posture with the most macabre title, the Corpse Posture (No. 112, Fig. 39).

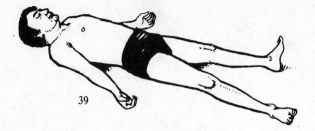

39

112. Corpse Posture: *Savasana* or *Mrtasana*

Of the classic texts, the *Hatha Yoga Pradipika* calls this pose
Savasana, and the *Gheranda Samhita* calls it *Mrtasana*. *Sava* and
mrta both mean 'corpse'; our words 'mort', 'mortal', and 'mortuary'
are related etymologically to the Sanskrit *mrta*. As the name suggests, you lie full length on your back on the floor (on a soft carpet
or folded rug), close your eyes, and stay still, as though playing
dead. If you do not care for the name 'Corpse', think of this asana
as the Total Relaxation Posture.

Lie full length on the back, legs stretched out (though not rigid),
with the feet a little apart and each foot falling limply outwards. The
arms, also extended without being rigid, should rest on the floor a
little way out from the sides. In most illustrat ons of this posture
the hands are shown with palms up, but a few teachers suggest
palms down, with the fingers spread a little apart, or that the sides
of the hands should rest on the floor. In the first and last of these
hand positions the fingers are limp and slightly curled up – note
that if you do straighten them it creates tensions in the hands and
forearms. In the second position the weight of the hands on the
floor straightens the fingers and the hand is supported without
creating tensions. Experiment and see which hand position suits
you best. Let go, so that the whole body goes limp and rests with
its full weight (Fig. 39).

Unless the nostrils are blocked, breathe through the nose quietly
and smoothly. Take a couple of deep breaths, as though into the
stomach, each time exhaling very fully and drawing the abdomen
in. The occasional involuntary deep breath and sighing exhalation
in the early minutes of relaxation are signs that tension knots are
unravelling. Soon the breathing should become quiet, smooth,
and even.

Now give all your attention to releasing from tension each part of the body in sequence from feet to scalp. The sensitive facial muscles, which are intimately associated with the emotions, provide a subtle task for relaxation, which is one reason why we leave them to the last. Send the message 'let go' to each part – muscles are yours to command, though most people today have to re-create the mind– muscle *rapport* that they had for a brief time in childhood.

First observe your breathing – nothing else – for a minute or two, until it settles into a smooth, light, relaxed, and rhythmic muscular action, free from constricting and cramping tensions. Then turn your full attention to letting go in each body part so that tension drains away from it and it rests with its full weight. Models in this respect are the baby in the cot and the sleeping cat. If your attention wanders, avoid the least trace of irritability and bring the attention back patiently to focusing on the selected body part. The sequence is as follows: left foot; left calf; left thigh, front and rear; right foot; right calf; right thigh, front and rear; pelvis; abdomen; lower back; chest; upper back; left hand; left forearm; left upper arm, front and back; left shoulder; right hand; right forearm; right upper arm, front and back; right shoulder; throat; neck; jaw; lips; tongue; eyes; brow; scalp.

Now observe your breathing again – thus quietening the mind and aiding relaxation. After a minute or two you can again let the attention roam like a torch beam over the body from feet to scalp. You can continue in this way for as long as the time given to relaxation permits. As you master the art of letting go with the body muscles you find that the mind relaxes concomitantly. The *Hatha Yoga Pradipika*, i, 34, says: 'Lying down on the ground like a corpse is called *Savasana*. It removes fatigue and gives rest to the mind.' And the *Gheranda Samhita*, ii, 19, says: 'Lying flat on the ground (on one's back) like a corpse is called the *Mrtasana*. This posture destroys fatigue, and quiets the agitation of the mind.'

113. Stick Posture: *Yastikasana*
Few books on Yoga give any specific posture for relaxation other than the Corpse Posture. There *are* others – the Stick Posture (*Yastikasana*) is one of them.

Lie full length flat on the back on the floor as in the Corpse Posture, except that the arms are extended above the head, resting on the floor with the palms of the hands turned up This is a pose of relaxation: so do not turn it into a stretching exercise by stiffening the arms or deliberately lengthening the body. The legs may be spread apart so as to form an angle symmetrical with that of the arms, which can, if you wish, be varied between straight up and the crucifix position. Fig. 4 (No. 30) could be depicting one Stick Posture position if the legs were spread apart.

The Stick Posture, when performed for a few minutes preceding a Yoga programme, has a benefit additional to that of rest and relaxation: the abdomen is flattened, imparting a sense of firmness, and the mild stretching action on the trunk, shoulders, and arms gives one a sense of being bodily and mentally alerted for the more deliberate stretching *asanas* to come.

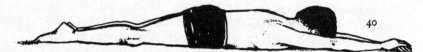

40

114. Crocodile Posture: *Makarasana*

The *Gheranda Samhita* gives this concise description of the Crocodile Posture: 'Lie on the ground face down, the chest touching the earth and both legs stretched out: catch the head with the arms.' B. K. S. Iyengar interprets this as clasping the back of the head and raising the upper body and legs off the floor, turning the pose into a variation of the Locust Posture. But most instructors treat *Makarasana* as a relaxation posture for relieving fatigue. Theos Bernard in his *Hatha Yoga* calls it the Dolphin Posture, but does not describe it.

Lie face down on the ground, with the arms stretched forward together, one palm on the back of the other hand. The legs are together, with the toes pointing, and the chin rests on the floor (Fig. 40). Breathe freely and relax for several minutes. This is the version given by Dhirendra Brahmachari, based on the *Gheranda Samhita* text quoted above.

Archie J. Bahm (*Yoga for Business Executives*), one of the few writers of Yoga text-books to provide a variety of relaxation postures, interprets the *Gheranda Samhita*'s 'catch the head with the arms' as 'folding arms and resting your head on them, on either cheek.'

115. Prone Posture: *Advasana*

This can be considered as similar to the Stick Posture (*Yastik-asana*. No. 113), except that you lie full length face down. The leg

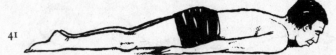

41

and arm positions can be varied in angle as in the Stick Posture.
It can also be a prone equivalent of the Corpse Posture (No. 112).

Lie face down, the legs extended either together or a little way apart,
the toes flat so that the fronts of the feet rest on the floor. The arms
are by the sides or a little way out from the sides, with the palms of
the hands turned either up or down. Experiment with the hand
positions and see which of the two alternatives suits you best.
The chin rests on the floor. This is the prone equivalent of the
Corpse Posture, and the body-part relaxation sequence described
for *Savasana* (No. 112) can again be utilized. You may prefer to
rest a cheek, rather than the chin, on the floor (Fig. 41). If you are
treating *Advasana* as the prone equivalent of the Stick Posture, the
arms are stretched overhead, with the palms of the hands flat on
the floor, at the angle or angles you find most restful. You can also
vary the angle made by the legs to match that of the arms, giving
what feels like an apt symmetry to the posture. You can rest either
the chin or a cheek on the floor. Breathe freely and relax for some
minutes. The pose may be used for taking a brief nap.

116.   Side Relaxation Posture: *Dradhasana*
Dradha means 'firm'. Like the Prone Posture (No. 115), the Side
Relaxation Posture can be used either for rest or for taking a nap.

You can lie on either side. If you lie on the left side, the left arm
is folded so that the palm of the hand is turned up and the head
rests on the wrist. The right leg rests directly on top of the left
leg. The right arm rests along the right side of the body with the
palm of the hand placed on the right thigh. It is important in this
posture that the spine should be straight. You may prefer lying on
the right side with the right cheek resting on the right wrist.

117.   Western Side Relaxation Posture
All the preceding relaxing and sleeping postures – the Corpse
Posture, Stick Posture, Crocodile Posture, Prone Posture, and Side
Relaxation Posture – were devised originally for rapid recuperation
from fatigue, by relaxing for a few minutes or taking a nap on the
ground, without the assistance of a mattress or pillow. Though the

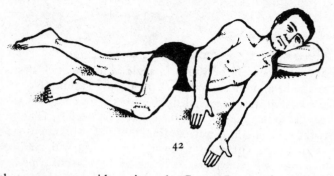

42

other postures provide variety, the Corpse Posture has been found the most beneficial for efficacious relaxation. All these postures may be used at times of fatigue for a few minutes' sleep, but in this writer's opinion none is ideal for that purpose, and the Western alternative described in *Yoga and Vitality* for relaxing and sleeping while lying on the side should be utilized when circumstances permit.

It is not ideal to sleep in any position that interferes with the circulation of the blood, and circulation will be affected after some time if you rest the head on the arm. Sleeping on the back in bed encourages mouth instead of nostril breathing, puts pressure from the blankets on the toes and feet, and may set up tensions in the lower back. Too high a pillow places a strain on the neck and shoulder muscles. Having one or both arms overhead retards the circulation and may cause a tingling sensation in the hands. Lying prone restricts breathing. For these reasons the writer feels justified in introducing an on-side position that avoids the dangers and tensions mentioned.

Use a pillow, cushion, or substitute to place the head in alignment with the spine. Only when nothing else suitable is available should you fold one arm and rest your head on the wrist. If you are lying on the right side, with the right cheek on a pillow, the right arm is stretched straight out in front, the palm of the right hand turned up. The left arm hangs limply across the diaphragm. The left leg is bent to a right angle and the left knee brought over to rest on the floor. The right leg is slightly bent. Keep the chin up enough to give good alignment between the head and the spine (Fig. 42).

This is a most restful position, either for relaxation or for sleeping, and a posture that repays every minute of practice. It is highly recommended to all readers, but has special value for those who suffer from backache or sleeplessness. It is also very restful for pregnant women.

118.   Rapid Relaxation Posture
There are times when only a few brief minutes are available for relaxation. At such times the letting-go relaxation method described for use in the Corpse Posture would take too long; but only if you have practised it for some time will the rapid method be effective.

Lie flat on your back in the Corpse Posture (No. 112, Fig. 39). Take a deep breath low down in the abdomen and raise the upper body, arms, and legs three or four inches from the floor, stiffening them as you do so. Hold the whole body tense for six seconds; then flop back into the starting position, exhaling, and letting go all tension so that it instantly dissolves. Breathe freely and smoothly and lie flat with your full weight (Fig. 39).

SUPINE POSTURES

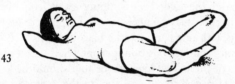

43

119.   Modified Fish Posture: *Matsyasana*
In the advanced version of this posture (No. 263, Fig. 121) the legs are interlocked in the Lotus position; bu this valuable posture is available in modified form to all who can cross their legs in the Easy Posture (No. 81, Fig. 22). Lie flat on the back with the feet crossed at the ankles and pulled as close as possible to the body. Spread the knees well apart and keep them as low as you can. Cross the wrists behind the neck and rest the head on the arms (Fig. 43). Breathe freely and deeply. Stay motionless in the posture for at least thirty seconds.

The Modified Fish Posture might almost have been included among the preceding relaxation postures, so restful is it. But in fact it is a useful stretching and limbering exercise, as well as relieving fatigue. The ankles and legs are limbered, and the hip joints loosened. Posture is improved – remember to keep the back

flat on the floor, from the shoulders to the lower back. Not least of
the benefits from this pose is the freedom given to respiration. The
pose encourages deep abdominal breathing, the diaphragm being
free to perform its piston-like movement, going down on each
inhalation, swelling out the lower abdomen, and going up on each
exhalation, so that the lower abdomen collapses inwards. Crossing
the hands behind the neck expands the thorax, giving the lungs
maximum freedom for their bellows-like action; and the bellows-
like action; and the upper body is mildly stretched.

120.   Supine Preparation for Perfect Posture I: *Siddhasana*
For this supine posture, first sit on the floor and pull the ankle of
one leg so that the leg is fully folded and the heel in against the
crotch as shown in Fig. 24 (No. 83). Retaining the leg positions –
one leg fully extended, the other fully folded with the sole of the
foot flat against the inside thigh of the other leg – lie flat on the back
with the wrists crossed behind the neck to support the back of the
head with the arms. The position of the upper body and arms is
that given for the Modified Fish Posture (No. 119, Fig. 43). To
prevent the foot of the folded leg slipping away from the body a
little as you lie back, it may be necessary to keep a grip on the ankle
of the folded leg with one hand and lie back gradually, adopting an
intermediate semi-reclining position, propped half up on one elbow.
The outer edges of the folded leg and the foot should be kept down
flat on the floor. Breathe freely and stay in the posture for at least
thirty seconds. Repeat, folding the other leg.
    This posture loosens the hip joints and limbers the legs, calms
and tones the nervous system, improves posture (keep the full
length of the back down flat), expands the thorax, encourages deep
abdominal breathing, and mildly stretches the upper body. It
conditions the legs and hips for sitting in the Perfect Posture
(*Siddhasana*, No. 195, Fig. 83).

121.   Supine Preparation for Perfect Posture II: *Siddhasana*
The pose is as for No. 120, except that instead of crossing the wrists
behind the neck you stretch the arms overhead, the backs of the
hands resting on the floor. Hold the pose for at least thirty seconds,
folding first one leg, and then the other. Breathe freely.
    The effects are much as for No. 120, but with a more powerful
stretching of the upper body. It is more difficult to keep the lower

back and the folded leg in contact with the floor. No. 120 and
No. 121 both have their distinct yet closely-related benefits; the
latter is not superior in all ways to the former. Both versions are
worth performing.

122.   Supine Preparation for Lotus Posture I: *Padmasana*
Sit on the floor with the legs spread apart. Fold one leg and grasp
the ankle. Draw the toes and instep of the foot on to the top of the
thigh of the extended leg, as high up the leg as possible. Keeping
the legs in the positions just described, lower the back to the floor.
Cross the wrists behind the neck and rest the head on the arms.
Keep the full length of the back flat on the floor. Breathe deeply
and freely, swelling out and drawing in the abdomen. Perform
folding first one leg, then the other, staying in the pose at least
thirty seconds.

The thigh and knee of the folded leg should be kept in contact
with the floor. This is more difficult to accomplish than in the
Supine Preparation for Perfect Posture (Nos 120 and 121). Whether
you manage it completely or not, this posture limbers the legs and
loosens the hip joints, conditioning both for the sitting Lotus
Posture (No. 199, Fig. 87). At the same time the posture expands
the thorax, encourages deep abdominal breathing, and mildly
stretches the upper body.

123.   Supine Preparation for Lotus Posture II: *Padmasana*
As in Supine Preparation for Perfect Posture II, this version differs
from the first version of this preparation by stretching the arms
overhead, the backs of the hands resting on the floor.

The effects are much the same as for No. 122, but with greater
stretching of the upper body. Both versions are worth performing;
No. 123 is not superior in every way to No. 122.

124.   Pumping
Lie flat on the back, the arms by the sides with the palms of the
hands turned up, the feet together or slightly apart. Relax completely. Give all your attention to the abdomen in this exercise:
shoulders, arms, legs – all other body parts in effect – stay immobile
and relaxed. Take a rapid deep breath, thrusting out the abdominal
wall; then immediately expel the air from the lungs in an exhalation
as rapid as the preceding inhalation, at the same time pulling the

abdominal wall back towards the spine. Keep the shoulders, the vack along its full length, the hips, and the legs firmly on the floor. This is an abdominal rather than a breathing exercise. There is only time for short sharp inhalations and exhalations, each resulting involuntarily from the rapid pumping action – one second for each in or out movement of the abdominal wall. Make ten of these in-and-out movements. Relax for about twenty seconds, breathing normally; then repeat the exercise. The posture and abdominal movements as shown for No. 125, Figs 44–5, except that the arms stay by the sides.

F. A. Hornibrook made this a key exercise in his best-selling book *The Culture of the Abdomen*, and called it 'Pumping'. It firms and tones the abdominal muscles, massages the abdominal viscera, and strengthens the abdominal wall and prepares it for *Uddiyana* (No. 162) and *Nauli* (No. 418). It also corrects constipation: 'the main object of this movement is to increase the peristaltic action of the bowels,' says Hornibrook.

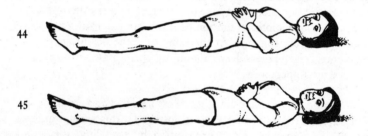

44

45

125. Abdominal Breathing

It is important that every person who takes up Yoga should acquire the habit of deep and healthful breathing. This means abdominal breathing, with the diaphragm free to perform its up-and-down, piston-like motion. Breathing shallowly with the chest muscles results in inadequate oxygenation of the blood, and deprives the abdominal wall and viscera of a continuous massage. Yoga breathing (*pranayama*) was fully discussed and described in *Yoga of Breathing*. The recumbent posture gives an opportunity to learn abdominal breathing, feeling the movements of the diaphragm and stomach on inhalation and exhalation.

Lie flat on the back, the legs extended together, the palms of the hands placed on the abdomen so that the tip of the second (longest) finger of the left hand meets that of the right hand over the navel. The forearms are held in against the ribs. In correct Yogic breathing the rib-box is felt to expand as you inhale, and at the same time the abdomen swells and rises against the hands, lifting them, the diaphragm having moved down (Fig. 44). As you exhale slowly and evenly, the abdomen is felt to subside and the rib-box gradually to move in (Fig. 45). Practise abdominal breathing for two or three minutes: breathe slowly, smoothly, and evenly, filling the lungs with air, but never to the point of discomfort. Make thorough exhalations. emptying the lungs so that the abdominal wall sinks in towards the spine, creating a hollow. The key muscle in respiratory action is the diaphragm, which moves down as we breathe in and moves up as we breathe out.

After four weeks' practice you can keep the hands on the floor and the arms by the sides and take note of the sensations of deep abdominal breathing as they occur purely with your kinesthetic sense and without the aid of the forearms or hands. Thereafter, in performing this recumbent abdominal breathing, record the muscular sensations with the palms of the hands and the forearms only during the first minute of breathing in and out. During the following one or two minutes take mental note only of the rise and fall of the abdomen and the out-and-in umbrella-like expansion of the rib-box.

The healthful habit of abdominal breathing is learned in this exercise and should become automatic at all times – standing, walking, and sitting, as well as lying on the back. Because of the more through emptying of the lungs, this exercise, even more than the preceding Pumping, trains the abdominal wall to relax and retract, due to the vacuum created, towards the spine – the key to success in the valuable Yogic muscle controls of *Uddiyana* (No. 162) and *Nauli* (No. 418).

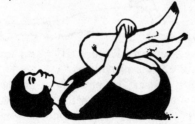

46

126.   Supine Knee Squeeze Posture I, also called Wind-relieving Posture: *Pavanmuktasana*

Lie flat on the back. Draw both knees up to the chest, having crossed the ankles. Clasp the arms around the knees, left hand gripping right wrist or right hand gripping left wrist. Keeping the knees together, press them firmly down towards the body, so that the fronts of the thighs press down on the abdomen. Keep the full length of the back flat on the floor. Keep the head down and look straight up (Fig. 46). Squeeze the knees firmly for ten seconds. Relax the pressure, but do not alter the pose, for ten seconds. Then again firmly press the legs against the body for ten seconds. Breathe freely in this exercise.

This posture limbers the hips and legs, and massages the abdominal wall and the abdominal viscera. It corrects indigestion and constipation. As the name 'Wind-relieving Posture' implies, intestinal gases may be released during the squeeze.

127.   Supine Knee Squeeze Posture II, also called Wind-relieving
       Posture: *Pavanmuktasana*
This time instead of raising and squeezing both knees together, lie flat on the back and raise each leg separately, clasping it with both hands, one hand on the knee and the other hand below the knee. Press the folded leg firmly down towards the body. Keep the full length of the back on the floor. Do not raise the head, but look straight up. Breathe freely. Squeeze firmly for ten seconds. Relax the pressure for ten seconds, without altering the pose. Press firmly again for ten seconds. Repeat, folding the other leg.

Benefits are as for No. 126.

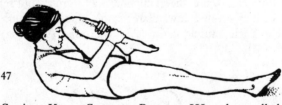

47

128.   Supine Knee Squeeze Posture III: also called Wind-
       relieving Posture: *Pavanmuktasana*
Begin as for No. 127, but as you press down on the folded leg, raise the head and shoulders and press the forehead and kneecap together. Hold the pose steadily for ten seconds as before (Fig. 47). At the end of the ten seconds, lower the head and shoulders back to the floor, but keep the knee drawn up to the body, though

relaxing the pressure for ten seconds. Raise forehead to kneecap again and press firmly for another ten seconds. Repeat, folding the other leg. Breathe freely.

The effects are as for No. 126, but in addition the neck and shoulders are strengthened.

129. Canoe Posture I
Lie flat on the back, the legs extended together, the palms of the hands placed flat on the tops of the thighs. Take a breath, and raise the head and shoulders just far enough to bring the feet into view. Do not sit up beyond that point. The hands will slide a few inches down the thighs. Hold the position reached for ten seconds, pressing down hard with the palms of the hands on the thighs and contracting and hardening the abdominal muscles. Hold your breath during contraction. Lower the head and shoulders to the floor; relax for fifteen seconds; then repeat the abdominal contraction, again for ten seconds.

This is a mild sit-up, but when combined with conscious contraction of the abdominal muscles and pressing down hard with the hands (arms straight), the Canoe Posture strengthens and tones the abdomen, chest, and shoulders.

130. Canoe Posture II
Begin as for Canoe Posture I (No. 129), but when raising the head and shoulders, lift the legs also, keeping them stiffly together, so that the heels are three inches off the floor.

The effects are as for No. 129, with intensified contraction of the lower abdomen and toning and firming of the legs and hips.

131. Back-stretching Posture: *Paschimottanasana*; also called
        Posterior Stretch Posture: *Ugrasama, Brahmacharyasana*
Alternative spellings of the Sanskrit title are *Paschimottanasana* and *Paschimatanasana*. *Paschima* means 'back' or 'posterior', and *tan* means 'stretch'. *Paschima* also means 'west', which B. K. S. Iyengar sees as a reference to the back of the body, the front of the body being the east, the head representing north, and the feet representing south. Alain Danielou links the 'west' with the rising of *kundalini* energy up the spine (see *Yoga of Meditation*). *Ugra* means 'formidable' or 'noble'. *Brahmacharya* means 'self-control', and the pose is associated with mastery over the sexual energies.

The fully-stretched position to aim for is shown in Fig. 97, and described in No. 221. However, beginners do well to grasp the ankles rather than the feet, and few can bring the face down to the knees. Stretch the spine gradually. The Standing Forward Bend Posture (No. 67, Fig. 14) helps limber the spine for the Back-stretching Posture, which is a sort of Supine Forward Bend. The version given here follows logically from Canoe Posture I (No. 129) and suits persons in the early months of Yoga practice.

Lie full length on the back, the legs outstretched together, the palms of the hands placed flat on the tops of the thighs. Breathing in, commence a slow curl up of the upper body, sliding the hands down the thighs towards the knees. Slowly bring up the head, shoulders, and back, the spine stretching vertebra by vertebra. On reaching a vertical position with the upper body, change from inhaling to exhaling and continue the body movement downwards, lowering the head as far as you comfortably can towards the knees. At the same time slide the hands down to the ankles, or to the feet if suppleness permits. For some weeks after beginning this posture stay in the stretched-forward position only ten seconds; later, add seconds as you become more comfortable in the pose. If you stay bent forward longer than ten seconds, breathe freely. Coming out of the pose is a slow unwinding, breathing in slowly.

The Back-stretching Posture promotes the strength and suppleness of the spine, and stretches the muscles of the back, arms, and legs. The hamstring muscles at the backs of the thighs may resist stretching, but loosen up with practice. The abdomen is contracted in the early states of the curl-up, and is squeezed in bending forwards. Digestion is improved and constipation corrected. The pelvis is stretched and improved circulation brought to it. The pose is said to lead to mastery over the sexual energies and to improve sexual fitness.

132. Ankle Grasp Posture
Lie flat on the back, the arms extended overhead, the backs of the hands resting on the floor (No. 30, Fig. 4). Inhale and slowly raise the left leg, without bending it, until it is perpendicular. Grasp the left ankle with both hands, keeping the back flat on the floor (Fig. 48). If you cannot hold the ankle without raising the shoulders from the floor, stretch the arms towards the ankle as far as you can. The right leg stays on the floor. Hold the pose for ten seconds; then

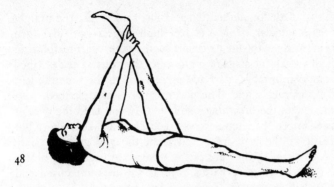

48

slowly lower the left leg and the backs of the hands to the floor, exhaling. Repeat raising the right leg and grasping the right ankle with both hands. If you hold the pose longer than ten seconds you should breathe freely after ten seconds.

The Ankle Grasp Posture firms and tones the abdomen, buttocks, and thighs, limbers the hips, and tones the nervous system. It reduces fat on the lower abdomen.

133. Foot Above Posture I: *Urdhva Prasarita Padasana*
Urdhva means 'above', *prasarita* means 'held out', and *pada* means 'foot'.

Lie flat on the back, the legs extended together, and the arms extended overhead, palms up (No. 30, Fig. 4). Keeping the knees together, draw them up to the chest; then straighten the legs to perpendicular and lower them slowly to the floor. Breathe in as you draw up the knees and straighten the legs, and breathe out as you lower the legs.

This posture removes fat from the abdomen, firms and tones the legs, limbers the hips, and strengthens the lower back. It aids digestion and corrects constipation.

134. Foot Above Posture II: *Urdhva Prasarita Padasana*
Lie flat on the back, the legs extended together, the arms stretched overhead with the backs of the hands flat on the floor (No. 30, Fig. 4). Take a deep breath. Without bending the legs and keeping the back flat on the floor, raise the legs from the floor to an angle of thirty degrees, exhaling. Hold the legs up for ten seconds. Then, still exhaling, move the legs higher to sixty degrees and hold them

steady at that angle for another ten seconds. Finally take the straight
legs to perpendicular. Hold the feet high for ten seconds; then
lower them slowly to the floor without bending the legs, breathing in.

When you reach the stage of performing the exercise as described
above quite comfortably, start adding seconds to the time the legs
are held up at each angle. The performance is as described, with
an adjustment to the breathing regulation. If you hold the pose at
each stage longer than ten seconds, you should take a short but
deep breath as the legs are raised from thirty degrees to sixty
degrees, and again as they are raised from sixty degrees to ninety
degrees. Otherwise you exhale slowly as the legs are raised and
held. As before, breathe in as the legs are lowered.

The benefits are as for No. 133, but intensified.

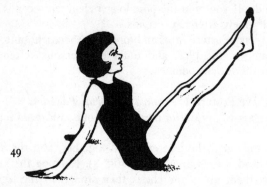

49

135. Angular Posture I
Of the two versions of the Angular Posture given here, version I is
the less difficult as regards balancing, and should be mastered fully
before tackling version II.

Lie flat on the back, the legs fully extended, the arms by the
sides, the palms of the hands turned down. Exhaling, raise the legs
stiffly and at the same time raise the upper body, with straight
back. Raise the trunk to an angle of forty-five degrees and the legs
to the same angle so that the upper body and the legs form a right
angle. As the back lifts clear of the floor, take the arms back and
support the balancing on the buttocks by placing the palms of the
hands on the floor behind and out from the shoulders, the fingers
pointing away from the body (Fig. 49). Hold the V position steadily
for at least ten seconds. If you hold it longer than ten seconds,

breathe freely after the first ten seconds. At the conclusion, return slowly to the starting position lying full length on the floor, breathing in.

The Angular Posture limbers the hips, strengthens and firms the abdomen, hips, and legs, improves balance, and tones the nervous system.

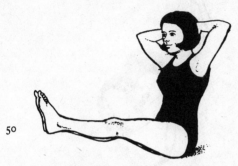

50

136. Angular Posture II
In version II of the Angular Posture you dispense with the support of the arms, instead clasping the hands behind the head, with the elbows spread wide. Breathing out, sit up slowly and raise the straight legs until trunk and legs form a right angle (Fig. 50). Balance steadily on the pelvis for ten seconds. Return slowly to lying full length on the floor, breathing in. If you stay in the V position longer than ten seconds, breathe freely after the first ten seconds.

The effects are as given for No. 135, but intensified due to the balance having to be maintained without the arm props of version I.

137. Buttocks Balance Posture: *Ubhaya Padangusthasana*
Ubhaya means 'both', and *padangustha* means 'big toe'. In the full version (No. 247, Fig. 111) you raise the legs and the torso to form the V position of the preceding Angular Postures, holding the big toe of each foot. Group A practitioners should be content with first achieving good balance while grasping the ankles rather than the toes.

Lie flat on the back. Sit up and flex the legs and grasp the ankles. Keeping a firm hold on the ankles, straighten the legs and balance steadily on the buttocks, the arms straight, forming a V with torso and legs. It will probably take some practice to judge correctly the extent to which you can lean back without toppling over.

The Buttocks Balance Posture limbers the hips, strengthens and firms the arms, legs, abdomen, hips, and back, improves balance, and tones up the nervous system. It also stimulates the circulation, aids digestion, and corrects constipation.

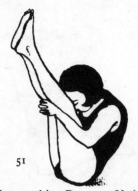

51

138. Balancing Back-stretching Posture: *Utthita Paschimottanasana*
This is a variant of the Back-stretching Posture *Paschimottanasana* (No. 221, Fig. 97), performed while balancing on the pelvis. Group A practitioners should use the following version.

Lie flat on the back, the arms by the sides, the legs fully extended together. Exhaling, curl up slowly, raising the head, shoulders, and back, and at the same time raising the legs stiffly. As you reach the right-angled V position of Figs 49 and 50, clasp the hands behind the knees and bring the knees and the forehead into contact. Press the forehead against the knees and balance steadily on the pelvis for ten seconds (Fig. 51). Return slowly to the starting position, breathing in. If you stay in the balancing position longer than ten seconds, breathe normally after ten seconds.

Beginners are likely to find it necessary to flex the knees slightly in order to rest the head against them. Perfect balance may take a little time to attain. Soon, however, the balance should be steady and the legs locked at the knees.

The Balancing Back-stretching Posture has all the effects described for the preceding posture (No. 137), with the additional benefits of limbering and strengthening the spine.

139. Supine Knees Spread Posture
Lie flat on the back, the hands clasped behind the head, the elbows

spread wide. Bring the soles of the feet together and draw the joined feet as far towards the body as you find possible, keeping the feet in contact with the floor. Spread the knees as wide apart and keep them as close to the floor as you can manage without discomfort. Keep the full length of the back flat against the floor. Breathe normally. Stay in the pose at least twenty seconds.

The Supine Knees Spread Posture increases the flexibility of the hip joints, limbers the legs, firms and tones the hips and legs, and sends blood to the pelvic area. It has therapeutic value in cases of sexual disorders and women's pelvic ailments.

140.   Supine Leg Stretch Posture
Lie flat on the back, the arms by the sides, the legs fully extended together. Slowly stretch one leg away from the body, pointing the toe, keeping the heel on the floor, and keeping the full length of the back pressed flat on the floor. Sustain the stretch for at least ten seconds, breathing freely. Repeat with the other leg.

The Supine Leg Stretch Posture firms and tones the feet, legs, hips, and lower back, stimulates blood circulation, tones the nervous system, and improves posture.

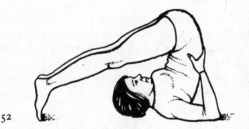

52

141.   Supported Plough Posture: *Halasana*
Hala means 'plough'. This graceful posture, which superbly stretches the whole body, is one of the most important basic poses of Yoga. It is often performed as a continuation of the Shoulder-stand Posture (*Sarvangasana*, No. 147, Fig. 55), to which it is closely related. In both the Shoulderstand and the Plough Posture the body is supported by the neck and shoulders, with steadying support from the arms in beginners' versions. In the Shoulderstand the legs are held straight up, perpendicular to the floor. In the Plough Posture the legs are lowered together overhead until the toes rest on the floor. As the Shoulderstand is described among the

inverted postures to follow, we give the Plough Posture here as a separate *asana*.

Lie flat on the back, the legs fully extended together. Swing the legs overhead, straightening them, and supporting the body on the neck and shoulders. Use the backs of the upper arms as props pressing the fingers on the backs of the ribs, with the thumbs separate and placed below the hips. Keep the elbows in close to the body (No. 147, Fig. 55). Now slowly lower the straight legs behind the head: their own weight should take them down until the toes rest on the floor (Fig. 52). Keep the toes down on the floor for at least six seconds. Respiration is restricted in the pose, so breathe without holding the breath, making short and rather rapid inhalations and exhalations through the nostrils.

Common faults: i. The elbows are placed too far out from the sides. ii. The trunk and legs are not in a straight line and perpendicular to the floor. iii. The toes are pointed, tensing the leg muscles; the legs should be relaxed. iv. The pose is not held steadily; legs and trunk are moving. v. The descent from the inverted position is too abrupt, so that the head lifts off the floor. Coming out of *asanas* should be given just as much care as going into them.

Common faults: i. Bending the legs. ii. Holding the elbows out too wide; keep them in against your sides. iii. Effortful, jerky movements. Performance of this pose should be graceful and flowing, both in going into the posture and in unwinding out of it. iv. Pushing the hips and legs beyond the head with the arms. The arms should serve only as props. Their support is dispensed with in Group B practice.

The posture is not suitable for persons with weak vertebrae. Do not force yourself in the early stages of practice. Let the feet fall only as far as the body finds comfortable. Practice soon brings correct performance and an accompanying sense of achievement in a posture that is not as difficult as it looks.

The Plough Posture keeps the entire spine supple and youthful, and stretches the whole body. It slims the abdomen, hips, and legs. It activates the circulation, nourishing the roots of the spinal nerves, the facial tissues, and the scalp. It aids digestion and bowel action. It is held to be excellent for the endocrine glands, the liver, the spleen, and the reproductive organs, and to correct menstrual disorders.

PRONE POSTURES

142. Cobra Posture: *Bhujangasana*

Bhujanga means 'cobra'. The posture takes its name from its resemblance to a cobra rearing, hood spread, to strike. It is one of the great classic poses of Yoga, and one that most beginners can accomplish in the modified form here to be described. The main difference between the adept's execution (No. 316, Fig. 147) and that of the tyro is twofold: i. To avoid back strain, the beginner needs to have his hands placed in front of the shoulders rather than below them, which means a less severe back bend when the body is raised. ii. Until the lower back becomes very strong the beginner relies on the arms to push the body up and bend the back; whereas the adept slowly raises the upper body mainly with back power, though he calls on the thrust of the arms in the final stages of bending the spine.

Lie flat on the abdomen, the legs stretched out together, the soles of the feet turned up and the toes flat. The arms are bent and the hands placed flat on the floor, the fingers pointing forward, five or six inches in front of the shoulders. The elbows are kept in against the sides of the body. The chin rests on the floor. To locate the correct position for the hands, place the palms flat on the floor in front of the shoulders, the fingertips in line horizontally with the chin.

Inhaling, slowly raise the head, neck, and upper back successively, straightening the arms. You should feel the spine bending vertebra by vertebra. In the final position the arms are either straight or almost straight, and the body from the navel down to the feet presses on the floor. Most Yoga teachers instruct their pupils to raise the chin and bend back the head at the peak of the back bend, but a few prefer the more formal keeping of the chin level, so that the eyes are looking straight ahead rather than diagonally upwards. Rely as far as possible on the lower back muscles at the start of raising the head, neck, and upper body, completing the back bend with the assistance of pressure from the straightening arms. In the Cobra Posture as described here for practice by Group A students the arms will slope away from the shoulders more than is shown in the illustration for Group B performance (No. 316, Fig. 147).

Hold the raised pose for ten seconds; then return slowly to the starting position, breathing out. If you stay in the pose longer than ten seconds, breathe freely after the first ten seconds.

The Cobra Posture, performed slowly and smoothly, exercises the spine, vertebra by vertebra, from the lumbar region to the neck, limbering and strengthening it. The front of the body – legs, abdomen, chest, throat, jawline – are all beneficially stretched. The circulation is stimulated, and the dense network of nerves in the spinal solumn receives an additional supply of blood. The pose improves digestion and relives constipation. It normalizes glandular activity, and is said to correct menstrual disorders and to be excellent for the reproductive organs.

143.   Bow Posture I: *Dhanurasana*

Dhanu means 'bow'. In this pose the spine, trunk, and legs take the shape of a bow, and the arms are pulled taut like a bow string.

Here is a case where merely attempting the posture, even if (literally) you never get it off the ground, will do you a lot of good. In time, and without straining, the thighs and chest will lift from the floor. As a result of spreading the legs wide, as recommended here in this modified version of the posture, success in 'lift off' is achieved before long, if not on the first attempt. When the muscles concerned in this somewhat vigorous posture have strengthened, the legs can be kept closer together, thus moving progressively nearer to the full version of the Bow (No. 322, Fig. 149).

Lie flat on the abdomen and chest, the chin on the floor, the knees spread well apart. Flex the legs and bring the heels back close to the buttocks. Grasp the ankles firmly, the thumbs and fingers side by side. Lift the head, neck, and shoulders as high as you can, at the same time pulling on the ankles strongly, the arms straight, and lifting the thighs and chest clear of the floor, so that you balance on the stomach. Hold the 'drawn bow' for six seconds at least.

Some authorities say that you should inhale as you pull; others say exhale; yet again, others recommend free breathing. The position makes regulated breathing difficult, and we side with the teachers who say 'breathe freely'. This means that your are free to give all your attention to 'drawing the bow'.

The tingling glow that is brought to the whole body by this posture testifies to a marked stimulation of circulation and stretching of the entire musculature. The spine, hip joints, and shoulder joints are all limbered, and the back muscles are strengthened. The front of the body, including legs, abdomen, chest, arms, throat, and jawline, is strongly stretched and firmed. The stomach muscles are massaged and the abdominal viscera stimulated and toned. Glandular functioning is regulated. The health and fitness of the pelvic area is improved.

144. Bow Posture II: *Dhanurasana*

Lie flat on the stomach and chest, the chin resting on the floor. Fold the legs and bring heels back towards the buttocks. Reach back the hands and grasp the ankles firmly, thumbs and fingers side by side. The legs can be close together or slightly parted. Raise the head and shoulders. Inhaling, pull the heels down strongly on the buttocks for ten seconds. Relax the pull without letting go of the ankles, exhaling. Rest for twenty seconds; then again pull the heels down on the buttocks.

This is a simplified form of the advanced variation of the Bow Posture depicted in Fig. 152 (No. 325), in which the heels are pulled down to the sides of the hips, not on the tops of the buttocks as here.

The back is not so strongly bent in this variation as in No. 143, but the legs are bent more strongly. This pose has most of the effects of No. 143.

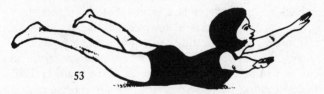

53

145. Boat Posture: *Navasana*

According to which authority on Yoga you follow, this pose and poses very similar to it may be treated either as variations of the Locust Posture or as variations of the Bow Posture. Strictly speaking, the Locust Posture involves the raising of the lower part of the body, and the Bow Posture the raising of both lower and upper parts to give the back-bending bow effect. We side with those who treat the Boat Posture as a variation of the Bow.

Lie flat on the floor, face down, the legs well spread, the soles of the feet turned up, the toes flat. The arms are fully extended in front at wider than shoulders' width, palms down. Match symmetrically the angles of the arms and legs. Rest the chin on the floor. Now raise simultaneously the head, chest, arms, and legs. Keep the arms and legs as high as possible without bending them (Fig. 53). Try to have only the stomach muscles on the floor. Maintain the position of contraction for at least six seconds. Breathe freely. As you become stronger, bring both the legs and the arms closer together, approaching the more advanced posture depicted in Fig. 155 (No. 330).

The beneficial effects are as for No. 143.

INVERTED POSTURES

The Headstand Posture (*Sirsasana* – *sirsa* means 'head') has been called 'the King of *Asanas*'. Its benefits arise from physiogical changes produced by reversing the normal pull of gravity on the body – we cannot change gravity's direction, but by standing on the head we subject our flesh and vital organs to a pull from feet to head instead of the customary pull from head to feet. The benefits claimed for the Headstand are given after the description of the last of the full Headstand Postures, No. 354. We spend most of out active day with gravity dragging in one direction on the muscle tissues and vital organs. The heart works to pump blood upwards to the brain. By inverting the body we provide a tonic rejuvenation. All those tissues and organs that had begun to sag are enabled to find correct and more youthful placement. The Headstand, even in the careful few seconds the beginner should stay in it, proves an exhilarating and rejuvenating experience.

However, the full version involves severe pressure on the top of the skull and an unfamiliar rush of blood to the head. It should be approached cautiously, in stages, and for some persons it is not advisable at all. It should be avoided by persons suffering from high blood pressure and ailments connected with the brain, eyes, and ears. If in doubt, consult your doctor. Indian experts tend to be less cautionary about age restrictions than Western teachers, but the full head balance has obvious dangers for elderly persons, whose bones are brittle and easily broken. After forty, especially if one is overweight, caution should be exercised. We give milder alternatives to the full topsy-turvy pose, the most prominent of which is the Shoulderstand (*Sarvangasana*), a great *asana* in its own right. If the Headstand is 'the King of *Asanas*', the Shoulderstand surely must the the 'Queen'.

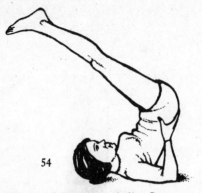

54

146. Half Shoulderstand Posture: *Ardha-Sarvangasana*
Persons who cannot immediately adopt the full Shoulderstand
Posture – perhaps because of obesity or muscular weakness – should
start with the Half Shoulderstand Posture.

Lie flat on the back, the legs extended together. Bending the
legs, draw back the knees, and raise the hips off the floor. Support
the hips with the hands, the thumbs separated widely from the
fingers. The elbows and the backs of the upper arms provide the
base support. The elbows should rest on the floor at shoulders'
width – not out wider as shown in a few books on Yoga. Upper and
lower arms form a right angle at the elbow. Straighten the legs
above the face at an angle to the floor of about forty-five degrees.
The trunk's slanting away from the floor at about the same angle
means that the abdomen and legs form a right angle (Fig. 54).
Breathe deeply into the abdomen. Hold the pose for at least twenty
seconds.

Regular practice of the Half Shoulderstand Posture should soon
lead to performance of the full posture, in which the legs are extended perpendicular to the floor. The benefits from the Half
Shoulder stand are similar to those for the full posture (No. 147),
but with milder effect.

147. Shoulderstand Posture: *Sarvangasana*
Sarva means 'all' or 'complete', and *anga* means 'body': hence the
Shoulderstand is sometimes called in English the All-body or the
Complete Posture. Another English title, because the legs and
trunk are held straight up, is the Candle Posture.

Lie flat on the back, the legs extended together. Bend the legs

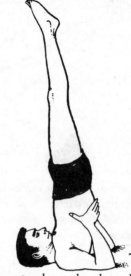

55

and bring back the knees to above the chest. Use the elbows and
upper arms as a base (elbows not wider apart than shoulders'
width) and prop the body by placing the hands against the small of
the back with the thumbs spread apart from the fingers. Note that
the hands could not be placed against the hips as in the Half
Shoulderstand Posture, because the hips are now to be raised much
higher. Bring the trunk to a vertical position and extend the legs
straight up so that the legs and trunk form a straight line perpendicular to the floor. In bringing the trunk upright the sternum
touches the chin. Bring the chest to the chin, not the chin to the
chest. Bodyweight is centred on the shoulders and neck (Fig. 55).
Breathe freely and deeply in the abdomen. Stay steadily in the
candle-like position for at least twenty seconds. Come out of the
pose slowly and smoothly.

The Shoulderstand or All-body Posture is not mentioned in the
traditional literature, but its history is a long one. It is a boon to
those who cannot master the Headstand, or who find the latter too
hazardous. Even those who are skilled in the Headstand should
never omit the Shoulderstand from regular practice.

Sarvangasana, by inverting the body, enables the venous blood
to flow to the heart without battling with gravity. Blood flows to
the brain, and to the scalp and facial tissues. The Shoulderstand has

the reputation of being a rejuvenator. Blood also flows to the neck, with a beneficial effect on the thyroid and parathyroid glands. The nervous system is calmed. The spine is strengthened, and the whole body firmed and toned. *Sarvangasana* relieves congestion in the legs, pelvis, and abdomen, and prevents or relieves varicose veins, asthma, insomnia, constipation, *prolapsus*, menstrual disorders, and menopause disturbances. It is said to increase sexual fitness in both men and women. It stimulates the endocrine glands, and invigorates the whole body in a harmonious way.

The Shoulderstand is unsuitable in cases of high blood pressure, spinal weakness, any disorder of the thyroid gland, chronic sinusitis or nasal catarrh, angina, otitis, sclerosis of the blood vessels of the brain – in short, severe ailments of the neck and head. Any reader with doubts about the suitability of the pose should take the advice of his doctor.

Learning the Headstand
The Headstand, in the fully inverted form, is a more severe posture than the Shoulderstand. Either the forearms, elbows, and sides of the hands, or alternatively the palms of the hands, provide an aid to steady balance – most Yoga instructors advise the former. Either way, much of the weight of the body is taken by the top of the skull. It is advisable, therefore, to exercise on a folded blanket or rug, a thick carpet, or some other soft surface which will cushion a roll over. In addition, a cushion or pad may be required to protect the head – this should be stable and of uniform thickness.

Like the person who takes up Judo, the person who wishes to master the Headstand Posture should first learn how to roll over without fear or discomfort. There should be a soft and even surface on which to land, and room to tumble over without the risk of painful knocks against furniture or other objects.

Take up the Quarter Headstand Posture (No. 148, Fig. 56). The hands cup the back of the head, with the fingers interlaced and interlocked. The inner edges of the hands rest on the floor, as do the forearms and elbows, the latter spread not wider than the shoulders. The top of the head rests on the floor. The trunk is vertical, and the legs are straight, with the toes resting on the floor. (The hand and arm position just described is that favoured by most Yogins in the headstand: the alternative is to place the palms of the hands flat on the floor at shoulders' width, the fingers pointing forward and spread. In both methods the arms are used to aid balance.) A sway forward or to one side will be detected by the clasped hands or the forearms respectively in the position we are here describing. Bring the knees forward towards the chest, hunching up the body into a relaxed ball. Then roll over, the way children delight in rolling on grass. As you roll over, always observe three rules: i Roll up into a *relaxed* ball. Have you noticed how young children and drunken men seem to be protected against falls? This is because they usually fall while relaxed. So make this rolling over practice child's play – or tipsy man's play if you prefer. ii. Unclasp the hands immediately you start to go over; otherwise the locked hands could receive a painful jerk. iii. Bend the legs so that the soles of the feet slap the floor and act as shock-absorbers.

Practise the roll over until it presents no problems. The principles just described apply equally to an overbalance from the full Headstand, which should be rare if one learns in stages as described here. The learning stages in themselves are valuable exercises, bestowing many of the physiological benefits claimed for the full Headstand Posture. The body should be conditioned by the Quarter Headstand; then by the Half Headstand; and finally by the Assisted Headstand. The Shoulderstand (No. 147, Fig. 55) also provides preparation for the full Headstand, for it accustoms the body to the inverted posture.

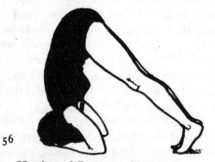

56

148. Quarter Headstand Posture: *Sirsasana*
Alternative spellings of *Sirsasana* (literally 'head posture') are *Sirshasana*, *Shirsasana*, and *Shirshasana*.

The Quarter Headstand is achieved by going into the Embarrassed Child's Posture (No. 104), and then straightening the legs and moving the feet forward cautiously until the trunk is perpendicular to the floor and supported by the top of the skull, the inner edges of the hands (which cup the back of the head with the fingers interlaced and interlocked), the forearms and elbows, and the toes of both feet (Fig. 56). Breathe freely and stay in the pose for six to ten seconds at first, increasing the duration of immobility as the body becomes more accustomed to the inverted position.

Following the pose, sit on the heels for a minute or so while the blood flows away from the head. Come out of the pose slowly – otherwise an abrupt reversal of the body position could cause giddiness.

A multiplicity of benefits are claimed for the Headstand, 'the King of *Asanas*'. The Quarter Headstand Posture shares some of these benefits, though reduced to some extent since some weight is taken on the toes and the legs slanting downwards. The back and neck are strengthened, and the legs firmed. The brain, scalp, neck, and facial tissues are nourished with blood.

Caution: the inverted postures are not suitable for persons suffering from high blood pressure, heart trouble, or ailments of the brain, eyes, nose, ears, and neck. Check with your doctor if you have any doubts in the matter.

149.   Quarter Headstand Posture II: *Sirsasana*
This is like No. 148, except that in this version you use the alternative placing of the hands. The palms of the hands are placed on the floor at each side of the head. The parted fingers point straight forward. The elbows are kept in towards the body and the hands are placed at shoulders' width. This hand position is shown in Fig. 159.

150.   Half Headstand Posture I: *Ardha-sirsasana*
This begins like the Quarter Headstand (No. 148), but has an additional stage. Having slowly walked forward until the back is vertical and the weight is centred on the top of the head, with balancing support from the clasped hands, the forearms, and the elbows, giving a little thrust with the toes and slowly raise the legs until they are parallel to the floor and at right angles to the torso (Fig. 57). Hold this position of balance steadily for a few seconds, breathing freely; then slowly lower the toes to the floor. Slowly come out of the inverted pose by bending the knees, and sit back on the heels for a minute or so while the blood flows away from the head.

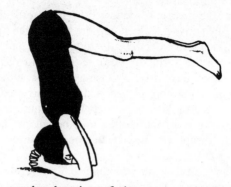

57

Add seconds to the duration of the pose as the body becomes accustomed to it.

For the beginner, this Half Headstand with straight legs is not as easy as it looks in an illustration. The neck muscles may require strengthening before success can be achieved. Neck and spine have to be in line. Easier for most beginners is the version of the Half Headstand Posture performed with bent legs, No. 152.

151. Half Headstand Posture II: *Ardha-sirsasana*
This is like the Half Headstand with straight legs brought parallel to the floor, as in No. 150, except that the weight is taken by the top of the head and the palms of the hands, which are placed at shoulders' width at each side of the head. This hand position is shown in Fig. 159.

152. Half Headstand Posture III: *Ardha-sirsasana*
Most beginners find it easier to attain the Half Headstand Posture if they bend their legs instead of keeping them straight. The knees are brought in close to the body. It is also easier for most people to go into the full Headstand Posture from this half-way stage with knees bent than it is with the legs straight.

You can begin in the Quarter Headstand Posture (No. 148, Fig. 56). Bend the knees and walk forward on the toes until the trunk is in a perpendicular position, neck and back in line, the weight taken on the top of the head, the hands, the forearms, and the elbows. Bring the knees inside the elbows and as close to the chest as possible. With neck and back solidly balanced, lift the toes simultaneously off the floor, bringing the knees up close to the

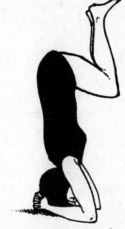

58

chest. Raise the feet slowly until the soles of the feet are pointing towards the ceiling with the legs half bent. and the lower legs from knee to ankle in a vertical position (Fig. 58). Breathe freely. Stay in the pose only a few seconds at first, but add seconds later. Balancing is usually found to be easier than in the version with straight legs.

Benefits are as for No. 148, but with only the thighs failing to achieve the vertical position, the effects are now moving nearer to those of the full Headstand, (described after No. 354.) Caution is as for No. 148.

153. Half Headstand Posture IV: *Ardha-sirsasana*
This is like No. 152, but the palms of the hands share the weight with the top of the head.

154. Inverted Crow Posture: *Kakasana*
Another way to strengthen the neck muscles and become accustomed to the inverted posture is to place the palms of the hands on the floor in the second of the alternative hand and arm positions, and then kneel on the backs of the upper arms, as in the Crow Posture (*Kakasana*, No. 397, Fig. 178), but with the top of the head placed on the floor. This looks more difficult than it actually is. It is more a matter of acquiring co-ordination than of strength.

155. Assisted Headstand Posture: *Sirsasana*
Just as the Half Headstand Posture should not be essayed until the

Quarter Headstand Posture has been fully mastered, so the Assisted Headstand should be performed only after the Half Headstand has become familiar and comfortable.

Go into the Half Headstand Posture and have a reliable assistant hold your ankles while you go into the full Headstand (Nos 338 and 339, Figs 159 and 160). If you move into the full Headstand from the Half Headstand with straight legs, the legs are simply swung up slowly together until legs and trunk are in a straight line. Most people find the bent-leg approach the easier. From the Half Headstand with legs half bent and the lower legs (from knees to ankles) in a vertical position, take the feet across the buttocks so that the soles of the feet point towards the wall behind the head – the lower legs are now horizontal instead of vertical. The legs are then straightened and legs, trunk, and neck brought into a straight line perpendicular to the floor.

The assistant keeps a light hold of the ankles, and when you are in the fully-inverted position lets go of the ankles, though he keeps his hands only inches away. Great care should be taken by both persons concerned. For a few seconds the Yoga student gets the feeling of balancing unaided in the full topsy-turvy pose. As in learning to ride a bicycle, there may be some moments of panic-wobble in early attempts. The first – perfectly steady – success gives great satisfaction.

The effects are those for the full Headstand, described after No. 354.

156. Wall-assisted Headstand Posture: *Sirsasana*
Once a measure of confidence has been gained, the Yoga student can practise the Headstand Posture using a wall for support. Utilizing the two walls of a corner is even better, for swaying to one side is then easily detected. The distance one places ones head from the wall or walls is important: twelve to fifteen inches is the correct range. When the beginner has gained confidence by using the two walls of a corner for support, he should utilize a single wall for a time; finally no wall at all and no other support will be needed.

Balance on the head and arms and bring the folded legs close in to the body. Find secure balance; then make a little hop from the toes, and go into the Half Headstand Posture with bent legs. (No. 152, Fig. 58). Once you feel stable in the Half Headstand, keep the legs bent and take the soles of the feet up and over to

rest flat against the wall, Breathe freely all the time. Do not arch
the back. From this inverted position with the soles of the feet flat
on the wall, slowly draw in the buttocks, carefully take the feet
away from the wall, and slowly straighten the legs so that the whole
body is perpendicular and balancing only on the head and arms
(Nos 338 and 339, Figs 159 and 160). You are not likely to be
successful at the first few attempts, and you may go into a panic-
wobble immediately you make the startling discovery that you are
standing on your head. When finally you balance easily for a few
seconds, without wobble, make do with that; add a second at a
time and make progress carefully until you can stay on your head
close to the wall for thirty seconds – that will be long enough for
the present. Care should be taken as the legs are lowered back to
the floor. Sit on the floor for a short time – do not stand upright
abruptly following a Headstand.

You may feel that it would be easier to walk your feet up the wall
until a Headstand has been simulated. This is what is against the
idea: it would be only a simulation. Whatever psychological satisfaction it would give, this method would lead to badly overbalancing
in the real thing. Stick to the method described in the previous paragraph.

The final stage is to practise straightening the legs slowly out of
the Half Headstand Posture without the feet resting on the wall. The
presence of the wall will provide security, but it should not be necessary. You will have mastered 'the King of *Asanas*'.

157.   Incline-board or Tilt-chair.
The beneficial principle of refreshing the body by placing the feet
higher than the heart and head need not be denied to those for whom
the Headstand and the Shoulderstand are too hazardous. Lying on
the back on the floor with the feet on a chair-seat is useful. Some
hospital beds can be tilted to put the patient on an incline, feet higher
than head. We can ourselves make use of a length of board, a little
longer than our height and about a foot wide. Set this *securely* at an
angle against a bed, office desk, or other suitable support. Lie full
length on the board with the feet higher than the head. Adjust the
angle of incline to suit your requirements and to provide variety.

Instead of using a board, you can purchase a tilt-chair on which
the body lies curved, but again with the feet higher than the head,
thus utilizing the valuable principle of giving the body a holiday

from its normal battle against gravity.

It should not be thought that the use of an incline-board or tilt-chair is recommended only for those who cannot invert the body more strongly in the preceding postures. Everyone will benefit from this milder method – especially if at the same time it is made an opportunity for relaxation, using the body-parts sequence of let-go relaxation described for No. 112 (Corpse Posture: *Savasana* or *Mrtasana*(. Five, ten, or fifteen minutes a day proves a tonic refreshment. Those whose occupations keep them standing for several hours a day should have an extra tilt-relaxation session.

SERIES POSTURES

Sun Salutations (*Surya Namaskars*)

A case can be made for including the graceful posture series *Surya Namaskars* in Group B rather than Group A, on the grounds that perfect performance requires advanced co-ordination and suppleness. On the other hand, if we had to wait for perfect performance of every stage of the series, many of us would never be able to garner its enormous benefits. Moreover, most stages of the Sun Salutations fall within the capacities of most students of Yoga, even if the linking of the positions by less advanced students lacks the fluidity of the adept. As to the most difficult stages, even the beginner can achieve an approximation of what is aimed at and benefit highly thereby, without having to omit any stages from the series. And practice through time makes, if not for perfection in every case, at least for progress towards it. One learns how to make the modifications that bring smoothness to the transitions – a slight bending of the legs as one bends forward, the fingers pressing on the floor instead of the palms of the hands, the head brought in the direction of the knees even if not resting on them. The important point is for the student to accept his physical limitations and not force himself to the point of strain.

This series is a Yoga programme in itself – a kind of concentrated Yoga potion. Some of the positions have already been given in Group A modifications – for example, the Standing Forward Bend (*Padastasana*) and the Cobra Posture (*Bhujangasana*). The great majority of Yoga postures require poised immobility. This is only momentarily true here: you pause only for a second or two in each completed stage before moving on to the next position. Adepts take only twenty seconds for a ten-position cycle – but most practitioners will find such a speed destroying the accuracy of performance, and should settle for a slightly slower rate. Nevertheless, several successive cycles should produce perspiration and quickened breathing. Commence with two cycles only, gradually adding two cycles until you are performing twelve, which is the most frequently advocated number, there being twelve names for the sun in the Sanskrit language.

Surya means 'sun', and *namaskars* means 'salutations', 'obeisances', or 'prayers'. The postures are performed traditionally at sunrise, when the air is deemed to be rich in *prana* (cosmic energy). The series is a proven vitalizer, bringing a youthful suppleness to the spine and firming and toning the entire body. Each position has its valuable physiological effects, some of which were described earlier. Though much more than just a warm-up, the Sun Salutations serve that function when performed at the start of a Yoga programme. My own preference is to treat them as separate from the main programme of the day, and to perform them on rising in the morning, when they sweep sleep from the limbs and provide an invigorating start to the day.

The first version we give is that most frequently found in Yogic literature. The second version is that taught and written about by Shrimant Balasahib Pandit Pratinidhi, the Raja of Aundh. The third version is that favoured by the author, combining stages of the first two. The fourth version is a shortened and simplified series suggested by Archie J. Bahm, in *Yoga for Business Executives*. Other variations are more concerned with the execution of the stages than with the overall design of the series. Each reader should experiment, decide on the version that best suits his or her build and degree of suppleness and co-ordination, and then give it an extended try-out. Eventually it should be found that the postures flow together and the series takes on the beauty and harmony of a fine piece of music or a work of art.

158. Sun Salutations I: *Surya Namaskars*

Position 1. Stand up straight in poised posture, the feet together, the fingers and the palms brought together in front of the chest, the fingers pointing upwards and thumbs touching the chest (the traditional Indian gesture of respect or homage). It will help if the big

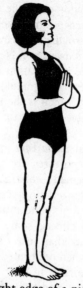

59

toes are touching the straight edge of a piece of cloth spread on the floor specially for this exercise, or if the edge or pattern of a carpet or rug provides a suitable guide-line. Pratinidhi's description of this stage advises stiffening the whole body in a wave-like action from the feet (pressing them down on the floor) to the scalp, flattening the stomach on the way (Fig. 59). It helps to think of the body being charged with solar energy. Breathe freely.

Position 2. Inhaling, raise the arms high and back, the palms facing forwards. Throw the head back, bending the spine back from the waist. (Fig. 1) depicts this stage, but the feet should be together.

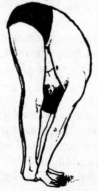

60

Position 3. Exhaling, bend forward from the waist and touch the hands to the floor beside the feet, the longest fingers in line with the toes. The adept places the palms of the hands flat on the floor, but the beginner may find it more convenient to touch down the spread fingers. Again: the adept keeps his knees locked and lowers his face against his knees. The beginner usually has to bend his knees a little, and he brings his face as close to his knees as he can comfortably manage. The hands now stay in place until near the end of the cycle (Fig. 60).

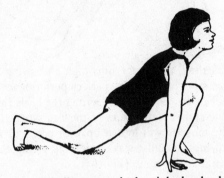

61

Position 4. Inhaling, stretch the right leg back and go down on the right knee, at the same time lifting the head up. The hands and the left foot stay in position. The toes of the right foot are bent to grip the floor (Fig. 61).

Position 5. Retaining the breath, straighten the right leg and take the left leg back alongside the right, supporting the body on the hands and toes. From the back of the head to the heels should be a straight line. This is the Wheelbarrow Posture (No. 107, Fig. 37).

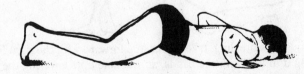

62

Position 6. Exhaling, bend the arms and lower the forehead, chest, and knees to the floor. Keep the pelvis raised, pulling in the abdominal muscles. Press the chin into the jugular notch. The hands press down firmly, and the elbows are kept high (Fig. 62). This is called the Eight Parts Posture (*Sastanganamasker*).

Position 7. Inhaling, straighten the arms and raise the upper body up and back, keeping the pelvis and legs on the ground (No. 136, Fig. 147). This is the Cobra Posture (*Bhujangasana*).

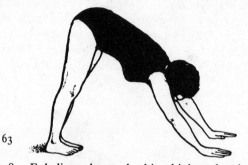

63

Position 8. Exhaling, thrust the hips high and swing the head down between the straight arms. In perfect performance the feet are flat on the floor from toes to heels. Getting the heels right down may not be possible at first if the backs of the legs signal resistance. Do not strain: the muscles will loosen up with practice. The back from shoulders to hips should be as straight as possible. Pull the abdomen back towards the spine (Fig. 63).

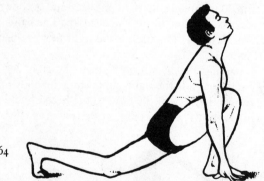

64

Position 9. Inhaling, take a long step forward with the right foot, bringing it in line with the hands, at the same time lowering the left knee to the floor and thrusting forward the chest (Fig. 64). This is Position 4 with the right knee now forward instead of the left.

Position 10. Exhaling, assume Position 3 again by bringing the left foot forward beside the right foot, raising the hips, and straightening (or nearly straightening) the legs (Fig. 60).

Position 11.   Straighten up from the waist and swing the arms high and back, inhaling (No. 8, Fig. 1). This is a repeat of Position 2.

Position 12.   Exhaling, lower the arms to the sides and stand up straight (No. 56, Fig. 8).

This completes one cycle. In performing the second cycle repeat the twelve positions, but take back the left leg at Position 4 and step forward with the left foot at Position 9. Thereafter continue to follow this alternating leg sequence.

When the reader has studied the above description of the twelve positions and consulted the illustrations, he should find the following list helpful for quick reference:

Position 1.   Stand upright, breathing freely.
Position 2.   Arms raised, breathing in.
Position 3.   Bend forward, breathing out.
Position 4.   Right leg back, breathing in.
Position 5.   Hands and toes, holding the breath.
Position 6.   Prone on floor, breathing out.
Position 7.   Cobra Posture, breathing in.
Position 8.   Inverted V, breathing out.
Position 9.   Right leg forward, breathing in.
Position 10. Bend forward, breathing out.
Position 11. Arms raised, breathing in,
Position 12. Arms by sides, breathing out.

The above guide describes performances of cycles 1, 3, 5, and so on. For even-numbered cycles, only Position 4 and Position 9 are different.

Position 4.   Left leg back, breathing in.
Position 9.   Left leg forward, breathing in.

159.   Sun Salutations II: *Surya Namaskars*

The following ten positions are those taught by Shrimant Balasahib Pandit Pratinidhi, the Raja of Aundh, as a complete form of Yoga exercise. For adults, he gives three hundred cycles daily as the target to aim for. Other Yoga teachers give *Surya Namaskars* as but one part of Yoga posturing, with twelve cycles daily the recommended quota.

Position 1.   As Position 1 of Sun Salutations I, (Fig. 59).

Position 2.   As Position 3 of Sun Salutations I, (Fig. 60), except that the wrists and not the longest fingers are in line with the big toes.

Position 3.   As Position 4 of Sun Salutations I, Fig. 61, except that the right leg has not been extended as far back. Upper and lower leg form a right angle, and the thigh is vertical in line with the arms. More of the trunk presses against the upper surface of the left thigh.

Position 4.   As Position 8 of Sun Salutations I, (Fig. 63), except that the angle of the inverted V is sharper, due to the legs not having been taken as far back as in the first version.

Position 5.   As Position 6 of Sun Salutations I, (Fig. 62).

Position 6.   As Postion 7 of Sun Salutations I, (No. 316, Fig. 147), except that the pelvis is also raised, so that the body is supported by the hands, knees, and toes. The shorter step back, as in Position 3, means that the arms are about vertical rather than slanting away from the body as in (Fig. 147).

Position 7.   The hips are thrust high – a return to Position 4.

Position 8.   A return to Position 3, except that the right and not the left knee stays forward. The position is as in (Fig. 64), but with the left leg extended less far back.

Position 9.   A return to Position 2.

Position 10.   A return to Position 1.

Pratinidhi gives the following breathing regulation for the above ten-position sequence.

Position 1.   Breathe in. Stand upright.
Position 2.   Breathe out. Bend forward.
Position 3.   Breathe in. Right leg back.
Position 4.   Hold. Inverted V.
Position 5.   Breathe out. Prone.
Position 6.   Breathe in. Cobra Posture.
Position 7.   Hold. Inverted V.
Position 8.   Hold. Right leg forward.
Position 9.   Breathe out. Bent forward.
Position 10.   Breathe in. Stand upright.

The author prefers breathing out on Positions 4 and 7, breathing in on Position 8 and holding the breath on Position 5.

160.   Sun Salutations III: *Surya Namaskars*
The author suggests and recommends the following combination of postures:

Position 1.   As Position 1 of Sun Salutations I, Fig. 59.
Position 2.   As Position 2 of Sun Salutations I, No. 8, Fig. 1.
Position 3.   As Position 3 of Sun Salutation I, Fig. 60.
Position 4.   As Position 4 of Sun Salutations I, Fig. 61.

Position 5.   As Position 8 of Sun Salutations I, Fig. 63.

Positions 6 to 12.   As Positions 6 to 12 of Sun Salutations I.

This follows Sun Salutations I, except that the inverted V position is performed twice, as it is in Sun Salutations II. This makes for a natural and easily-remembered in-out breathing sequence, with only one holding of the breath in position. For quick reference:

Position 1.   Stand upright, breathing freely.

Position 2.   Arms raised, breathing in.

Position 3.   Bend forward, breathing out.

Position 4.   Right leg back, breathing in.

Position 5.   Inverted V, breathing out.

Position 6.   Prone on floor, holding the breath.

Position 7.   Cobra Posture, breathing in.

Position 8.   Inverted V, breathing out.

Position 9.   Right leg forward, breathing in.

Position 10. Bend forward, breathing out.

Position 11. Arms raised, breathing in.

Position 12. Arms by sides, breathing out.

161.   Sun Salutations IV: *Surya Namaskars*

Archie J. Bahm, in *Yoga for Business Executives* (Stanley Paul, 1967), suggests a ten-position cycle in which the legs are kept together at all times. It can be summarized as follows:

Position 1.   Stand upright, breathing freely.

Position 2.   Arms raised, breathing in.

Position 3.   Bend forward, breathing out.

Position 4.   Inverted V, breathing in.

Position 5.   Prone on floor, breathing out.

Position 6.   Cobra Posture, breathing in.

Position 7.   Inverted V, holding the breath.

Position 8.   Bend forward, breathing out.

Position 9.   Arms raised, breathing in.

Position 10. Arms by sides, breathing out.

This has the merit of simplicity, and avoids the rather awkward leg-split changes and postures. But it also misses their physiological benefits, stretching the whole body and massaging through thigh pressure the abdomen and its contents. However, readers who find difficult the leg positionings of the first three series of *Surya Namaskars* could perhaps with advantage use version IV for conditioning purposes, incorporating the leg-bending later. Mr Bahm suggests varying the distance of the hands from the feet.

Dhirendra Brahmachari introduces an entirely new stage into *Surya Namaskars*. In the leg back position, lean as far back as you can and stretch the arms up and back, the palms of the hands turned up with the thumbs touching (No. 78, Fig. 19).

MUSCULAR LOCKS (*BANDHAS*)

Bandhas are muscular locks, seals, or restraints applied in Yoga breathing (*pranayama*) during the pauses between inhalation and exhalation and exhalation and inhalation. The Sanskrit word *bandha* is linked etymologically with such English words as 'band', 'bind', 'bond', and 'bound'.

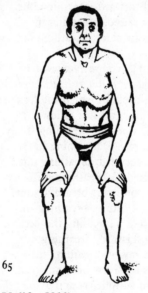

65

162. Abdominal Uplift: *Uddiyana*

Uddiyana – one of the three main *bandhas* of Hatha Yoga – means 'flying up'. It is associated with the most esoteric of Yoga practices – the control of the flow of energies (*prana*) and their movement ('flying') up the central channel of the spine to the brain. Though classified as a *bandha*, *Uddiyana* or abdominal uplift is one of the most valuable exercises of Yoga in its own right, and unequalled for the culture of the abdomen.

Stand with the feet spread about one foot apart. Stoop forward slightly, bend the knees a little, and place the palms of the hands and the spread fingers on the thighs just above the knees, with the fingers turned inwards. Using both nostrils and mouth for maximum speed and effect, empty the lungs of air – some residual air will always remain, but you will not be aware of it. Pressing the hands down on the thighs and, concentrating on the solar plexus, draw the abdominal wall back and up into the thoracic cavity. In time, provided there has been a thorough exhalation, the retraction will be effortless (Fig. 65).

Perform this on an empty stomach, and after emptying the bladder (bowels too if possible). As breathing has been 'locked', the control should not be held longer than five seconds at first, increasing gradually to ten seconds. Perform three times, increasing to six times after some weeks.

Uddiyana strengthens the abdominal muscles, removes superfluous fat, provides an internal massage as the abdominal viscera are drawn back and squeezed, and improves digestion and elimination from the bowels. The raised diaphragm is said to massage and tone the muscles of the heart. It has been found to correct menstrual irregularities, but should *not* be performed *during* menstruation or pregnancy.

Once a deep and easily-held retraction is achieved, you may consider mastering the spectacular muscle control of isolating the central recti muscles. This is called *Nauli* (No. 418, Figs. 191 and 192).

V Group A Postures: Programme Planning

Yoga practice is a continual process of discovery – about one's body, one's mind, and the integral relationship of the two. One moves towards re-establishing the kind of body-mind *rapport* one had in childhood and the retraining of kinesthesis, the sense by which one perceives one's posture, weight, pressure, muscle tone, and so on. This sense is the surest guide to planning posture programmes. Detailed schedules – day to day, week to week, month to month – recommended by writers on Yoga are of little use, and can sometimes be harmful, for readers are certain to find that some of the postures indicated go against the body's wisdom. But guide-lines for shaping a daily programme may be indicated. The following rules should be observed:

1. No forcing of joints or limbs beyond capacity, as signalled by discomfort or pain.

2. Do not carry a programme to the point of fatigue. It is better to perform a small number of postures well, smoothly, and with good form, than to tackle double or treble the number with awkward form, discomfort, or strain. Clumsy or painful performance disrupts the calm, attentive attitude that is an essential part of Yoga practice.

3. Finish a programme with the feeling that all parts of the body have been exercised, and feeling refreshed and well-toned: for Yoga is relaxation as well as exercise.

4. If the spine is bent in one direction in a group of *asanas*, bend it in the opposite direction during the next few postures.

5. Beginners and intermediate students should precede the main programme with five or ten minutes of warming up and limbering up, as indicated at the end of that section.

6. Once comfortable mastery of Group A postures is achieved,

explore Group B postures and see if you can formulate a programme of the more advanced *asanas*.

7.   The best sequence in terms of utilizing energy is from standing postures to sitting and kneeling postures; then to supine and prone postures. The inverted poses may be split if desired, a few near the beginning of a programme and a few at the end. A few minutes of relaxation should precede and conclude a programme. The Abdominal Uplift may be performed at a separate time of day: on rising is a good occasion, for the stomach is then empty. The Sun Salutations may also be performed separately.

8.   A satisfactory Yoga programme should include relaxation, warm-ups, all-body stretches, forward bends, backward bends, spinal twisting, poised sitting or kneeling, leg limbering, abdominal squeezing and contracting, inverted postures, and abdominal muscle controls.

Relaxation: mainly Corpse Posture, No. 112. Occasionally Nos. 113, 114, 115, 116, 117, or 118.

Warm-ups and limber-ups: as indicated following that section.

One to five postures should then be selected from each of the following sections:

All-body stretches: Nos 56-65, 78-9, 95-8, 101, 106-8, 119, 131, 138, 141, 158-61.

Forward bends: Nos 66-70, 85, 99-101, 103-5, 131, 138.

Backward bends: Nos 71-2, 105, 109-110, 142-5.

Spinal twisting: Nos 73, 91.

Sitting or kneeling: Nos 81-4, 90, 92-4.

Leg limbering: Nos 74-7, 83-4, 86-7, 11, 120-3, 139-40.

Abdominal squeezing and contracting: Nos 80, 88-9, 102, 126-30, 132-8.

Inverted: Nos 146-56.

Abdominal muscle controls: Nos 124-5, 162.

Conclude with a few minutes of relaxation.

VI Group B Postures

GROUP B POSTURES

Here we have most of the great basic *asanas* of Hatha Yoga, with their many variations. Their antiquity is shown by the Sanskrit names, based often on the natural stretching movements of animals, birds, and reptiles. This is certain: a number of these poses will prove too difficult for all but a few remarkably supple practitioners. So be patient and make progress slowly, smoothly, and carefully. Do not force or take risks when a pose proves beyond the body's suppleness, strength, or co-ordination. With the huge repertory of poses offered on these pages there should be no difficulty in devising programmes to meet your needs and physical capabilities. Programmes should be planned on the lines suggested following the description of the postures.

STANDING POSTURES

163.   Tree Posture 1: *Vrksasana*
Stand upright. Flex the left leg and, pulling on the ankle, upturn the left foot high up on the right thigh. Keep the back straight. Bring the palms of the hands together a little above the head with the arms half bent, the fingers pointing upwards and the albows held out wide. It will assist good balance to fix the gaze on a point level with the eyes on the wall ahead (Fig. 66). Breathe freely and deeply, staying in the pose at least ten seconds. Repeat, balancing on the left leg.

The Tree Posture limbers the hips, strengthens the ankles, firms

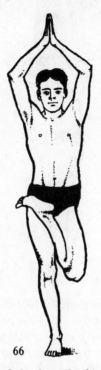

66

and tones the muscles of the legs, back, and chest, expands the thorax, and improves balance, posture, and concentration.

164.   Tree Posture II: *Vrksasana*
An alternative placing of the raised foot – corresponding to Perfect Posture (*Siddhasana*) rather than to Lotus Posture (*Padmasana*) – is to rest the sole of the foot against the inside of the thigh with the heel pulled far up against the crotch, and the knee drawn out wide. The beginners' version, with the sole of the foot placed against the inside of the knee is given in No. 57, Fig. 9.

165.   Eagle Posture I: *Garudasana*
Garuda means 'an eagle'.
Stand upright. Bend the left knee slightly and twist the right leg over the left leg so that the right instep is tucked behind the left calf. The arms are crossed in front of the chest so that the left elbow rests on the right biceps against the elbow joint, and the left fist is

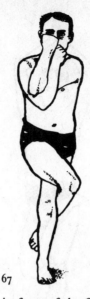

67

kept above the right fist in front of the face (Fig. 67). Stay steady
at least ten seconds, breathing freely. Then repeat the pose, balancing
on the right leg and reversing the arm and leg positions.

The Eagle Posture promotes suppleness in the legs and shoulders,
strengthens the knees, ankles, and calf muscles, develops co-ordination and balance, and improves concentration.

166.   Eagle Posture I: *Garudasana*

In this version bend forward from the complete pose above so that
the lower elbow rests on top of the upper thigh a little above the
knee.

The effects are as given for No. 165, with more pressure on the
abdominal muscles and organs.

167.   Eagle Posture III: *Garudasana*

In this very advanced version you keep the arms entwined and bend
forward so that the chest rests on the upper thigh.

The benefits are as for No. 165, with additional pressure on the
abdominal muscles and organs, and on the sex glands.

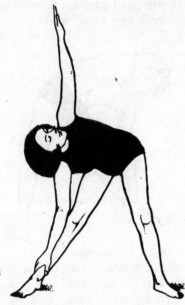

68

168. Triangle Posture 1: *Trikonasana*

Tri means 'three', and *kona* means 'angle'.

There are two main versions of the Triangle Posture: one in which the legs are kept straight, and a more difficult version in which the feet are spread further apart at the start and the leg is flexed on the side to which you bend. In both versions the arms are kept straight throughout.

Stand erect, the feet spread wide apart. Breathe in deeply and extend the arms sideways in line with the shoulders and parallel to the floor, the palms of the hands turned down. Keeping both arms and legs straight, bend to the right from the waist and grasp the right ankle or foot with the hand. The left arm swings straight up until perpendicular to the floor. Twist your head to look up at the up-raised hand (Fig. 68). Stay bent over at least ten seconds. Repeat to the other side.

Our illustration shows the ankle being grasped, which is the formal requirement, but you may prefer to place the hand on the foot or even flat on the floor beside the foot.

The Triangle Posture firms and tones the leg muscles, removes superfluous fat from the waistline, expands the chest, stretches the arms, shoulders, and back, and massages the abdominal organs. It nourishes the spinal nerves with extra blood.

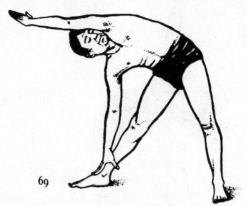

69

169.   Triangle Posture II: *Trikonasana*
This has an additional stage beyond the position shown in Fig. 68. Carry the raised arm over the head until it is parallel to the floor, with the upper arm pressing against the ear (Fig. 69). Keep the head level in this version and look straight ahead. Bend over to each side.

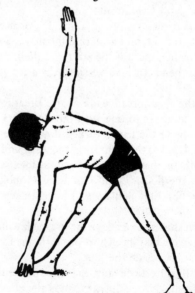

70

170.   Revolved Triangle Posture: *Parivrtta Trikonasana*
Parivrtta means 'turned round' or 'revolved'
Stand erect as at the start of Nos 168 and 169. As you bend to the
right side, twist round and bring the left hand to the right ankle or
foot, or touch the floor beside the foot. The right arm is stretched
straight up perpendicular to the floor, and the head is twisted to
gaze at the uplifted right hand (Fig. 70). Stay bent over at least ten
seconds, breathing freely. Repeat to the other side.
    The benefits are as given for No. 168, with an additional twisting
of the waistline.

171.   Stretched Lateral Angle Posture: *Utthita Parsvakonasana*
Utthita means 'extruded' or 'stretched', *parsva* means 'side' or
'flank', and *kona* means 'angle'.
B. K. S. Iyengar gives a variation of the Triangle Posture in which
one leg is bent to form a right angle between upper and lower leg
and the side presses down on the thigh. The feet are spread four to
four and a half feet apart, with the foot on the side to which you
bend turned to ninety degrees and the other foot turned slightly in
the same direction. The wide foot placement and the bending of the
leg to a right angle mean that the trunk can be stretched low to the
side and the palm of the hand can be placed on the floor behind the
foot, with the armpit and side against the top of the thigh. The other
arm is brought across above the ear and kept locked at the elbow.
    The benefits are as for No. 168, with additional pressure on the
abdomen, stimulating peristaltic activity in the intestines. The
posture is thus a cure for constipation. Extra blood flows to the
abdominal organs. The ankle and knee of the bent leg are strengthened.

172.   Revolved Lateral Angle Posture: *Parivrtta Parsvakonasana*
This requires considerable suppleness. In No. 171 the right hand
was placed behind the right foot or the left hand behind the left foot.
In the revolved version you twist round so that the right palm is set
on the floor behind the left foot or the left plam placed on the floor
behind the right foot. You are now looking in the opposite direction
to that in No. 171. Again the bend over is so deep that armpit and
flank press down on the top of the thigh of the bent leg.
    The effects are as for No. 171, but intensified.

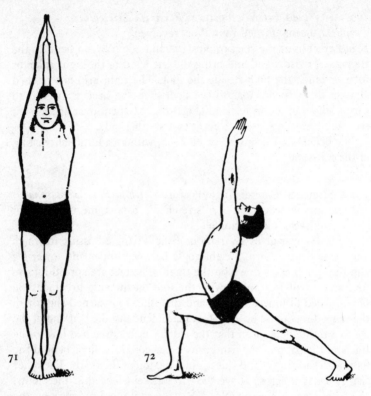

71   72

173. Virabhadrais Posture I: *Virabhadrasana*
Virabhadra is one of the intrepid heroes of Hindu legend.
Stand upright with the feet and knees together, the arms extended
overhead, covering the ears, the palms of the hands joined together
(Fig. 71). Spread the legs wide apart and turn to the right so that
the right foot has turned ninety degrees, and the left foot just slightly,
to the right. Both legs and both arms are straight at this stage. Now
bend the right knee and take it forward until it is above the heel,
ankle to knee being vertical, and upper and lower leg forming a
right angle. The left leg stays locked at the knee and the arms are
still together and locked overhead. Complete the pose by throwing
the head back and gazing up at the hands, which are still pressed
together (Fig. 72). Hold the pose for at least ten seconds, breathing
freely. Repeat, turning to the left and flexing the left leg.
   This pose limbers and strengthens the ankles, knees, hips, and

shoulders, and firms and tones the legs, hips, chest, back, and neck. The chest is expanded. The hamstring muscles at the backs of the thighs are loosened. Balance and concentration are improved. The concomitant psychological tone is one of heroic strength and compact power.

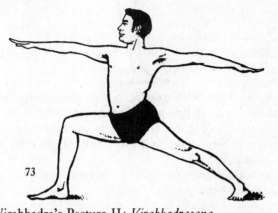

73

174. Virabhadra's Posture II: *Virabhadrasana*
Stand upright with the feet spread wide apart and the arms extended in line with the shoulders, palms down. Turn the right foot fully ninety degrees to the right and the left foot slightly to the right. Flex the right knee until the knee is over the heel and the lower and upper leg form a right angle. Stretch the right arm strongly to the right and the left arm strongly to the left in line with the shoulders. Turn the head to the right and gaze at the back of the right hand (Fig. 73). Hold the pose for at least ten seconds, breathing freely and deeply. Return to the starting position; then repeat, bending the left knee and gazing at the left hand.

175. Virabhadra's Posture III: *Virabhadrasana*
This is a continuation of the final position of Virabhadra's Posture I, turning it into a balance on one leg with the arms, trunk, and one leg in line parallel to the floor.
  Stand upright as shown in Fig. 71. Spread the legs widely apart, turn to the right, bend the right knee, and take up the final position of version I (Fig. 72). Bring the arms down to a position parallel to the floor. Gazing at the hands, bring the trunk down over the right thigh. Lift the left leg off the floor, at the same time straightening

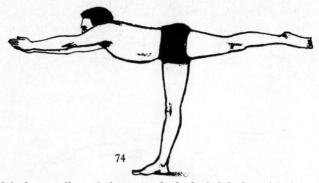

74

the right leg, until you balance on the locked right leg with the arms, trunk, and left leg all in line parallel to the floor, the instep of the left foot facing down (Fig. 74). Breathing freely, hold the pose for at least ten seconds. Repeat the pose through its stages until you are balancing on the left leg.

The benefits are as given for No. 173, but the pose requires greater co-ordination and balance.

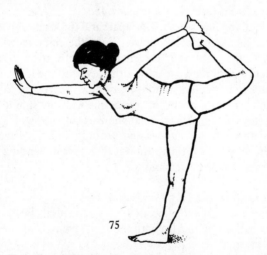

75

176. Toppling Tree Posture I: *Vrksasana*
The starting position is that shown in Fig. 10 (No. 58). Standing upright with the feet together, fold the left leg, taking the heel back and grasping the foot with the left hand. Hold the right arm straight up alongside the right ear, the palm of the hand forward.

Keeping the back straight and the right leg locked at the knee, tilt forward until the right arm, trunk, and left thigh are in line parallel to the floor and you balance on the straight right leg (Fig. 75). Balance steadily for at least ten seconds, breathing normally. Repeat, balancing on the left leg.

The Toppling Tree Posture limbers, strengthens, and firms the legs, reduces fat on the waistline, aids digestion and elimination, tones up the nervous system, and improves balance and posture.

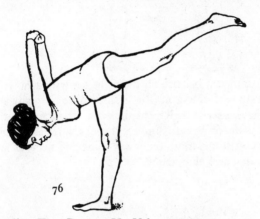

76

177. Toppling Tree Posture II: *Vrksasana*
Stand erect with the feet and knees together. Interlace and interlock the hands behind you. Take a deep breath. Exhaling, tilt forward, at the same time raising the left leg straight up behind you, until head, trunk, and left leg are in a straight diagonal line with the head lower than the foot. The arms are straight up perpendicular to the floor, and you are balancing on the straight left leg (Fig. 76). Balance steadily for at least ten seconds, breathing normally. Then repeat, balancing on the left leg.

178. Half-moon Posture: *Ardha-chandrasana*
Ardha means 'half', and *chandra* means 'moon'.
Stand upright, the arms by the sides, the feet spread about three feet apart. Turn the right foot to the right ninety degrees and the left foot slightly to the right. Bend the right leg, lean over to the right, and place the palm of the right hand on the floor about a foot in front of the toes of the right foot. Raise the left leg straight up from the floor without bending it and at the same time straighten the

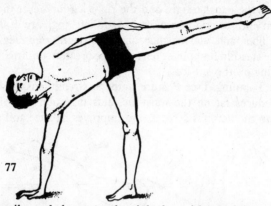

77

right leg until you balance on the right leg with steadying support from the straight right arm (Fig. 77). Breathe normally and balance for at least ten seconds. Repeat the pose, balancing on the left leg.

The Half-moon Posture limbers the legs, hips, and spine, reduces fat on the waistline, tones the lower spine and nervous system, and aids digestion and elimination.

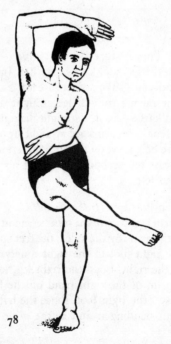

78

179.   Lord of the Dance Posture I: *Natarajasana*
Nata means 'dancer', and *raja* means 'lord' or 'king'. This posture
is frequently seen in Hindu sculpture depicting Siva as Lord of the
Dance. Nataraja is one of the names of Siva.
Balance on the slightly-bent left leg. The right leg is bent and held
across to the left. The right arm forms a right angle just above the
head, the palm turned up. The left arm is curved to the right in
front of the diaphragm, the palm down and the fingers held loosely
(Fig. 78). Breathe normally and balance for at least ten seconds.
Repeat, reversing the roles of the arms and the legs.
    The Lord of the Dance Posture strengthens and firms the legs,
tones the nervous system, and improves physical and mental poise.
The accompanying feeling tone is that of poised balance and the dance
of life.

180.   Lord of the Dance Posture II: *Natarajasana*
Another frequent depiction of the pose is with the upper arm curved
across the front of the chest, rather than above the héad as described
in No. 179.

181.   Lord of the Dance Posture III: *Natarajasana*
B. K. S. Iyengar gives a very advanced posed which is more gymnastic than dance, though graceful-looking if you can do it. The left
arm is extended straight out in front parallel to the floor. The right
leg is flexed behind the buttocks and the big toe is grasped between
the thumb and the index and middle fingers of the right hand. By
a rotation of the right elbow and shoulder the right arm is stretched
up behind the head, the right leg is pulled up until the lower leg
and instep form a perpendicular line, and you are balancing on the
straight left leg. Breathe freely and hold the pose for ten to fifteen
seconds. Repeat, balancing on the straight right leg.

182.   Lord Kalabhairava's Posture: *Kalabhairavasana*
This pose is named after one of the Hindu deities.
Stand with the spine straight and place the right foot directly in
front of the left foot, the toes of both pointing forward. The right
arm is stretched out stiffly in front slanting diagonally downwards,
and the left arm similarly is held stiffly behind. The palms of both
hands are turned down. Open the eyes and the mouth as wide as
possible and thrust the tongue out and down strongly. Both legs are

locked at the knees. Take a deep breath. Gaze straight ahead and tense the muscles for ten seconds. Repeat, reversing the roles of the arms and the legs.

Lord Kalabhairava's Posture depends for its effects on the amount of energy with which you charge the nerves and body. It strengthens and tones the eyes, jaw muscles, tongue, and throat. Extra blood is brought to the facial tissues. The difficulty is in maintaining perfect immobility. Balance, posture, and concentration are improved, and the nervous system is toned:

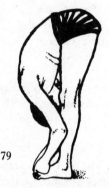

79

183.   Standing Forward Bend: *Padahastasana*
Padahastasana means 'foot-hand posture'. The beginners' version was described in No. 67 Fig. 14.
Stand erect with the legs together. Breathing in deeply, raise the hands high overhead, palms forward and the upper arms covering the ears. Exhaling and keeping the legs locked at the knees, fold forward from the waist, stretch down, and grasp the feet, keeping the elbows pulled in close to the legs. Press the face against the knees (Fig. 79). Stay bent forward ten to fifteen seconds.

The Standing Forward Bend Posture stretches, strengthens, and limbers the spine, loosens the hamstrings, firms and tones the legs, massages the abdominal muscles and organs, tones the nervous system, and stimulates the circulation. Additional blood flows to the brain, scalp, and face.

184.   Alternate Leg Standing Forward Bend Posture: *Padahastasana*
Stand upright with the feet spread wide apart. Clasp the hands

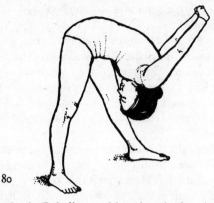

80

behind the back. Exhaling and keeping the legs locked at the knees, bend forward from the waist and press the face to the left knee, swinging the arms over the back and forward as far as possible (Fig. 80). Keep the head lowered ten to fifteen seconds. Then stand up straight, breathing in. Exhaling, bend forward and lower the face to the right knee. Again stay down ten to fifteen seconds. Alternatively, the hands may be held against the lower back.

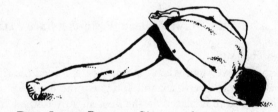

81

185. Deep Lunge Posture: *Sirsangusthasana*
Sirsa means 'head', and *angustha* means 'big toe'. The head is brought deep down to the toes.

Stand with the legs wide apart and the hands clasped behind the back. Exhaling, bend forward and, bending the left leg, lower the forehead down to the left big toe. (Fig 81). Stay down ten to fifteen seconds; then stand up and repeat to the other side.

This pose brings great suppleness to the legs and waist, massages the abdominal region, and improves balance.

186. Balancing Forward Bend Posture: *Padahastasana*, or *Urdhva Prasarita Ekapadasana*

Urdhva means 'above', *prasarita* means 'extended', *eka* means 'one', and *pada* means 'foot'.

Stand upright, the feet and the knees together. Take a deep breath. Exhaling, bend forward from the waist and catch the right ankle with the left hand, placing the palm of the right hand on the floor alongside the right foot. Lower the face to the right knee. At the same time swing the left leg back and up as high as possible. Balance on the right leg ten to fifteen seconds. Repeat, balancing on the left leg.

187.   Half-lotus Forward Bend Posture: *Ardha-padmottanasana*
Ardha means 'half', *padma* means 'lotus', and *uttana* means 'stretch'.
Stand upright. Bend the left knee, grasp the foot and pull it high, sole up, on the right thigh in the half-lotus position. Exhaling, bend forward and place the right palm on the floor alongside and outside the right foot and the left palm flat on the floor to the left of the right foot and in line with it. Press the face against the right knee. Stay down ten to fifteen seconds. Repeat to the other side.

The abdominal wall and organs receive a strong massage. The pose removes superfluous fat from the waistline, tones and firms the legs, limbers the legs and hips, aids digestion and elimination, and improves balance.

188.   Bound Half-lotus Forward Bend Posture: *Ardha-baddha Padmottanasana*
Baddha means 'bound'.
In this more difficult version, when the right leg is folded the right arm is taken across the lower back and you grasp the big toe of the right foot. The left palm is placed on the floor slightly to the left of the left foot. Then reverse the roles of the arms and the legs to balance on the right foot.

189.   Hand-to-Big-Toe Posture I: *Hasta Padangusthasana*
Hasta means 'hand', and *padangustha* means 'big toe'.
Stand upright with the legs together. Shift your weight on to the left leg. Flex the right leg in front and grip the big toe with your right hand. Pause a moment, breathing evenly, and securing good balance. Then slowly straighten the right leg out to the side. Extend the left arm from the shoulder to aid balance (Fig. 82). Keep upright and steady for ten to fifteen seconds, breathing evenly. Repeat, balancing on the right leg.

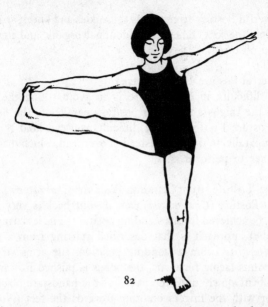

82

This posture limbers, strengthens, and tones the legs, hips, and lower back, and increases physical and mental poise.

190.   Hand-to-Big-Toe Posture II: *Hasta Padangusthasana*
Proceed as for No. 189, except that the raised leg is straightened directly in front instead of to the side.

191.   Hand-to-Big-Toe Posture III: *Hasta Padangusthasana*
If you are very supple, after you have adopted the final position of No. 190 you can grasp the foot with both hands, pull it higher, and press the face against the raised leg.
The effects are as for No. 189 but intensified.

192.   Powerful Posture I: *Utkatasana*
Stand erect with the feet and knees together, the arms extended overhead, covering the ears, the palms of the hands pressed together (No. 173, Fig. 71). Exhaling, and keeping the spine as upright as possible, bend the knees and slowly lower the buttocks, as though on to the the seat of an invisible chair, until the thighs are parallel to the floor. Hold the sitting-on-air position for ten to twenty seconds, and then stand upright, inhaling.

The Powerful Posture strengthens the ankles and knees, strengthens and firms the legs, tones the abdominal organs, and improves balance and posture.

193. Powerful Posture II: *Utkatasana*
The main difficulty in this posture is to avoid tilting the trunk forward as the thighs approach a position parallel to the floor. If Powerful Posture I is found very difficult, you can hold the arms straight out parallel to the floor instead of overhead, which makes the posture easier to perform.

194. Wheel Posture, from Standing Position: *Chakrasana*
The Wheel Posture (*Chakrasana*) can, if your back is very strong and supple, be achieved from a standing position. The less dangerous (to the spine) approach is that described starting from a supine position, No. 301. From a standing position, the arms stretched overhead, palms facing forwards, the pelvis is pushed forward and the back is bent slowly until the palms of the hands are placed flat on the floor with the fingers pointing towards the feet (No. 301, Fig. 138). In early practice it is advisable to have an assistant to support the back or you can stand near to a wall, bend backwards, and slide the hands down the wall.

The benefits are as described for No. 301. Variations of the posture are described following No. 301.

SITTING AND KNEELING POSTURES

The sages who formulated the Yoga system found that certain sitting postures in which the legs are crossed and locked brought stability, compactness, and concentrating and harmonizing of the psycho-physical energies. This meant that these sitting postures were ideal for meditation, during which the body needs to be perfectly secure and immobile, with the spine straight and vertical, so that there is no danger of the meditator falling forwards, backwards, or to one side. These meditative *asanas*, described below, are valuable postures in themselves, apart from their use in mastering the mind's turbulence. Once mastered they provide a unique feeling of firmness, stability, compactness, balance and poise, promoting qualities of inner poise and self-mastery. The vital energies are gathered and contained. The blood circulates freely in the spine, abdomen, and brain. It becomes easy to breathe deeply and freely. The legs and hips are limbered, and pelvic mobility is increased. The ankle, knee, and hip joints are strengthened. Rheumatism and arthritis are countered. The lumbar region receives a therapeutic stretch and the spine is strengthened. The nervous system is toned. The abdomen is free of harmful pressures and deep abdominal breathing is encouraged. The centre of gravity is felt to be in the abdomen, a little below the solar plexus.

Each pose should be held for at least a minute. Breathe freely, unless otherwise instructed. In Buddhist and Tibetan Yoga the hand and arm positions assume great symbolic importance and variety, but for our purposes there are only two positions: one hand on top of the other in the lap, the lower palm cradling the back of the hand above; or the palms resting lightly on the knees, thumb and forefinger brought together to make a circle – the other fingers may be loosely curled or pointing straight out in a more dramatic gesture.

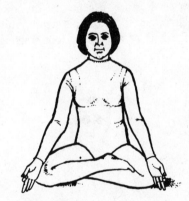

83

195.   Perfect Posture: *Siddhasana*
Siddha means 'adept', and *siddhas* are 'perfected' Yogins.
Sit on the floor with the legs extended. Bend the left leg and, pulling on the ankle, place the heel against the perineum, the soft flesh between genitals and anus. The right leg is then folded and the heel is pulled back against the pubic bone. The outer edge of the foot, sole upturned, is inserted in the fold between the calf and thigh of the left leg. Buttocks, thighs, and knees rest on the floor

288   THE COMPLETE YOGA BOOK/II: POSTURE

(Fig. 83). The position is one of great stability. The roles of the legs should be reversed regularly, left over right, right over left. This applies to all the cross-legged postures.

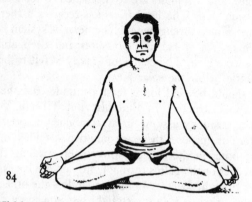

84

196. Hidden Posture: *Guptasana*
Sometimes this is called Free Posture or *Mukthasana*. It resembles the preceding Perfect Posture, except that the lower leg is against the opposite thigh rather than the perineum, and the ankles are crossed so that the heel of the upper foot rests against the pubis (Fig. 84).

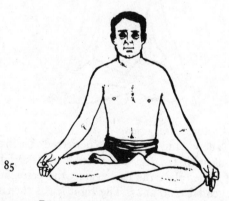

85

197. Prosperous Posture: *Swastikasana*
The swastika is a well-known 'good fortune' symbol. This is also called the Ankle Lock Posture.

Cross the ankles so that each foot is inserted between the thigh
and calf of the opposite leg. The knees are kept down on the floor.
(Fig. 85). Note that both feet are visible in frontal view. They are
not in the Hidden and Perfect Postures.

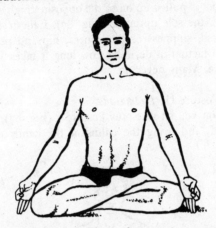

86

198.   Half-lotus Posture: *Ardha-padmasana*
This resembles the Perfect Posture, except that one foot is upturned
on top of the opposite thigh and against the groin. The other foot
is pulled in against either the perineum or the root of the opposite
thigh (Fig. 86).

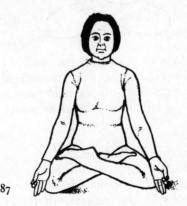

87

199.   Lotus Posture: I: *Padmasana*
This is the classic posture of meditation in the East and the very

symbol of the meditating Yogin. Sometimes it is called the Buddha Posture.

The body is supported firmly on the buttocks and thighs, the spine is erect, and the neck and head are poised in line with the spine. Each foot is pulled up on to the opposite thigh and in against the groin with the sole upturned (Fig. 87). Length of leg in proportion to torso, slimness or plumpness, hip and pelvic mobility – these are all factors in deciding how long it takes Westerners to attain this pose. Many never do.

200. Lotus Posture II: *Padmasana*
In this variation you sit in Lotus Posture I (Fig. 87), stretch both arms overhead, and bring the palms of the hands together.

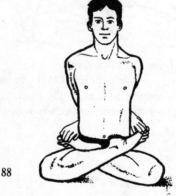

88

201. Bound Lotus Posture: *Banda Padmasana*
In the Lotus Posture (Fig. 87), cross the arms behind the back and grip the toes of the right foot with the right hand and the toes of the left foot with the left hand. The chest moves forward and expands (Fig. 88).

202. Auspicious Posture I: *Bhadrasana*
In this sitting position, traditionally adopted by Indian çobblers, the knees are spread wide out to the sides and the soles and heels are brought together with the heels against the perineum. The knees touch the floor and feet are pulled together and held captive between the hands. Spine and head are in vertical line (Fig. 89).

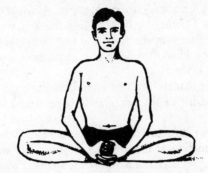

89

The hands may be placed on the knees when the posture is employed for meditation.

Practice of this pose, with its wide-apart pull on the pelvis, makes for easier childbirth. It also tones the reproductive organs and the urinary system.

203.   Auspicious Posture II: *Bhadrasana*
Auspicious Posture I (Fig. 89) can be combined with a forward bend by leaning forward from the waist and lowering the forehead to the floor, exhaling. Stay in the head-down position ten to fifteen seconds, breathing normally.

204.   Cowherd Posture: *Gorakshasana*
Goraksh means 'cowherd'.
From Auspicious Posture (Fig. 89) move the body slightly forward and sit with the perineum (between genitals and anus) placed over the heels.

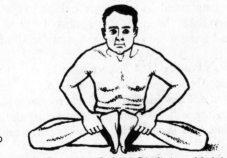

90

205.   Nerve-power Posture: *Sakthi Chalini* or *Mulabandhasana*
This requires more advanced ankle flexibility than *Bhadrasana*

(Fig. 89), which one needs to master first. Again the soles of the feet are brought together by fully folding the legs, but the feet are vertical with the toes on the floor and the heels pointing towards the chin (Fig. 90). Hold the pose fifteen to thirty seconds, breathing normally.

Yogins believe that this posture stimulates the body's main nerve centres. The health of the sex glands is enhanced.

206.   Ankle-twist Posture: *Khandapitasana* or *Mulabandhasana*

This is a continuation of the previous posture, and more difficult; great care should be taken not to injure the ankles. From the position shown in (Fig. 90), place the hands on the floor behind the hips, lift the buttocks a little, and move forward until you are sitting over the feet, whose toes are pointing *backwards*. Stay in the pose fifteen to thirty seconds, breathing normally.

These postures in which the perineum (*khanda*) is against the feet have connections with the arousal and control of the sexual energies and the nerve force known as *kundalini* or serpent power, gathered in the Root centre (*Muladhara chakra*).

The *chakras* are energy centres of the subtle body – see the chapter on Kundalini (Serpent Power) Yoga in *Yoga of Meditation*.

207.   Vamadeva's Posture I: *Vamadevasana*

Vamadeva is one of the many names of Siva, third god of the Hindu trinity.

The incredibly supple B. K. S. Iyenger is shown in his Plate 465 sitting on one foot in the Ankle-twist Posture and folding the other leg with the foot upturned on the opposite thigh in the Half-lotus position. He then holds the upper foot against the groin with both hands, one arm having to be brought across the small of the back.

208.   Vamadeva's Posture II: *Vamadevasana*

In this variation Mr Iyengar pulls the soles of the feet together against the side of one hip (his Plate 466). He recommends *Vamadevasana* for removing stiffness from the legs, toning the spine, improving digestion, and keeping the genital organs healthy.

209.   Upward Ankle-twist Posture I: *Nabhipedasana* or *Kandasana*

Adopt the feet-together position shown in (No. 202, Fig. 89). Then

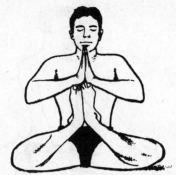

91

use the hands to bring the heels against the abdominal wall, the toes pointing upwards. When the feet are firmly in position, the hands may be brought together in a homage gesture above the feet and against the chest (Fig. 91). An alternative position for the hands is on the knees as depicted for such meditative *asanas* as the Perfect Posture (No. 195, Fig. 83), and the Lotus Posture (No. 199, Fig. 87). Hold the pose fifteen to thirty seconds, breathing normally. *Kanda* is one of the nerve power centres connected with awakening serpent power or *kundalini*. It is situated about a foot above the anus.

210.   Upward Ankle-twist Posture II: *Nabhipedasana* or *Kandasana*

Proceed as for No. 209, but stretching the arms overhead, either at shoulders' width with the palms facing forwards or bringing the palms together. In both cases the arms are locked at the elbows.

211.   Thunderbolt Posture I: *Vajrasana*

Group A practitioners were instructed to sit on the inner edges of the heels and soles (No. 92). For advanced practice you should sit on the floor *between* the feet, keeping the back perfectly straight and placing the palms of the hands on the knees (No. 92, Fig. 27). Sit for at least twenty seconds, breathing normally. In this sitting position it is possible to lean back until you are lying flat on the back, without the position of the legs having changed (No. 295, Fig. 135).

212.   Thunderbolt Posture II: *Vajrasana*

Sitting between the feet as just described in No. 211, stretch both arms overhead and press the palms of the hands together with the arms fully extended. Hold the pose for twenty to sixty seconds, breathing freely.

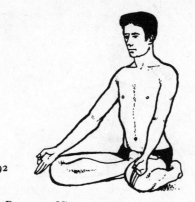

92

213. Hero's Posture: *Virasana*

This is the main version of the Hero's Posture and the one given in the *Gheranda Samhita*. One leg is folded with the upturned foot brought back to rest against or slightly below the buttock on its own side of the body. The other leg is folded and the foot upturned on top of the opposite thigh and against the groin. The hands rest on the knees and the spine is kept straight (Fig. 92). Stay in the pose at least twenty seconds, breathing normally. Repeat, reversing the roles of the legs.

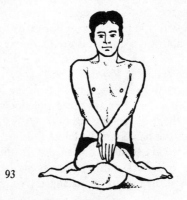

93

214. Dangerous Posture: *Samkatasaa*

The name refers to the formidable appearance of the pose rather than to the dangers of practice.

The legs are crossed, the left heel is brought against the right buttock, and the right heel is brought against the left buttock.

The back is kept straight, and the back of one hand is placed against the upper knee. The palms of the hands are together (Fig. 93). Stay immobile in the pose for at least twenty seconds, breathing normally. Sir Paul Dukes calls this the Bull Posture, because of the bull's horns appearance of the crossed legs.

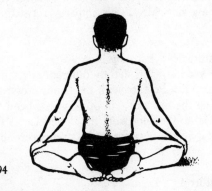

94

215. Frog Posture: *Mandukasana*
In this sitting posture the knees are spread very wide on the floor. Each leg is folded back and the sole upturned behind the buttock on its own side of the body. The big toes are touching. The palms of the hands rest lightly on the knees and the spine is kept erect and the head level (Fig. 94). Stay in the pose for at least twenty seconds, breathing deeply.

Pelvic mobility and health benefits result from the wider spacing of the knees.

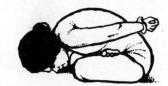

95

216. Yoga Posture I: *Yogasana*
Sit in the Lotus Posture (No. 199, Fig. 87). Take a deep breath; then exhale, bend the trunk forward, and lower the forehead to the floor. Hold the arms behind the back (Fig. 95). Stay in the pose for ten to twenty seconds, breathing normally.

The abdominal muscles and organs receive considerable massage in the bent-forward position; digestion and elimination are improved.

217.   Yoga Posture II: *Yogasana*
Proceed as in No. 216, but rest the chin first on one knee and then on the other knee. Stay bent forward each time for ten to twenty seconds, breathing normally. This imparts a twist to the basic posture.

218.   Yoga Posture III: *Yogasana*
A more difficult version, with slightly different effects on the body, is to perform the Yoga Posture with the hands crossed behind the back and grasping the big toes – in other words bend forward and touch the forehead to the floor from the Bound Lotus Posture (No. 201, Fig. 88). Stay in the pose for ten to twenty seconds, breathing normally.

219.   Yoga Posture IV: *Yogasana*
From the Bound Lotus Posture (No. 201, Fig. 88), lower the chin first to one knee, and then to the other knee. Stay in the bent-forward pose each time for ten to twenty seconds, breathing freely.

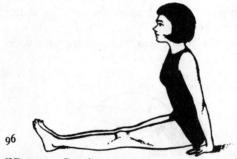

96

220.   Staff Posture: *Dandasana*
This is a simple-looking pose, but difficult in correct performance. Sit on the floor with the legs extended together, forming a right angle with the upright trunk. Place the palms of the hands on the floor, right palm by the right hip, left palm by the left hip, the fingers pointing towards the feet. Keeping the back straight, press down strongly with the arms, locking them at the elbows. Expand

the chest and pull in the abdomen (Fig. 96). Breathing freely, maintain the downward pressure of the arms for fifteen seconds.

The Staff Posture expands the chest and strengthens the arms, shoulders, and back. It is the starting position for several other postures.

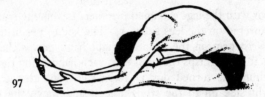

97

221. Back-stretching Posture I: *Paschimottanasana*
This time we include this posture among the sitting poses because we begin by sitting on the floor with the legs extended together (No. 220, Fig. 96). Take a deep breath; then exhale and bend forward, sliding the palms down the legs to the feet and lowering the face to the knees. The forearms and elbows lie on the floor close to the legs. You can pull the trunk down gently with the arms (Fig. 97). Stay in the pose for ten to twenty seconds, breathing freely.

If the posture is correctly performed, the back should feel stretched but relaxed. The hamstrings at the backs of the legs loosen with practice and cease to protest. There is a stimulated traffic of blood along the spine, nourishing its complex network of nerves. Fresh blood is also brought to the pelvis – one factor in this pose's reputation for increasing sexual vigour and control and improving the health of the reproductive organs. The abdomen and its contents are squeezed, encouraging good digestion and efficient elimination.

222. Back-stretching Posture II: *Paschimottanasana*
Here you sit with the legs spread wide apart. Reach out and grasp the toes of the right foot with the right hand and the toes of the left foot with the left hand. Exhaling, lean forward and lower the forehead to the floor. Very advanced performance is to perform the full splits, grasp each foot, and lower the face and chest to the floor. Duration and benefits are as given for No. 221.

223. Back-stretching Posture III: *Paschimottanasana*
Again sit on the floor with the legs spread apart to their limit and locked at the knees. With both hands grasp one foot or the toes of

one foot. Exhaling, lower the face and the chest on to the leg.
Repeat to the other side. Duration and benefits are as given for No.
221.

224. Twisting Back-stretching Posture: *Paraivrtt Paschimottan-asana*

Sit on the floor with the legs extended together. In this the trunk is
twisted and lowered on the legs sideways. The key to performance
is a crossed-wrist grip on the feet: the right hand grasps the left
foot and the left hand grasps the right foot, each hand being twisted
so that the thumb is turned down. Twist the trunk to the left,
lower the right side on to the straight legs, and move the head
between the spread elbows. The left elbow is raised and the right
elbow is lowered to outside the left knee. The back of the right upper
arm rests on the left knee. Fig. 103, No. 233 shows the Twisting
Back-stretching Posture performed with the trunk lowered on to
one extended leg instead of both legs. Hold the pose for ten to twenty
seconds, breathing normally. Then repeat to the other side.

The effects are as for No. 221, but with a lateral twisting action
on the abdomen.

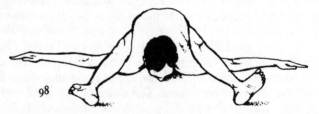

98

225. Tortoise Posture: *Kurmasana*

This time you sit on the floor with the legs spread apart slightly.
Draw up the knees, bend forward, and slip the arms below the knees.
Stretch the arms fully out sideways, the palms flat on the floor.
Straighten the legs and press the chin, shoulders, and chest to the
floor (Fig. 98). Hold the pose for ten to twenty seconds, breathing
normally.

The effects are as given for No. 221.

226. Leg-lock Tortoise Posture: *Kurmasana*

This is a continuation of No. 225. The first requirement, having
taken the pose shown in (Fig. 98), is to turn the palms up and then

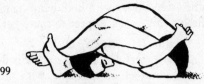

99

move the arms back alongside the hips. The knees are then bent
and the chest is lifted slightly. The hands are now clasped behind
the back. Next cross the feet at the ankles. Finally, push the head
down on to the floor below the ankles (Fig. 99). Hold the pose for
ten to twenty seconds, breathing normally. In spite of the tied-in-a-
knot appearance, Yogins consider the pose to be highly refreshing.
The other benefits are as described for No. 221.

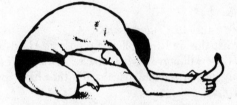

100

227. Head–Knee Posture I: *Janu Sirsasana*
Janu means 'knee', and *sirsa* means 'head'.
Sit on the floor with the legs extended together (No. 220, Fig. 96).
Bend the right leg and place the sole of the foot flat against the
inside of the left thigh at its root in such a way that the right knee,
the right leg, and the outer edge of the right foot all rest on the
floor. Take a deep breath. Exhaling, bend forward from the hips
and with both hands grasp the left foot and lower the face and
chest on to the leg. The elbows are lowered to the floor (Fig. 100).
Stay in the pose for ten to twenty seconds, breathing freely. Repeat
to the other side. Effects are as given for No. 221.

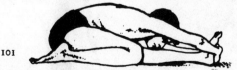

101

228. Head–Knee Posture II: *Janu Sirsasana*
This time one leg is extended as you sit on the floor and the other is
folded back with the foot by the hip. Exhaling, bend forward,

grasp the foot of the extended leg with both hands, and lower chest and chin on to the leg (Fig. 101). Repeat to the other side.

229.   Head–Knee Posture III: *Janu Sirsasana*

In this variation one leg is extended, and the other is flexed and the heel drawn back to the buttock on that side, with the sole flat on the floor and the knee pointing up. Reach forward, grasp the foot of the extended leg with both hands, and lower the chest and chin on to the leg. Repeat to the other side.

230.   Head-Knee Posture IV: *Janu Sirsasana*

This is like the preceding posture, except for a different placing of the arms. Again the chin is lowered to the extended leg, but instead of grasping the foot you clasp the hands behind the back, enfolding the flexed leg and drawing it firmly in against the side. Repeat to the other side.

231.   Heron Posture I: *Krounchasana*

Rather than list this and the following pose as Head-Knee Postures V and VI, we will borrow Mr Iyengars' name, Heron. Postures are more easily memorized and visualized if they have appropriately descriptive names.

This can be visualized as Fig. 100 (No. 227) with the trunk kept erect and the extended leg brought to a position perpendicular to the floor. Abdomen, chest, and chin are pressed against the raised leg, whose foot is grasped by both hands. You sit on the buttocks, and the leg that is not raised is flexed with the heel against the opposite thigh at its root (Fig. 102). Hold the pose for ten to twenty seconds, breathing normally. Repeat, reversing the roles of the legs. The effects are as given for No. 221.

102

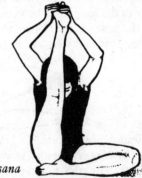

232.   Heron Posture II: *Krounchasana*

This is like Heron Posture I, Fig. 102, except that the leg that is not raised is folded back so that the instep rests on the floor by the buttock on its own side, as in Fig. 101. Duration, breathing, and benefits are as given for the preceding Heron Posture I.

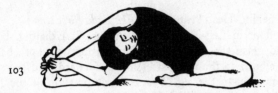

103

233.   Twisting Head-Knee Posture: *Parivrtta Sirsasana*
Sit and fold one leg and extend the other as shown in Fig. 100 (No. 227). Cross the wrists, twisting the hands so that the thumbs are turned down, and grasp the outside of the foot of the extended leg. Spread the elbows, resting the lower elbow on the floor, and lower trunk sideways on to the straight leg, at the same time twisting the trunk and bringing the head between the elbows (Fig. 103). Stay in the pose for ten to twenty seconds, breathing normally. Repeat to the other side. Benefits are as given for No. 221.

234.   Leg-behind-Head Posture I: *Eka Pada Sirsasana*
Sit on the floor with the legs extended together (No. 220, Fig. 96). Bend one knee and use both hands to pull the leg behind the shoulder and head. Now sit as erect as possible. The palms may be placed by the hips as in the illustration for *Omkarasana*, (No. 249, Fig. 113), or brought together in front of the chest. Hold the pose for fifteen to thirty seconds, breathing deeply. Repeat to the other side.

The legs are limbered and stretched by this pose, which also strengthens the back and neck and contracts the abdomen, enhancing abdominal health.

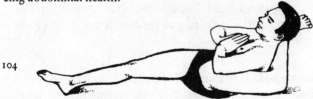

104

235.   Leg-behind-Head Posture: *Eka Pada Sirsasana*
Sitting in the preceding posture, lean right back without raising

the extended leg off the floor. The palms of the hands are held together before the chest (Fig. 104). Stay in the pose for fifteen to thirty seconds, breathing deeply. Repeat to the other side. Benefits as given for No. 234.

236. Leg-behind-Head Posture III: *Eka Pada Sirsasana*
Sit on the floor in Leg-behind-Head Posture I. Exhaling, bend-forward and grasp the foot of the extended leg with both hands. Lower the elbows to the floor, stretch well forward, and press the chest and chin on to the leg. This is a combination of the Leg-behind-Head Posture and the Head–Knee Posture, and can be visualized as Fig. 100 (No. 227) with the flexed leg placed behind the shoulder and head. Stay in the pose for ten to twenty seconds, breathing normally. Repeat, reversing the roles of the legs. This pose combines the effects of Nos. 221 and 234

237. Leg-behind-Head Posture IV: *Eka Pada Sirsasana*
Sit on the floor with one leg extended and the other flexed and placed behind the shoulder and head in Leg-behind-Head Posture I (No. 234). Reach back, enfolding the flexed leg with both arms, and link the fingers behind the back. This pulls the flexed leg lower down the back. Hold the pose for ten to twenty seconds, breathing freely. Repeat to the other side. The effects are as given for No. 234.

238. Leg-behind-Head Posture V: *Eka Pada Sirsasana*
Adopt the preceding posture, No. 237. Exhaling, lower the chin to the knee of the extended leg. Repeat to the other side. Duration and benefits are as for No. 234.

239. Leg-behind-Head Posture VI: *Eka Pada Sirsasana*
This is like Leg-behind-Head Posture IV, except that instead of one leg being extended, it is flexed and the foot is upturned on the opposite thigh.

240. Leg-behind-Head Posture VII: *Eka Pada Sirsasana*
This is like the preceding posture, No. 239, except that the lower leg is folded back with the foot upturned by the hip as in the Thunderbolt Posture (No. 92, Fig. 27).

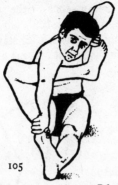

105

241. Shooting Bow Posture I: *Akarna Dhanurasana*

Sit on the floor with the legs outstretched together (Fig. 96).
Reach forward and grasp the big toe of the right foot with the
left hand. Bend the right knee and draw the right foot up to a
position by the left ear as though drawing a bow. As you do so, reach
over the bent right leg with the right arm and grasp the big toe of the
left foot, keeping the left leg straight (Fig. 105). Hold the 'drawn
bow' for ten to fifteen seconds, breathing normally. Repeat, reversing the roles of the arms and the legs.

The three versions of the Shooting Bow Posture keep the spine
and the leg and hip joints supple, take fat from the waistline, stretch
the thigh muscles, massage the abdomen and its viscera, correct
constipation, and aid digestion.

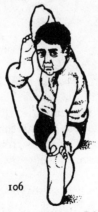

106

242. Shooting Bow Posture II: *Akarna Dhanurasana*

This time the right big toe is grasped by the right hand and drawn back by the right ear. Simultaneously, reach forward with the left hand and grasp the left big toe, the left leg staying at the knee (Fig. 106). Duration and benefits are as for No. 241.

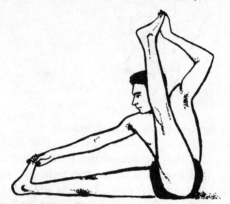

107

243. Shooting Bow Posture III: *Akanra Dhanurasana*
This like No. 242, except that the foot of the raised leg is pulled up high, straightening the leg and bringing it alongside the ear (Fig. 107).

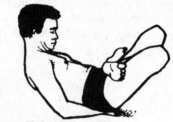

108

244. Balance Posture: *Tolangulasana*
Sit on the floor in the Lotus Posture (No. 199, Fig. 87). Lower the elbows and the forearms to the floor behind the hips, and balance with the buttocks on the forearms, the chin pressed down on the chest (Fig. 108). Sit for fifteen to thirty seconds, breathing freely.

The Balance Posture takes stiffness from the hip and shoulder joints, contracts the abdomen, and tones the thyroid gland.

245. Fore and Aft Leg Splits Posture: *Anjaneyasana* or
       Hanumanasana
Swami Vishnudevananda names this pose after Anjana, the mother

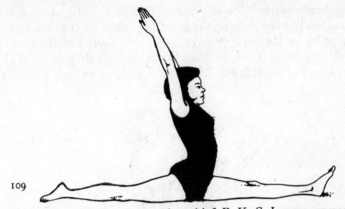

109

of Hanuman, a powerful monkey chief. B. K. S. Iyengar names the
pose after Hanuman.

Kneel with the palms of the hands on the floor beside the hips.
Then slide the left leg forwards and the right leg backwards to the
full extension of both legs. Raise the palms off the floor and bring
them together overhead with the arms fully extended (Fig. 109).
Hold the pose for ten to twenty seconds, breathing deeply, before
returning to the kneeling position and repeating the splits with the
right leg stretched forwards and the left leg stretched backwards.

This pose stretches, limbers, and tones the leg muscles, and
brings blood to the pelvis. It prevents sciatica.

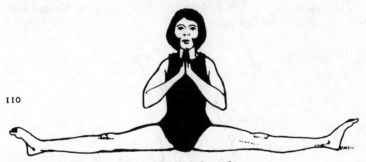

110

246.   Sideways Leg Splits Posture: *Samakonasana*
Samakona means 'same angle'.
This is a more difficult posture than the preceding splits. You
should lower yourself into it from a standing-upright position,
spreading the feet slowly apart. Reach down and place the palms

of the hands on the floor on front at shoulders' width, until the backs of the legs rest fully on the floor. The palms are then brought together before the chest (Fig. 110). Hold the pose, with the back straight, for ten to twenty seconds. Come out of it by pressing the palms on the floor in front. The benefits are as given for No. 245.

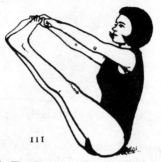

111

247.   Balancing Big Toe Posture: *Utthita Padangustasana*
          Padangusta means 'big toe'.
Start from the sitting-on-floor position shown in No. 220, Fig. 96. Bending the knees, draw back the feet and catch the right big toe with the right hand and the left big toe with the left hand. Straighten the legs and arms so that you balance on the buttocks, the trunk and the legs forming a V shape (Fig. 111). Hold the pose for at least fifteen seconds, breathing normally.

The Balancing Big Toe Posture stretches and firms the legs and improves abdominal fitness.

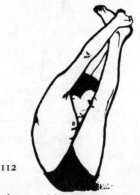

112

248.   Balancing Back-stretching Posture: *Utthita Pashimottanasana*

Fig. 51 (No. 138) shows a simplified version of this posture, which can be a continuation from the preceding Balancing Big Toe Posture, Fig. 111 Clasp the hands around the soles of the feet and press the face against the knees (Fig. 112). Hold the pose for ten to twenty seconds, breathing freely. The benefits are as described for No. 221.

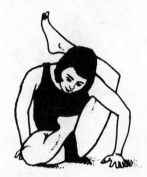

113

249.   OM Posture: *Omkarasana*

Sometimes this is called the Prana Posture (*Pranasana*). *Prana* is cosmic energy. The appearance of the pose resembles the written Sanskrit syllable OM, sacred to the Hindus, which represents the Absolute.

Upturn the right foot on the left thigh against the groin. Grasp the left foot and place the left leg behind the left shoulder and the head. Place the palms of the hands flat on the floor by the hips (Fig. 113). Stay in the pose for at least fifteen seconds, breathing freely. Change sides and repeat.

The OM Posture massages the abdomen and tones the abdominal organs, loosens the hip joints, the nervous system, firms the legs, aids digestion, and encourages regular elimination.

250.   Foetus Posture: *Garbhasana*

Sit in the Lotus Posture (No. 199, Fig. 87). Thrust the arms between the calves and thighs. Lean back slightly and balance on the coccyx. A nonchalant air is given by resting the chin on the hands (Fig. 114). An alternative hand position is holding the ears. Stay in the pose for ten to twenty seconds, breathing freely. Repeat, reversing the leg crossing. Theos Bernard calls this *Uttanakurmasana*.

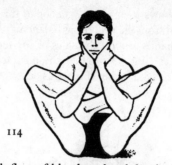

114

There is a rich flow of blood to the abdominal viscera due to the strong contraction of the abdominal wall. Pelvic health also benefits.

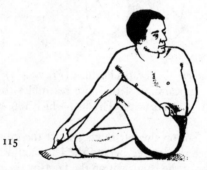

115

251. Spinal Twist Posture: *Matsyendrasana*

Matsyendra was one of the founders of Hatha Yoga. This is one of those poses to which applies the Chinese saying that a good picture is worth a thousand words. So study Fig. 115 carefully. Sit, bend the right knee, and place the right foot high up on the left thigh. Then place the sole of the left foot on the floor on the right side of the right knee, the ankle bone against the knee and the foot pointing in the same direction as the right upper leg. The left knee is almost in the right armpit. Reach out with the right arm and grasp the left foot or ankle— the arm is outside the left leg with the back of the arm against the left side of the left knee. Finally, twist the trunk to the left, hold the left arm across the lower back, and gaze over the left shoulder. The twist begins at the sacrum and climbs gradually up the spine until with the turn of the head it reaches the neck. It is important to sit solidly on the buttocks and to keep the spine as straight and as relaxed as possible. Hold the pose for fifteen to thirty seconds. Repeat to the other side. Breathe freely.

The Spinal Twist prevents backache and lumbago, tones the liver and spleen, massages the kidneys, and makes the spine more elastic. It squeezes the abdominal viscera, aids digestion, and encourages natural peristaltic action in the intestines.

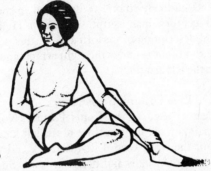

116

252. Half Spinal Twist Posture: *Ardha-Matsyendrasana*
This gives the spine a useful twisting and its benefits are much more than half those given for the full Spinal Twist above. If you find the full version too difficult, use *Ardha-Matsyendrasana*. It differs from the pose shown in Fig. 115 only in one respect: the lower leg rests on the ground, flexed, with the heel back against the opposite buttock (Fig. 116).

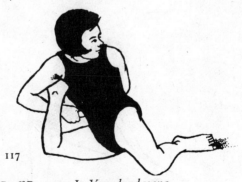

117

253. Yogin's Staff Posture: I: *Yogadandasana*
Sit on the floor. The left leg is folded back so that the foot is near the left hip. The right leg is bent and the sole of the right foot is

placed under the right armpit rather like a crutch. Finally, the hands are clasped behind the lower back (Fig. 117). Stay in the pose for at least fifteen seconds, breathing normally. Repeat to the other side. Despite its appearance, this is held by advanced Yogins to be a pose of rest and relaxation.

254. Yogin's Staff Posture II: *Yogadandasana*
Though you are unlikely to find it illustrated in modern manuals, an eighteenth century manuscript written in Hindi contains an illustration and description of performance of this posture in which the sole of the right foot is under the right armpit and the sole of the left foot under the left armpit.

255. Advanced Lion Posture: *Simhasana*
Sit with the legs crossed in the Lotus Posture (No. 199, Fig. 87). Place the left palm on the floor in front of the left knee and the right palm in front of the right knee. Lift the trunk and balance on the knees. Then lower the thighs and pelvis in front. Support yourself on the knees and straighten arms. The back is stretched and the chest pushed forward between the arms. Keeping the chin level, open wide the eyes and the mouth, and thrust the tongue out and down as far as possible. Hold the pose for ten to twenty seconds, taking short breaths through the mouth. The effects are as given for the easier Group A version, No. 93, plus limbering and stretching of the legs, pelvis, and trunk.

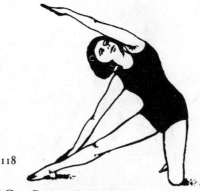

118

256. Locked Gate Posture I: *Parighasana*
Parigha is Sanskrit for a bar which secures a gate. The starting

position is kneeling on the floor with the knees and feet together and the arms extended to the sides in line with the shoulders, the palms turned down. The right leg is then stretched out direct to the right and straightened. Exhaling, dip the trunk to the right and bring the right hand to the right ankle, twisting the hand so that the palm is turned up. At the same time the left arm, kept straight, swings overhead beside the left ear (Fig. 118). Stay bent over to the right side for ten to twenty seconds, breathing normally. Repeat to the other side.

This pose strengthens the muscles at the sides of the waist, removes superfluous fat from the waistline, and tones the abdomen and the spinal nerves.

257. Locked Gate Posture II: *Parighasana*

From the position shown in Fig. 118, lower the trunk further and bring the palms of the hands together on the foot, the straight arms pressing against the ears. Hold the pose for ten to twenty seconds, breathing normally. The benefits are as for Locked Gate Posture I, but intensified.

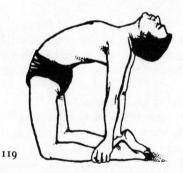

119

258. Camel Posture: *Ustrasana*

Kneel on the floor, the knees and ankles together, the toes flat on the floor. Bend back and grasp the ankles, the thumbs to the inside of each ankle. Push the pelvis forward, throw the head back, and arch the spine strongly (Fig. 119). Stay in the Pose for ten to twenty seconds, breathing freely.

The Camel Posture strongly stretches the spine and feeds the spinal nerves with blood. It stretches the whole front of the body, stimulates the circulation in all parts, and corrects rounded shoulders and a hump at the base of the neck.

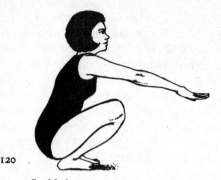

120

259.   Garland Posture I: *Malasana*

Middle Eastern and Eastern people have the ability to squat down with the soles and heels flat on the ground. Westerners tend to go up on to their toes when attempting this position. It is best to approach from squatting on the haunches with the knees, and ankles together and the feet flat on the floor. Assist with the hands if necessary, pushing up and raising the buttocks to balance with the arms stretched out in front (Fig. 120). Hold the pose steadily for fifteen to thirty seconds.

We are here treating the first stage of the Garland Posture as a posture in itself. Parts II and III will reveal why this pose has been so named. The squatting balance described above strengthens the legs, improves balance, and tones the nervous system.

260.   Garland Posture II: *Malasana*

Squatting on the heels (Fig. 120), spread the knees and thighs apart. Then lean forward and bring the shoulders and arms in front of the knees, resting the palms on the floor in front. Now take the arms back, enfolding the legs, and link fingers against the lower back. Exhaling, lower the forehead to the floor in front of the toes. Keep the forehead down on the floor for fifteen to thirty seconds, breathing normally.

261.   Garland Posture III: *Malasana*

This is like No. 260, except that one holds the backs of the ankles, which means that the forehead can be brought closer to the toes.

Garland Postures II and III impart a strong massage to the abdominal muscles and viscera, send a rich flow of blood to the pelvic region, enhance sexual fitness, and correct constipation and indigestion. The pose takes its name from the positioning of the arms.

262. Noose Posture: *Pasasana*

Again one sits on the heels with the feet flat on the floor and the ankles and knees together. The palms are on the floor at the sides of the hips. Twist the trunk to the right and take the left shoulder and arm outside the right knee. Turn the left arm up and wrap the left arm around the shins. Exhaling, twist the right shoulder back and turn the head to look over the right shoulder; at the same time link the fingers of the right and left hands against the side of the left thigh. Stay in the pose for fifteen to thirty seconds, breathing normally. The legs have been encircled as though by a noose. Repeat to the other side.

The spine has been given a lateral twist by this pose. Its other benefits are those given for the Garland Postures II and III (No. 261).

SUPINE POSTURES

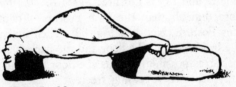

121

263. Fish Posture I: *Matsyasana*

This pose is so named because it is an excellent pose for floating in water, the centre of gravity having shifted towards the middle of the body.

Sit on the floor with the legs flexed and the feet crossed on to the thighs in the Lotus Posture (No. 199), Fig. 87. Supporting the body with the hands or elbows, lie back on to the floor. Keep the legs crossed and the knees down on the floor. Arch the back and throw back the head, pressing the crown of the head on the floor, so that the shoulders and back are off the floor. Finally, grasp the toes with the hands (Fig. 121). Stay in the pose for fifteen to thirty seconds, breathing freely.

In addition to the benefits to the legs and pelvis resulting from the Lotus Posture, the thorax is here expanded and made more mobile. The spine is strengthend and a rounded back is corrected.

The spinal nerves are irrigated and nourished with fresh blood. The abdomen is stretched and decongested, and its viscera and the pelvic organs are toned, as are the endocrine glands. Stimulation of the pancreas aids digestion. A rich supply of blood is directed to the pituitary and pineal glands located in the brain, and also to the thyroid and parathyroid glands. Painful piles are relieved.

264. Fish Posture II: *Matsyasana*
Having adopted the orthodox position (Fig. 121), take the hands away from the feet and fold the arms behind the head, resting the forearms on the floor. The benefits are as given above, but with an even deeper stretch and expansion of the thorax.

265. Fish Posture III: *Matsyasana*
A less strenuous variation consists of keeping the legs crossed, but lying flat on the back instead of forming a 'bridge' by arching the back. The arms are here extended over the head at shoulders' width to rest on the floor.

266. Supine Bound Lotus Posture: *Supta Baddha Padmasana*
This is more difficult than the Fish Posture. Adopt the sitting Bound Lotus Posture (No. 201, Fig. 88). Then lie back until the crown of the head rests on the floor and the back is arched. Lower the knees as far as possible towards the floor. Stay in the pose for ten to twenty seconds, breathing freely.

The effects are a combination of those of the Bound Lotus and those for the Fish Posture.

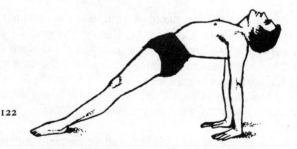

122

267. Front-stretching Posture I: *Purvottanasana* or *Katikasana*
Purva means 'the East', symbolizing the front of the body. The pose

is called the Inclined Plane Posture (*Katikasana*) in some manuals. This posture begins with lying flat on the back, though the final pose is as near as one comes to levitation in Hatha Yoga. The front of the body is stretched along its full length. The soles and heels are flat on the floor. The legs are straightened, as are the arms, vertically. Head and trunk are parallel to the floor (Fig. 122). Hold the pose for fifteen to thirty seconds, breathing freely. The Front-stretching Posture stimulates the circulation, and stretches the legs, abdomen, chest, shoulders, throat, and jaw. It limbers the shoulder joints, improves pelvic mobility, and tones the nervous system.

268.   Front-stretching Posture II: *Purvottanasana* or *Katikasana*
From the position shown in Fig. 122, raise the left leg as high as possible. Hold the leg up for ten to twenty seconds, breathing freely. Then lower the leg slowly to the floor and repeat, raising the right leg. Benefits are as given for No. 267.

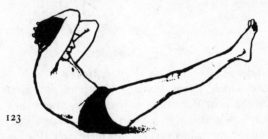

123

269.   Half-boat Posture: *Ardha-Navasana*
Lie flat on the back with the legs extended together. Interlace the fingers against the back of the head. Exhaling, curl up the head, neck, shoulders, and upper back, simultaneously raising the legs, which are kept locked at the knees. In the final position you balance on the buttocks with the tips of the toes level with the top of the head (Fig. 123). Hold the pose steadily for ten to twenty seconds, breathing rapidly.

    This pose strengthens the back, firms the abdomen and legs, and tones the nervous system, liver, spleen, and gall-bladder.

270.   Boat Posture: *Navasana*
Now we add the oars to the Half-boat Posture, take the feet higher, and make a more pronounced V of the trunk and legs. The head and

trunk are in line. Lie flat on the back with the legs outstretched together and the arms by the sides on the floor. Exhaling, sit up, keeping the head and back in line, and simultaneously raise the legs, which are also kept straight, taking the feet up above the level of the head. Finally, stretch the arms straight out parallel to the floor, the palms facing each other. Hold the pose for ten to twenty seconds, taking rather quick breaths. The effects are as given for the Half-boat Posture, but with stronger squeezing of the abdomen and its organs.

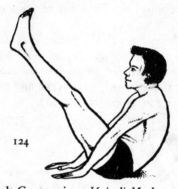

124

271. Thunderbolt Contraction: *Vajroli Mudra*
The posture which Theos Bernard illustrates as *Vajroli Mudra* differs from the Boat Posture in only one way: the palms stay flat on the floor beside the hips, and in the final stage the arms are straightened and the palms pressed down strongly (Fig. 124). Hold the pose for ten to twenty seconds, breathing as for the Boat Posture. The benefits are as given for the Boat Posture, No. 270.

272. Supine Back-stretching Posture: *Supta Paschimottanasana*
We have already had the Back-stretching Posture from a sitting and bending-forward approach (No. 221, Fig. 97) and balancing on the buttocks (No. 248, 112 Fig.). Now we perform it lying flat on the back throughout. Raise the legs, stiffly, exhaling, until the feet are above the face. Then reach up, grasp the feet with both hands, and pull the legs down until the knees are against the face. Keep the back as flat on the floor as possible and bring the elbows and backs of the upper arms to the floor. Hold the pose for ten to twenty seconds, breathing normally. The benefits are as given for No. 221.

125

273. Supine Head–Knee Posture: *Supta Janu Sirsasana*

Now we perform the head-to-one-knee posture lying on the back. It will be found that if face and knee are to come into contact it will be necessary to lift the head and the shoulders off the floor. The lower back, pelvis, and one leg stay flat on the floor. The arm not being used lies alongside the body. The left hand may pull down the left foot and the right hand the right foot; but it is also permissible to grasp the left foot with the right hand or the right foot with the left hand (as in our illustration, Fig. 125). Hold the pose for ten to twenty seconds, breathing normally. Then repeat to the other side. The benefits are as given for No. 221.

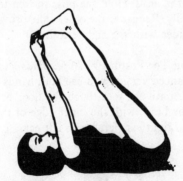

126

274. Supine Big Toe Posture I: *Supta Padangusthasana*

Lie flat on the back with the legs extended together, arms by sides. Exhaling, raise both legs stiffly until the feet are directly above the face. Reach straight up and grasp the right big toe with the right hand and the left big toe with the left hand (Fig. 126). Hold the toes for fifteen to thirty seconds, breathing freely. (In subsequent versions you grasp only one big toe at a time, and use only one hand.)

This posture removes tension and stiffness in the hip joints, stretches and firms the legs, prevents sciatica, and strengthens the lower abdomen.

275. Supine Big Toe Posture II: *Supta Padangusthasana*
This is like version I, but the legs are raised alternatively. The right toe is grasped with the right hand and the left toe with the left hand. One leg and arm stay flat on the floor. Duration and benefits are as for version I.

276. Supine Big Toe Posture III: *Supta Padangusthasana*
From position II, the right hand grasping the right big toe above the face, move the straight right leg and arm out to the right side until both rest on the floor. The right arm should be in line with the shoulders. The back and the left leg and arm stay flat on the floor. Stay in the pose for ten to twenty seconds. Repeat to the other side.

277. Supine Big Toe Posture IV: *Supta Padangusthasana*
In this version you bend the upraised left leg and bring the left foot across to the right shoulder without releasing the grip on the big toe. This means lifting the head slightly and taking the left forearm behind the head. Hold the pose for ten to twenty seconds, breathing normally. Repeat to the other side, bringing the right foot to the left shoulder with the right hand.

278. Supine Big Toe Posture V: *Suptà Padangusthasana*
In this very advanced version you use both hands and pull each leg down alternately until the toes touch the floor behind and slightly to one side of the head, with the inner edge of the calf against the ear – right leg to right ear, left leg to left ear.

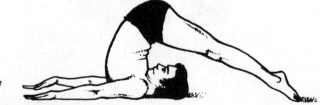

127

279. Plough Posture I: *Halasana*
The resemblance to a plough (*hala*) in this pose is unmistakable. In

Group A we gave the orthodox version in which the arms act as a support prop (No. 141, Fig. 52). Now we dispense with this prop and place the arms elsewhere in the final stages. First, exhaling, lower the legs from the Shoulderstand Posture (No. 147, Fig. 55) into the Supported Plough Posture (No. 141, Fig. 52). Pause a few seconds, breathing freely. Then, take the palms from the back and press them down on the floor with the arms fully extended in the opposite direction to the legs. Only the hands and forearms need move: the upper arms stay in the same position (Fig. 127). Hold the final pose for fifteen to thirty seconds, breathing freely.

The benefits given for No. 141 apply to this and to the following versions, intensified in some aspects.

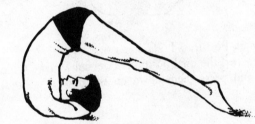

128

280. Plough Posture II: *Halasana*
This is like version I, except that when the hands cease acting as a prop for the trunk they are clasped behind the neck (Fig. 128).

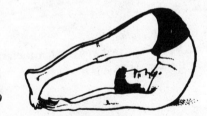

129

281. Plough Posture III: *Halasana*
This is like version I, except that the arms are stretched to touch the toes (Fig. 129).

282. Plough Posture IV: *Halasana*
This is like version I, except that as the straight legs are lowered above the head you reach out and grasp the toes as they approach

the floor. The backs of the hands rest on the floor. Holding the toes gives the pose a certain immobility.

283.   Plough Posture V:*Halasana*
In this version the legs are spread as wide as possible. Prop the back with the palms of the hands as shown in (No. 141, Fig. 52.)

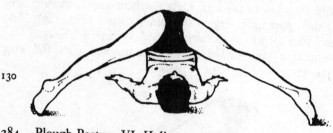

130

284.   Plough Posture VI:*Halàsana*
Having reached the final position of version V, take the palms from the back and press them down on the floor (Fig. 130).

131

285.   Plough Posture VII:*Halasana*
This is like version VI, except that you stretch the arms out wide and touch or grasp the toes (Fig. 131).

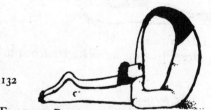

132

286.   Ear-press Posture I: *Karnapidasana*
Karna means 'ear' and *pida* means 'pressure'. This variation of the

Plough Posture is called the Choking Posture or Ear–Knee Posture in some manuals.

As the legs are brought above the head, bend and spread the knees a little, and lower the knees until they rest on the floor by the ears. The arms may be placed in three different positions. The first is to use them to pull behind the knees and hold them firmly against the floor, squeezing the ears (Fig. 132). Stay in the pose for fifteen to thirty seconds, breathing freely and rather rapidly. The benefits are as given for No. 141.

287. Ear-press Posture II: *Karnapidasana*
This is like the preceding version, except that the palms are placed against the lower back as in (No. 141, Fig. 52).

288. Ear-press Posture III: *Karnapidasana*
This is like version I, except that the palms are pressed on the floor and the arms fully extended in the opposite direction to the head, as shown in (No. 279, Fig. 127).

289. Lateral Plough Posture I: *Parsva Halasana*
Having reached the Supported Plough Posture position shown in (No. 141, Fig. 52), move the legs either to the right or to the left until the toes rest on the floor in line with the head. Make the lateral twist from the hips, keeping the head, shoulders, trunk, and arms firmly in position. Hold the pose for fifteen to thirty seconds, breathing freely. Repeat to the other side.

The benefits are as given for No. 141, with a lateral movement of the spine and a slightly different squeezing action on the abdominal viscera.

290. Lateral Plough Posture II: *Parsva Halasana*
Having reached and stabilized the final position of version I, take the palms off the back and press them on the floor with the arms extended in the opposite direction to the head, as shown in (No. 279, Fig. 127). Be content with version I if attempting version II means any loss of hip, trunk, or leg position. Duration and effects are as for version I, slightly intensified.

291. Noose Posture I: *Pasini Mudra*
Mudra is another word for 'posture'.

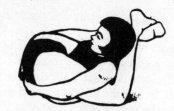

133

Swami Vishnudevananda calls this *Dwipadasana* (Two Feet Pose
or Two Legs Pose) and B. K. S. Iyengar calls it *Yoganidrasana*
(Sleeping Yogin's Posture). It might also be called Tortoise-on-
Back Posture, for one can go into it by leaning back from the
Balancing Tortoise Posture (No. 407, Fig. 183). It can also be
performed as a continuation from the Ear-press Posture (No. 286,
132). Or sit and place first one leg behind the shoulder and head,
and then the other leg in the same position on its side, cross the
ankles, and lie back. Finally, clasp the hands against the sacrum
(Fig. 133). Hold the pose for fifteen to thirty seconds, breathing
freely.

The spine is strengthened and the abdominal muscles are contracted, toning such vital organs as the liver, spleen, and kidneys.
The intestines are squeezed, preventing constipation. The pose is
restful for a supple person. It is used by Yogins in North India and
in Tibet to generate heat in icy conditions at high altitudes.

292. Noose Posture II: *Pasini Mudra*
This is like version I, except that instead of clasping the hands
against the lower back you press the palms down on the floor by
the hips.

293. Belly-turning Posture: *Jathara Parivartanasana*
Lie flat on the back, the legs extended together. Stretch the arms
out to the sides in line with the shoulders. Exhaling, raise the legs
together to a vertical position. Take a deep breath. Then, exhaling,
lower the straight legs to the right until the feet are beside the
right hand. This means moving from the hips and turning the
abdomen. Hold the pose for ten to twenty seconds, breathing
normally. Inhaling, raise the legs to perpendicular. Exhaling, repeat
to the other side.

The main difficulty in this posture is to keep the back and the
shoulders flat on the floor. The greater the success in this the more

beneficial the exercise, which strengthens the back and tones the abdominal organs. It also removes fat from the hips and waistline.

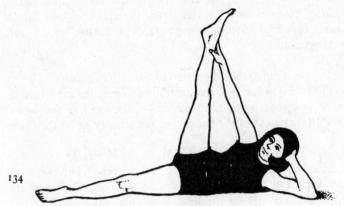

134

294.   Ananta's Posture: *Anantasana*
Ananta is one of the names of Vishnu.
Lie on the left side, the right leg lying along the left leg, and resting the left side of the head on the palm of the folded left arm. Now bend the right knee, catch either the ankle or the big toe, and straighten the right leg and right arm vertically (Fig. 134). Repeat to the other side.

The hips are limbered by this pose and the hamstrings loosened. Superfluous fat is taken from the abdomen and waistline, and pelvic health is enhanced.

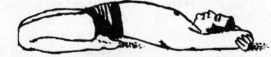

135

295.   Supine Thunderbolt Posture I: *Supta Vajrasana*
Sit with the buttocks on the floor between the heels in the Thunderbolt Posture (No. 92, Fig. 27). Exhaling, lean back slowly and lower first one elbow and then the other to the floor. Support the trunk for a few seconds on the elbows and forearms, and then lower the head and the back slowly to the floor. Keeping as much of the back as possible flat on the floor, fold and lock the arms above the head (Fig. 135). Lie still for fifteen to thirty seconds, breathing deeply.

This is said to be one of the most therapeutic postures in Yoga. It takes stiffness from the knee-joints, enlarges the rib-box, increases thoracic mobility, stretches the whole body, stimulates the circulation, removes unwanted fat from the abdomen and thighs and has a beneficial effect on the glands, reproductive organs, and nervous system.

296. Supine Thunderbolt Posture II: *Supta Vajrasana*
This is like version I, except that instead of folding the arms behind the head you stretch the arms out above the head at shoulders' width with the backs of the hands and the arms lying on the floor.

297 Supine Thunderbolt Posture III: *Supta Vajrasana*
This is like version I, except that the back is arched, and the head thrown back and the crown placed on the floor. The arms are folded and locked behind the head as in (Fig. 135.)

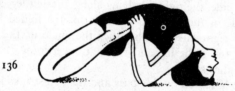

136

298. Supine Thunderbolt Posture IV: *Supta Vajrasana*
Sit between the feet in the Thunderbolt Posture (No. 92, Fig. 27). Exhaling, lean back on to the elbows and forearms and push the palm of the right hand below the right foot and the palm of the left hand below the left foot. Pull the feet and the lower legs off the floor. Now arch the back and lower the crown of the head on to the floor. The knees, the elbows, and the crown of the head now rest on the floor (Fig. 136). Hold the pose for ten to twenty seconds, breathing deeply.

The benefits are as given for No. 295, but intensfied in several respects.

299. Pigeon Posture I: *Kapotasana*
The starting point is the Supine Thunderbolt Posture (No. 295, Fig. 135). Bending the elbows so that they point upwards, place the palms flat on the floor by the shoulders with the fingers pointing

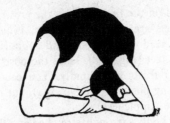

137

towards the feet. Exhale, and press up raising the pelvis, back, shoulders, and head off the floor. The body is now supported by the knees, lower legs, and palms. The whole front of the body is strongly stretched. Move the hands in until they are holding the toes and lower the forearms and elbows to the floor. Push the pelvis higher, move the hands to the ankles, and bring the crown of the head on to the soles of the feet (Fig. 137).

The entire body receives a powerful stretch and the spine becomes more flexible. The circulation is stimulated and many vital organs are nourished and toned. The health of the pelvic area is enhanced.

300.   Pigeon Posture II: *Kapotasana*
This is like the final position of the preceding version, but instead of holding the ankles you grip the left and right knees with the left and right hands respectively.

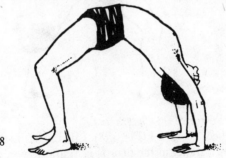

138

301.   Wheel Posture I: *Chakrasana*
Lying flat on the back, bend the knees and place the feet flat on the floor with the heels up against the buttocks and the lower legs vertical. Now bend the elbows, pointing them upwards, and place the palms on the floor by the shoulders with the fingers pointing towards the feet. Exhaling, raise the pelvis and trunk and place the

crown of the head on the floor. Palms, the crown of the head, and the soles and heels are now on the floor. Finally straighten the arms, raising the head off the floor, and support the arched body on the hands and feet (Fig. 138). Hold the pose for ten to twenty seconds, breathing freely and rapidly. You can also go into this pose from a standing position (see No. 194), but this requires great spinal strength and suppleness.

The front of the body is strongly stretched and the spine is strongly arched. The wrists and the ankles are strengthened. The circulation is stimulated and many glands and organs benefit.

302.   Wheel Posture II: *Chakrasana*
This is like version I, except that you lift the heels and support the body on the toes and palms, allowing a higher arching of the body.

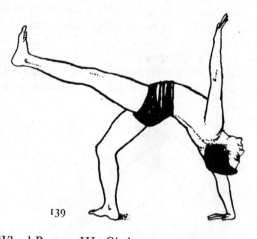

139

303.   Wheel Posture III: *Chakrasana*
Start from Wheel Posture I (Fig. 138). Lift the left foot and stretch out the left leg parallel to the floor (Fig. 139). Stay in the pose for ten to twenty seconds, breathing freely. Repeat, lifting the right leg.

304.   Wheel Posture IV: *Chakrasana*
This is like version III, except that you raise the left leg as high as possible and rise on the toes of the supporting right leg. Repeat to the other side.

305.   Wheel Posture V: *Chakrasana*
This is like version IV, except that when you lift the left leg as high
as possible, you take the left hand from the floor and place the palm
on the left thigh. Repeat to the other side.

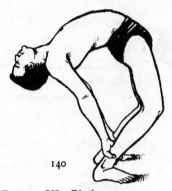

140

306.   Wheel Posture VI: *Chakrasana*
Start from Wheel Posture I (Fig. 138). Move the hands in gradually
until you grasp the ankles and stand with a powerful back bend (Fig.
140). Hold the pose for ten to twenty seconds. The benefits are as
given for No. 301.

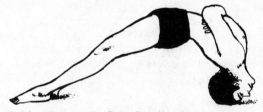

141

307.   Bridge Posture I: *Setu Bandhasana*
Lie flat on the back with the legs extended together. Draw the heels
back a little way towards the buttocks. Take the arms back over
the head and rest the palms on the floor by the head with the fingers
pointing towards the legs. Exhaling, press with the hands, arching
the back, and throw the head back so that the crown rests on the
floor. Fold the arms across the chest. Finally, straighten the legs
so that the body is arched and supported only by the soles and heels
and the crown of the head (Fig. 141). Hold the pose for ten to twenty
seconds, breathing freely.

The Bridge Posture series strengthens the neck and the spine, and brings fresh blood to the pineal, pituitary, and thyroid glands.

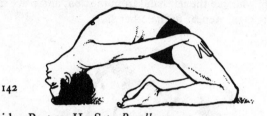

142

308. Bridge Posture II: *Setu Bandhasana*
One can attain a slightly different form of 'bridge' starting from the Supine Thunderbolt Posture (No. 295, Fig. 135). Lying flat on the back with the buttocks between the feet, push the pelvis up, arch the back, and support the body on the crown of the head and the fronts of the feet and lower legs (Fig. 142).

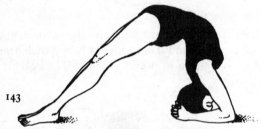

143

309. Bridge Posture III: *Setu Bandhasana*
This is like version I, except that the hands are clasped behind the head, with the elbows and forearms on the floor. The back bend is more pronounced (Fig. 143).

310. Bridge Posture IV: *Setu Bandhasana*
Starting from the preceding position (Fig. 143), raise one leg stiffly to as near perpendicular as possible. Hold the leg up for ten to twenty seconds. Lower the leg to the floor and repeat to the other side.

311. Bridge Posture V: *Setu Bandhasana*
From the 'bridge position, shown in Fig. 143, move the feet carefully back towards the head. Still resting the elbows and forearms on the floor, release the hands from their clasp behind the head and raise the head off the floor. Bring the feet closer to the head and grasp

the left ankle with the left hand and the right ankle with the right hand. You are now supported on the feet, elbows, and forearms near the elbows. The pelvis is raised very high and the trunk and upper arms are vertical. Stay in the pose for ten to twenty seconds, breathing freely.

312. Bridge Posture VI: *Setu Bandhasana*
An advanced continuation of the preceding pose is to release the grip on one ankle and raise that leg to perpendicular for ten to twenty seconds. Lower the raised leg and repeat with the other leg.

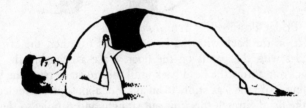

144

313. Bridge Posture VII: *Setu Bandhasana*
Less strenuous versions of the preceding 'bridges' can be achieved by keeping the back of the head, the neck, and the shoulders on the floor. The equivalent of version I can be reached by lowering the legs, one at a time, from the Shoulderstand Posture (No. 147, Fig. 55) and continuing to support the lower back with the hands (Fig. 144).

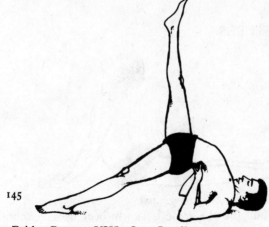

145

314. Bridge Posture VIII: *Setu Bandhasana*

From the above position (Fig. 144) raise one leg stiffly to vertical. Hold it straight up for ten to twenty seconds, breathing freely. Lower the leg to the floor and repeat with the other leg (Fig. 145).

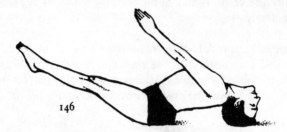

146

315. Bridge Posture IX: *Setu Bandhasana*
Lie flat on the back with the legs extended together, the arms by the sides with the palms on the floor. Take a deep breath. Arch the back and throw the head back until the crown rests on the floor. Exhaling, raise the legs stiffly to an angle of about forty-five degrees with the floor. Stretch the arms out straight and parallel to the legs and press the palms together (Fig. 146). Stay in the pose for ten to twenty seconds, breathing normally.

The spine is limbered and strengthened in its dorsal parts, and the abdomen is strengthened and toned. The neck, too, is strengthened, and the thyroid gland benefits from an increased circulation of blood.

PRONE POSTURES

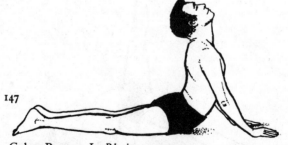

147

316. Cobra Posture I: *Bhujangasana*
In this graceful pose the spine is slowly bent back vertebra by vertebra and the body is supported on the legs, pelvis, and palms.

In the Group A version the palms were placed on the floor five or
six inches in front of the shoulders, but here they are placed *below*
the shoulders. Inhaling, raise the head and trunk slowly until the
arms are straight or almost so (Fig. 147). Give most of the work to
the spine rather than to the arms, and concentrate the full attention
on the slowly-bending spine. Hold the final position, which resembles a cobra rearing to strike, for ten to twenty seconds, breathing freely.

The benefits from the Cobra Posture series are as given for No.
142.

317. Cobra Posture II: *Bhujangasana*
In this version the palms are placed at the sides of the waist level
with the navel, the fingers pointing forwards. Inhaling, raise the
head and trunk into Cobra Posture I, but at the final stage fully
straighten the arms and lift the pelvis and the legs off the floor.
Throw the head back and look up at the ceiling. Support the body
on the palms and the toes for ten to twenty seconds, breathing
freely.

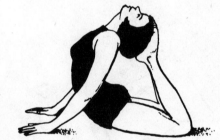

148

318. Cobra Posture III: *Bhujangasana*
From Cobra Posture I (Fig. 147), bend the knees and raise the lower
legs vertically. Then move the feet towards the head. Arch the
spine strongly, stretch the neck, and bring the head back against
the soles of the feet (Fig. 148). Hold the pose for ten to twenty
seconds, breathing freely and rapidly.

Some manuals call this the Swan Posture (*Swandasana*).

319. Cobra Posture IV: *Bhujangasana*
Perform the orthodox Cobra Posture I (Fig. 147). Stay in the pose

a few seconds, breathing normally. Then bend the knees and raise
the lower legs vertically. Take the left arm back and grasp the left
knee. Pause a few seconds; then take the right arm back and grasp
the right knee. Hold the final position for ten to twenty seconds,
breathing freely.

320. Cobra Posture V: *Bhujangasana*
Begin by performing the preceding version IV. Still holding the
kneecaps, slowly straighten the legs, so that the feet return to the
floor.

321. Cobra Posture VI: *Bhujangasana*
Begin from position V, and bend the spine and head as far back as
possible, assisted by pulling with the arms on the kneecaps. At the
same time bring the feet towards the head and rest the crown of
the head on the soles. Balance on the pelvis and thighs for ten to
twenty seconds, breathing rapidly. To come out of the pose safely,
straighten the legs and release the grip on one kneecap at a time.
Bring the palms to the floor in front, ending up in Cobra Posture I
(Fig. 147).

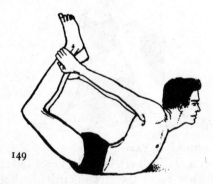

149

322. Bow Posture I: *Dhanurasana*
Lie on the stomach, bend the knees, and reach back and firmly
grasp the left and right ankles with the right and left hand respectively, thumbs and fingers on the same side. Pull on the ankles
strongly, lifting the thighs and chest off the floor and balancing
on the stomach. The feet are pulled higher than the head and the
body is bent into a bow shape. Hold the head level (Fig. 149). Hold

the pose for ten to twenty seconds. breathing freely. One gains
optimum height by holding the knees and ankles slightly apart at
'lift-off'; they are brought together once maximum height has been
reached. An important point is that the back stays relaxed during
the Bow exercise.

The benefits for the Bow series are as given for No. 143.

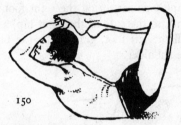

150

323.   Bow Posture II: *Dhanurasana*
In this version you reach back with the right hand and grasp the
right big toe, and then with the left hand and grasp the left big toe.
Take a firm grip. Balancing on the stomach, pull the feet to above
or on the head. The upper legs are parallel to the floor (Fig. 150).

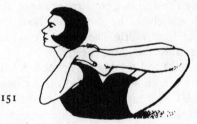

151

324.   Bow Posture III: *Dhanurasana*
This is like the preceding version II, but instead of pulling the feet
to the head you bring them down on to the shoulders (Fig. 151).

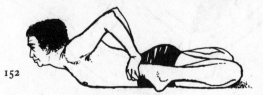

152

325.   Bow Posture IV: *Dhanurasana*

This is the full version of the beginner's pose, No. 144. Balancing on the stomach, grasp the right foot with the right hand and the left foot with the left hand. With a twist of the wrists bring the palms of the hands against the toes and press down the feet to the sides of the hips (Fig. 152).

326.   Bow Posture V: *Dhanurasana*
If one is very supple one can bring the right foot, pressing down with the right hand, to the side of the right hip, as shown in Fig. 152, and then pull the left foot, grasped by the big toe, either to the head or to the shoulder.

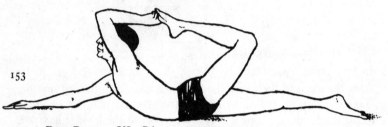

153

327.   Bow Posture VI: *Dhanurasana*
In this version only one leg and one arm are bent at a time. Lie flat on the stomach and chest, the chin on the floor and both arms extended straight in front of the shoulders. Bend the left elbow and the left knee, and lift the head, chest, and left leg. Reach back and grasp with the left hand the big toe of the left foot. The right arm and the right leg both stay extended on the floor. Raise the left elbow and the left foot high, making a bow of the left side of the body (Fig. 153). Repeat to the other side.

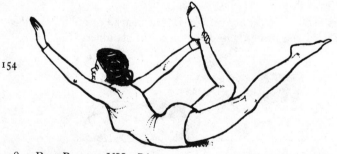

154

328.   Bow Posture VII: *Dhanurasana*

This is like version VI, but you balance on the stomach and both arms and both legs are lifted. The right hand grips the right ankle and pulls the right leg off the floor. Both left arm and left leg are raised (Fig. 154). Repeat, holding the left ankle with the left hand.

329. Sideways Bow Posture: *Parsva Dhanurasana*
First go into the orthodox Bow Posture (No. 322, Fig. 149). Then roll over on to the left side, without releasing the grip on the ankles. Stay on the left side for ten to twenty seconds, breathing freely; then roll back on to the stomach. Pause a few seconds, and then repeat to the right side.

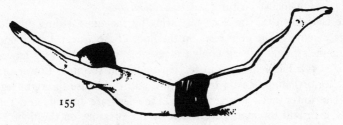

155

330. Boat Posture I: *Navasana*
Lie face down on the floor, the arms fully extended in front with the palms on the floor and the thumbs touching. The legs are also extended on the floor, the ankles together. Keeping the arms and legs together and as straight as possible, simultaneously lift them off the floor and balance on the stomach (Fig. 155). Hold the pose tautly for ten to twenty seconds, breathing normally. The effects are similar to those given for No. 143.

331. Boat Posture II: *Navasana*
This is like version I, but the arms are held stiffly wide and back as though you were completing a breast stroke in swimming.

332. Boat Posture III: *Navasana*
This is like version I, except that the hands are clasped at the back of the head and the elbows are pulled out wide.

333. Boat Posture IV: *Navasana*
This is like version I, but the arms are folded behind the back, placing additional pressure on the lower back.

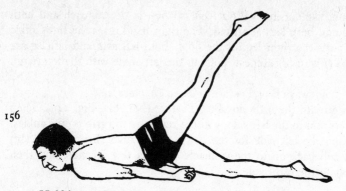

334. Half-locust Posture: *Ardha-salabhasana*
Lie face down on the floor, the arms by the sides, palms up, the
legs together. The chin rests on the floor. Take a deep breath and
raise the straight left leg as high as possible. Only the left leg moves
(Fig. 156). Hold the leg up for ten to fifteen seconds. Lower the
left leg, exhaling. Rest a few seconds, and then raise the right leg.
  The lower back is strengthened, the legs are firmed, and the
abdomen and its organs are toned by the pressure on the floor.

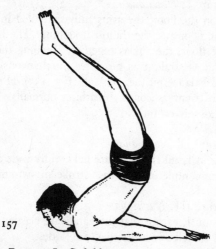

335. Locust Posture I: *Salabhasana*
The full Locust Posture is a much more vigorous exercise then the
Half-locust just described. The hands are brought together beneath
the groin and both legs are taken up as high as possible. The pelvis,

abdomen, and lower chest are also lifted and the support for this gymnastic pose comes from the arms, shoulders, and chin. Press down strongly with the arms (Fig. 157). Hold the raised pose for ten to fifteen seconds. In very advanced performance the Yogin balances on the chin, shoulders, and arms, and the legs and trunk are almost vertical. Lower the legs slowly and smoothly to the floor.

This gymnastic exercise irrigates the spine with blood, nourishing the spinal nerves. The back is strengthened, especially the lower portion. Blood is brought to the neck and brain. The health of the pelvic organs is enhanced.

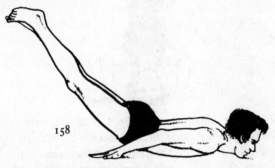

158

336. Locust Posture II: *Salabhasana*
The Locust Posture can also be performed without bringing the hands together below the body. Instead, press the palms down by the hips. One does not obtain so full a leverage for the arms in this position and one should be content to raise the legs stiffly together to an angle of forty-five degrees with the floor (Fig. 158).

337. Locust Posture III: *Salabhasana*
The full Locust Posture can also be performed with the palms flat on the floor by the chest, the elbows bent and held in close to the body.

INVERTED POSTURES

338. Headstand Posture I: *Sirsasana*
The full Headstand Posture should only be performed after its preparatory stages (Nos. 148 to 156) have been mastered. In Group

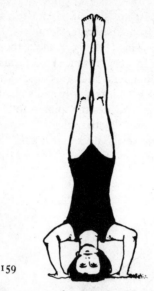

159

A instruction two approaches to the Headstand were indicated: first, by keeping the legs straight; and second, by bending the knees and bringing them close to the chest, and then raising the feet up and over until the soles faced the wall behind the head, whence the legs were straightened and the legs, trunk, neck, and head brought into vertical line. Two methods of arm support were also taught earlier. In the first of these the palms were flat on the floor, one at each side of the head, the fingers pointing in the opposite direction to the gaze (Fig. 159).

339. Headstand Posture II: *Sirsasana*
The second main placing of the arms in the Headstand is to form a triangle in which the hands are clasped at the back of the head with the fingers interlaced and interlocked. The inner edges of the hands rest on the floor, as do the forearms and elbows, the latter spread not wider than the shoulders (Fig. 160).

340. Headstand Posture III: *Sirsasana*
A rarer placing of the arms – not to be attempted until the two main placings are familiar and comfortable – is to turn the hands so that they point in the same direction as the gaze. Lower and upper arms

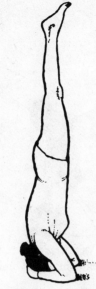

160

form a right angle. The hands and elbows can be brought close
together in front of the face. (Other very advanced arm placements
are Bound Hands and Freehand, described below.)

341.   Headstand Posture IV: *Sirsasana*

Most variations of the Headstand are concerned with changes in
leg position. One can make them either from Headstand I or from
Headstand II (Figs. 159 and 160). For this posture, spread the legs
as wide apart as possible – into topsy-turvy splits if the legs are
flexible enough.

Nos. 342-7 describe other variations of the leg position made
while in Headstand I or Headstand II.

342.   Headstand Posture V: *Sirsasana*

Balancing on the head, split the legs forwards and backwards as
far as you can with comfort (Fig. 161). Keep the legs apart at least
twenty seconds. Then bring them together again, and immediately
perform the fore and aft splits again, but reversing the earlier
direction of each leg.

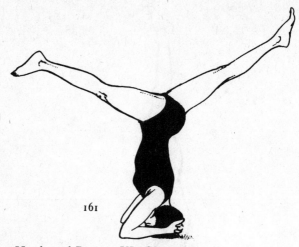

161

343. Headstand Posture VI: *Sirsasana*
Balancing on the head, bend the knees and press the soles of the feet together.

344. Headstand Posture VII: *Sirsasana*
From full Headstand Posture Nos. 338 or 339, lower the straight legs together slowly until they are at right angles to the trunk and parallel with the floor. This is a variation of the Half Headstand taught in Group A posturing, where the legs were raised from the floor.

345. Headstand Posture VIII: *Sirsasana*
From a full Headstand (Nos. 338 or 339), lower the left leg until the toes touch the floor in front of the face. Keep the leg down for at least twenty seconds; then bring it back to perpendicular. Now lower the right leg until the foot rests on the floor in front of the face. The trunk stays vertical (Fig. 162).

346. Headstand Posture IX: *Sirsasana*
Begin as the preceding No. 345, but lower the legs alternately so that each foot touches the floor as far out to its own side as possible, right foot wide to the right and left foot wide to the left.

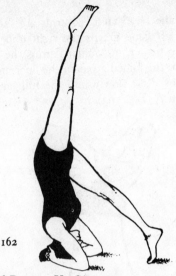

162

347.   Headstand Posture X: *Sirsasana*
From a full Headstand (No. 338 or 339), keeping the head, trunk, and legs perpendicular to the floor, interlock the legs in the manner of the Eagle Posture, (No. 165, Fig. 67).

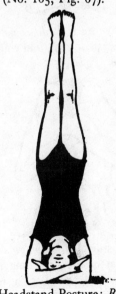

163

348.   Bound Hands Headstand Posture: *Baddha Hasta Sirsasana*

In this version of the Headstand the arms are folded in front of the forehead: the left hand grasps the right upper arm near the elbow joint and the right hand similarly grips the left upper arm. You kneel and place the folded arms on the floor and the head just in front of the arms. Rise slowly into the fully inverted position as taught in Section A (Fig. 163).

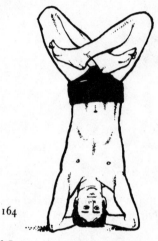

164

349.   Headstand Lotus Posture I: *Padmasana* in *Sirsasana*
In the full Headstand (No. 338 or 339), fold your legs into the Lotus position (Fig. 164).

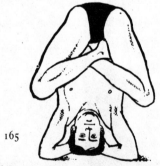

165

350.   Headstand Lotus Posture II: *Padmasana* in *Sirsasana*
From the inverted position of the preceding posture (Fig. 164), lower the legs until the crossed ankles are against the diaphragm (Fig. 165). Continue the Headstand in this position.

351. Headstand Lotus Posture III: *Padmasana* in *Sirsasana*
It is possible to lower the crossed legs even further than is shown in
Fig. 165. Bending from the waist, bring the legs down until the
knees rest on the upper arms, right knee on right upper arm and
left knee on left upper arm.

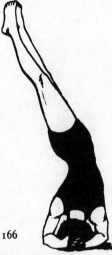

166

352. Twisting Headstand Posture: *Parava Sirsasana*
In the full Headstand Posture (No. 338 or 339), twist the pelvis
and legs first to the right and then to the left (Fig. 166). Exhale as
you twist, and inhale as you level up. Keep the legs and pelvis
turned for ten to twenty seconds each time, breathing freely.

353. Twisting Headstand Lotus Posture: *Parsva Padmasana* in
Sirsasana
Proceed just as described in No. 352, but with the legs crossed in
th Headstand Lotus Posture.

354. Freehand Headstand Posture: *Mukta Hasta Sirsasana*
This is a very advanced version, only to be attempted after more
basic versions have been mastered. Kneel and place the top of the
head on the floor. Stretch both arms straight out in front of the
shoulders, palms up. The trunk is brought to a perpendicular
position. Then, pressing down with the backs of the hands, raise

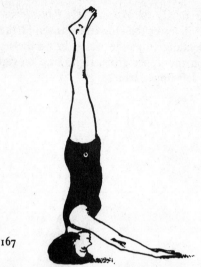

167

the legs slowly to form a vertical line with the trunk (Fig. 167).

The various Headstands described above should be sustained for only a few seconds to begin with, two seconds being added as comfort permits until inversion lasts for from one to five minutes. Persons who find the Headstand a strain should perform instead the milder Shoulderstand series.

The main physiological benefits from Yoga's inverted poses are produced by reversing the customary pull of gravity on the body. During the bodily inversion the tendency for the abdomen, abdominal viscera, and other tissues and organs to sag is countered. The blood circulates in a new way. Blood is drawn away from the congested feet and ankles and arterial blood flows to the neck, face, and brain. Hence the claim that the inverted poses create both beauty and intellect. The spinal nerves also benefit, and the heart receives a kind of holiday. The leg veins are rested, and the inverted poses counter varicose veins, piles, and prolapse of the abdominal organs. Therapeutic benefits are claimed in disorders of the uterus and ovaries. However, these poses should not be performed during menstruation or pregnancy. The important pituitary gland receives an increased flow of blood, and other glands also benefit. Sexual fitness and health are said to be enhanced. Posture is improved, and psycho-physical poise is increased.

Contra-indications: the inverted postures could be dangerous for

persons suffering from high blood pressure, or such eye disorders
as glaucoma and conjunctivitis, or where there is a risk of detachment of the retina. (Eyesight and hearing are often improved in
persons in normal health.) Nor are the postures safe for people
suffering from brain disease or injury. Medical advice should be
sought and taken when there is any doubt as to the safety of the
inverted poses. Some milder inverted poses will now be taught.

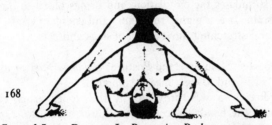

168

355.   Spread Legs Posture I: *Prasarita Padottanasana*
Spread the legs widely apart, the toes pointing forwards. Keeping
the legs locked at the knees, bend forward and place the palms on the
floor at shoulders' width, in line with the toes. Bend the elbows and
lower the top of the head on to the floor between the hands (Fig.
168). Stay in the pose for at least fifteen seconds, breathing freely.

In addition to the benefits described earlier for the inverted
postures, the legs and pelvis are strongly stretched.

356.   Spread Legs Posture II: *Prasarita Padottanasana*
Once version I has been mastered, you can move on to this more
advanced version, which differs from it only in one respect: the
hands are lifted from the floor and the arms are folded behind the
back.

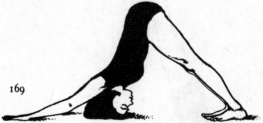

169

357.   Dog Stretch Posture: *Adho Mukha Svanasana*
This is a milder posture than the full Headstand. You make an
inverted V of the body, and then lower the front of the head on to

the floor and edge the hands forward until the arms are fully
stretched. Alternatively, you can move into the Dog Stretch from
Spread Legs Posture I (Fig. 168). Move the legs back gradually
until they are together, and simultaneously move the hands forward.
Two important points to observe: keep the back straight, and press
the soles and heels flat on the floor (Fig. 169).

The Dog Stretch removes stiffness from the legs, back, and
shoulders, stimulates the circulation, and brings blood to the neck,
face, and brain. It is a highly refreshing and energizing pose based
on the natural stretching movements of dogs and cats.

358.   Supported Shoulderstand Posture: *Salamba Sarvangasana*
Sa means 'with' and *alamba* means 'support'.
The orthodox prop was provided by the upper arms, elbows,
forearms, and the hands, placed on the lower back (No. 147, Fig.
55). But here the support is given by taking the hands away from
the back and stretching the arms fully along the floor, palms down,
in the opposite direction to the head – the position shown for the
arms in the illustration of Plough Posture I (No. 279, Fig. 127).
Hold the trunk and legs perpendicular to the floor and immobile
for fifteen to thirty seconds, breathing freely. If you wish to continue longer in the Shoulderstand Posture, return the hands to the
lower back (No. 147, Fig. 55).

The effects are as described for No. 147.

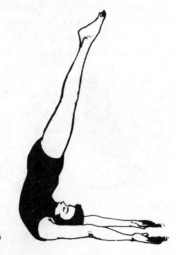

170

359. Unsupported Shoulderstand Posture: *Niralamba Sarvang-asana*
First adopt the supported Shoulderstand Posture shown in Fig. 55
(No. 147). Then stretch the arms above the head and along the
floor, palms up, at shoulders' width. Do not expect the legs to stay
vertical: they will tilt slightly towards the arms (Fig. 170). Hold the
pose steadily for fifteen to thirty seconds, breathing freely. If you
wish to keep the trunk and legs up longer, transfer your hands back
to the lower back (No. 147, Fig. 55).
   Benefits are as given for No. 147.

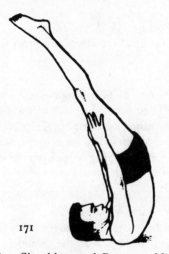

171

360. Balancing Shoulderstand Posture: *Niralamba Sarvangasana*
First achieve a steady performance of the Unsupported Shoulderstand Posture (Fig. 170). Then lift the arms from the floor and place
them along the body with the palms against the thighs. The raised
body is supported only by the head, neck, and shoulders (Fig. 171).
Hold the pose fifteen to thirty seconds, breathing freely. The legs
have to tilt slightly over the face.
   The Balancing Shoulderstand Posture shares the benefits given
for No. 147, with additional strengthening of the back muscles.

361. Shoulderstand Posture I: *Sarvangasana*
A range of variations is possible in the Shoulderstand Posture in
which the arms act as a prop for the back (No. 147, Fig. 55). They

are mainly leg movements, corresponding to the series given for the Headstand. First, spread the legs as widely apart as possible. Breathing freely, hold the leg position for at least fifteen seconds.

Breathe freely and hold the leg positions for at least fifteen seconds in the variations II to VI which follow.

362. Shoulderstand Posture II: *Sarvangasana*
This is like variation I, except that the legs are split fore and aft, as shown for the Headstand variation (No. 342, Fig. 161). Repeat, reversing the earlier direction of each leg.

363. Shoulderstand Posture III: *Sarvangasana*
Begin as for No. 361, but bend the knees and press the soles of the feet together.

364. Shoulderstand Posture IV: *Sarvangasasana*
Begin as for No. 361. Then lower one foot to the floor above the head, while keeping the other leg upright. Keep both legs locked at the knees. Bring the lowered leg back to perpendicular and, repeat with the other leg. No. 345, Fig. 162 shows the leg movement, but performed in the Headstand.

365. Shoulderstand Posture: V *Sarvangasana*
This is like the preceding posture, but lower each leg to the side and rest the toes on the floor level with the shoulders.

366. Shoulderstand Posture VI: *Sarvangasana*
Begin as before. Interlock the legs in the manner of the Eagle Posture (No. 165, Fig. 67).

367. Twisting Shoulderstand Posture: *Parsva Sarvangasana*
Starting in the supported Shoulderstand Posture (No. 147, Fig. 55), twist the trunk and legs first as far as possible to the left, and then as far as possible to the right, as shown in the Twisting Headstand Posture (No. 352, Fig. 166). Exhale as you twist, and inhale as you level up. Hold each twist for ten to twenty seconds, breathing freely.

172

368. Sideways Shoulderstand Posture: *Parsva Sarvangasana*
This is more difficult than the preceding twisting. First twist
trunk and legs to the left. Move the right palm against the right hip
with the wrists turned against the bottom of the spine. Shift the major
weight of the body on to the right wrist and the lower right arm.
Finally, swing the straight legs together diagonally out to the right
(Fig. 172). Hold the pose for ten to twenty seconds, breathing
normally. Then return to the basic posture (No. 147, Fig. 55) and
repeat to the left side.

369. Shoulderstand Lotus Posture I: *Padmasana* in *Sarvangasana*
In the propped Shoulderstand (No. 147, Fig. 55), cross the legs
into the Lotus position, as shown for Headstand Lotus Posture I
(No. 249, Fig. 164). Breathing freely, hold the pose steadily for at
least fifteen seconds.

370. Shoulderstand Lotus Posture II: *Padmasana* in *Sarvangasana*
In the Shoulderstand-combined-with-Lotus pose, lower the knees
to the floor behind the head. Keep them down for ten to twenty
seconds, breathing freely.

371. Shoulderstand Lotus Posture III: *Padmasana* in *Sarvangasana*
In the same posture, lower the knees to the floor in the direction
away from the head. Hold the pose for ten to twenty seconds,
breathing freely.

372. Shoulderstand Lotus Posture IV: *Padmasana* in *Sarvangasana*
In the same posture, lower the knees to the floor, first to the right,
and then to the left of the head. Duration and breathing are as for
above.

373. Twisting Shoulderstand Lotus Posture: *Parsva Padmasana* in *Sarvangasana*

In the same Shoulderstand Lotus Posture (No. 369), perform to each side the twist described in No. 367. Duration and breathing are as for III above.

374. Sideways Shoulderstand Lotus Posture: *Parsva Padmasana* in *Sarvangasana*

In the Shoulderstand Lotus Posture, perform the sideways swing described in No. 368 and shown in Fig. 172. Duration and breathing are as for III above.

BALANCING POSTURES

Under this heading we include some postures that are uncharacteristic of Yoga in that they are of a gymnastic nature, requiring considerable muscular strength or exceptional co-ordination.

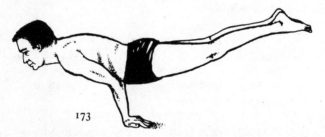

173

375. Peacock Posture I: *Mayurasana*

Kneel. Place the palms on the floor in front of the knees with the fingers pointing back towards the feet and the wrists and forearms touching. Lower the abdomen and chest on to the elbows and upper arms. Exhaling, bring the bodyweight forward and straighten the legs until the body balances in a straight horizontal line on the palms. Keep the elbows as close together as possible (Fig. 173). Balance for ten to twenty seconds, breathing freely. Some readers will find it helpful to rest the forehead on the floor at first and to raise the head simultaneously with the legs.

The Peacock Posture strengthens the back, and the abdominal muscles and organs are toned. It aids digestion and stimulates peristaltic activity in the intestines. The circulation is invigorated.

*Due to the considerable intra-abdominal pressure, this pose and its
variations are not suitable for women.*

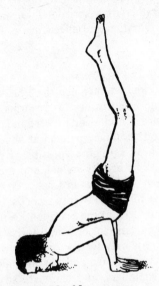

174

376.   Peacock Posture II: *Mayurasana*
The resemblance to a peacock displaying its feathers is more pronounced in this variation. From the horizontal posture (Fig. 173),
lower the forehead to the floor and swing the legs up high (Fig. 174).
An alternative method is to kneel and rest the forehead on the floor
from the beginning. Duration, breathing, and effects in these
variations are as given for No. 375.

377.   Peacock Posture III: *Mayurasana*
This is like the preceding posture, but you balance on the fists
instead of on the palms of the hands.

378.   Peacock Posture IV: *Mayurasana*
This is like No. 375, but you balance with the fingers pointing
towards the head instead of back towards the feet.

379–382.   Peacock Lotus Posture: *Padmasana* in *Mayurasana*
In this the Lotus leg crossing is combined in turn with each of
the preceding Peacock Postures.

383.   Modified Peacock Posture: *Hamasana*

Swami Sivananda teaches a preparatory stage as an *asana* in itself, calling it *Hamasana*. The toes and instep stay on the floor, so that the body is inclined rather than horizontal, with the head a little higher than the feet. Duration and effects are as for No. 375, but less intense.

384.   Scorpion Posture I: *Vrschikasana*

The Scorpion Posture looks rather like the Peacock Posture with the legs raised, but one balances on the forearms and there is no intra-abdominal pressure. Kneel. Bend forward and place the elbows, forearms, and palms on the floor, parallel at shoulders' width or slightly less. Lift the head as high as possible. Exhale and swing the legs and trunk up. The back is arched, and the legs swung up and angled forward over the head as in Locust Posture I (No. 335, Fig. 157). Hold the pose for ten to twenty seconds, breathing freely. In early practice you can go into the Scorpion Posture slowly from the Headstand, or use an assistant or a wall for safety purposes.

The Scorpion Posture is only for the most athletic Yogins. The spine is limbered and strengthened and the abdominal muscles are stretched. The arms, shoulders, and chest are strengthened.

385.   Scorpion Posture II: *Vrschikasana*

Begin as No. 384. The legs and the trunk in this variation are taken to a vertical balance with no arching of the back or angling forward of the legs.

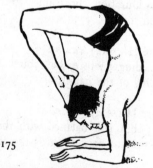

175

386.   Scorpion Posture III: *Vrschikasana*

From the final position of version I, slowly lower the soles of the feet on to the crown of the head (Fig. 175).

387.   Scorpion Posture IV: *Vrschikasana*

An even more advanced variation is to perform the preceding posture balancing on the palms of the hands instead of on the forearms. In other words, this is a gymnastic hand-balance from which the soles of the feet are slowly lowered on to the crown of the head.

388.   Repose Posture: *Sayanasana*

Begin by performing variation II of the Scorpion Posture. Then raise first one hand and then the other and cup the chin in the palms of the hands, balancing on the elbows. Stay in the posture as long as is comfortable.

This shares most of the benefits of Scorpion Posture I (No. 384).

389.   Balancing Tree Posture I: *Vrksasana*

Balance on the palms with straight arms, angling the legs forward over the head as in Scorpion Posture I, the lower legs parallel with the floor. Duration and benefits are as given for No. 384.

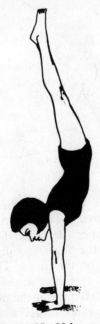

176

390.   Balancing Tree Posture II: *Vrksasana*

This is like the preceding posture, but the legs are taken overhead vertically (Fig. 176). This is the handstand of Western gymnastics.

391. Formidable Posture I: *Bherundasana*

In this very advanced pose you curve the back and the legs in a rearing-scorpion manner, but from a starting position lying full length on the stomach, with the palms flat on the floor by the chest, the fingers pointing towards the head. The arms are kept in against the sides. Bodyweight is taken mainly on the palms and the chin, and the feet are brought overhead with the toes pointing upwards. Hold the pose for ten to twenty seconds, breathing freely.

392. Formidable Posture II: *Bherundasana*

This is like version I, but the soles of the feet are lowered on to the crown of the head.

393. Formidable Posture III: *Bherundasana*

This is like version I, but the soles of the feet are lowered on to the floor in front of the face.

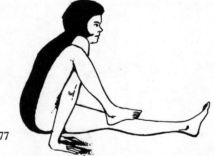

177

394. Arm Posture I: *Bhujasana*

Sit on the floor with the legs outstretched. Bend the right knee and place the right leg over the right arm, the back of the knee against the rear of the upper arm. Place the palms on the floor by the roots of the thighs, the fingers pointing forwards. Raise the body and balance solely on the palms. The left leg is extended parallel to the floor (Fig. 177). Stay in the pose for ten to twenty seconds, breathing freely. Repeat to the other side.

This pose contracts the abdomen and strengthens the wrists and arms.

395. Arm Posture II: *Bhujasana*
Balance on the palms as in the preceding version (Fig. 177), but wrap *both* legs over the upper arms, the left leg over the left arm and the right leg over the right arm. This is best approached from a standing position, hunkering and placing the palms on the floor between the knees. Duration, breathing, and effects as for No. 394.

396. Arm Posture III: *Bhujasana*
This is like version II, but the feet are locked by crossing the ankles.

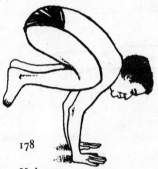

178

397. Crow Posture: *Kakasana*
Squat on the toes with the knees held apart. Place the palms on the floor between the knees, the fingers spread for optimum purchase. Placing the inner edges of the knees against the backs of the upper arms, lean forward until the feet lift off the floor and you balance on the palms. The elbows are slightly bent (Fig. 178). Hold the pose for ten to twenty seconds, breathing normally.

This pose strengthens the arms and shoulders, and massages the abdominal wall and the organs of the abdominal cavity.

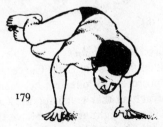

179

398. Sideways Crow Posture: *Parsvakakasana*
Begin as for No. 397, but in this version of the Crow Posture both

knees rest on one upper arm (Fig. 179). Balance for ten to twenty seconds, breathing normally.

399. Crow Lotus Posture: *Padmasana* in *Kakasana*
This is like No. 397, but the legs are crossed in the Lotus position. The elbows are slightly bent to provide a platform for the legs to rest on.

400. Sideways Crow Lotus Posture: *Padmasana* in *Parsvakak-asana*
This is like No. 398, but the legs are crossed in the Lotus position.

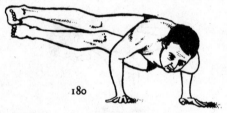

180

401. Curved Posture I: *Vakrasana*
The starting position is the Sideways Crow Posture (No. 398, Fig. 179). Slowly straighten the legs until they are extended parallel to the floor (Fig. 180). Perform to both sides. Duration and effects are as for the Crow Posture, No. 397.

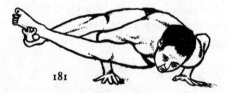

181

402. Curved Posture II: *Vakrasana*
Sometimes this is called the Pose of Eight Curves. It can be thought of as the preceding posture with one arm between the thighs. You make the same approach as that given for the Crow Posture, but bring the right leg over the right arm just above the elbow and the left leg below the slightly-bent right arm. Raise the legs off the floor and lock the legs by crossing the ankles (Fig. 181). Balance on the

hands for ten to twenty seconds, breathing freely. Repeat to the other side.

The effects are as for the Crow Posture, No. 397.

403.   One Leg Crow Posture I: *Eka Pada Kakasana*

In the Crow Posture (No. 397, Fig. 178), lift one knee from the back of the upper arm and stretch and straighten the leg behind. The extended leg will be at an angle slightly above horizontal. Repeat to the other side. Duration and effects are as for the Crow Posture, No. 397.

404.   One Leg Crow Posture *Eka Pada Kakasana*

Begin as in the previous version. One folded leg continues to kneel on the back of the upper arm, while the other leg is stretched fully forward parallel to the floor, with the back of the knee over the upper arm. Repeat to the other side.

405.   Balancing Leg-behind-Head Posture: *Utthita Eka Pada Sirsasana*

Sit on the floor with the right leg pulled behind the right shoulder and the head and the palms on the floor by the hips. Raise the hips off the floor and balance on the palms. Lift the extended left leg up to form a V shape with the trunk and legs. Hold the balance for ten to twenty seconds, breathing normally. Repeat to the other side.

This posture strengthens the wrists, arms, and shoulders, limbers the hips and legs, contracts and tones the abdomen, massages the adbominal viscera, aids digestion, corrects constipation, stimulates the circulation, and tones the nervous system.

406.   Krishna Posture: *Krishnasana*

Sit on the floor with the left leg extended and the right leg flexed and pulled behind the right shoulder and the head. Place the palms on the floor by the hips. Move the left leg to the left. Raise the body off the floor so that you are supported by the left foot and both palms. Twisting the trunk slightly to the left, raise the left arm straight up perpendicular to the floor. Balance on the left palm

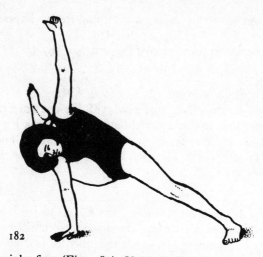

182

and the right foot (Fig. 182). Hold the balance for ten to twenty seconds, breathing freely. Repeat to the other side. Benefits are as for No. 405.

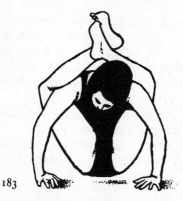

183

407. Balancing Tortoise Posture: *Utthita Kurmasana*
Sit on the floor. Pull the left leg behind the left shoulder and pull the right leg behind the right shoulder. Cross the ankles behind the head. Place the right palm near the right hip and the left palm near the left hip. Press down with the hands, straighten the arms, and balance on the palms with the hips off the floor (Fig. 183). Duration, breathing, and effects are as for No. 405.

408. Firefly Posture: *Tittibhasana*

This continues from the final position of the preceding Balancing Tortoise Posture (Fig. 183), and is attained by straightening both legs behind the upper arms. Duration, breathing, and benefits are as given for No. 405.

409. Swing Posture: *Lolasana*

Sit with the ankles crossed underneath the body, the right sole under the left buttock and the left sole under the right buttock. Press down firmly with the palms, which are by the hips, and raise the trunk and legs off the floor. Balance on the palms for ten to twenty seconds, breathing freely and holding the legs clear of the floor. Benefits are as for No. 405.

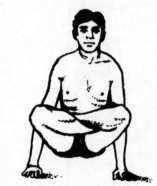

184

410. Scales Posture: *Tolasana*

Sit on the floor in the Lotus Posture (No. 199, Fig. 87), but with the right palm on the floor by the right hip and the left palm by the left hip. Straighten the arms, raise the trunk and legs, and balance on the palms for ten to twenty seconds, breathing freely (Fig. 184). This pose is compact and evenly balanced. It strengthens the wrists, arms, neck, shoulders, and abdomen, in addition to giving the usual benefits of the Lotus Posture.

411. Cock Posture: *Kukutasana*

Sit in the Lotus Posture (No. 199, Fig. 87). Insert the arms between the thighs and the calves up to the elbows. Then rock forward and balance on the palms with the body lifted off the floor (Fig.

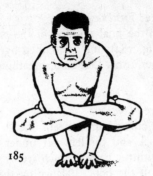

185

185). Hold the balance for ten to twenty seconds, breathing normally.
Benefits are as for No. 410.

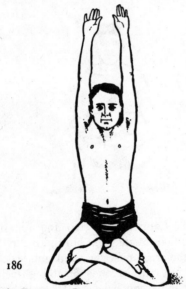

186

412. Mountain Posture: *Parvatasana*

In the Lotus Posture (No. 199, Fig. 87), place the palms on the
floor in front of the knees. Now lift the trunk straight up and balance
on the knees with the legs still crossed. Having found balance,
bring the palms of the hands together above the head (Fig. 186).
Hold the pose for ten to twenty seconds, breathing freely.

The benefits are those associated with the Lotus Posture, plus
work for the muscles that keep the body balancing in this posture.

413.   One Leg Posture I: *Eka Pada Hastasana*
Stand on the left leg with the right leg pulled behind the right
shoulder and the head. Bring the palms together in front of the
chest. Hold the pose for fifteen to thirty seconds, breathing freely.
Then repeat, balancing on the right leg.

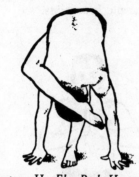

187

414.   One Leg Posture II: *Eka Pada Hastasana·*
Exhaling, bend forward from the preceding posture, bring the face
against the left knee, and press the palms flat on the floor, one to the
right of the supporting left leg and the other in line to the left (Fig.
187). Repeat to the other side.

One Leg Postures I and II limber, firm, and tone the spine and
the legs, massage the abdomen, tone the nervous system, and improve balance and concentration.

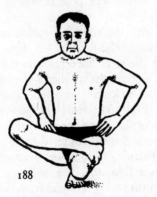

188

415.   Tiptoe Posture: *Padangusthasana*
The hands on the hips, the legs together, squat right down on the

toes. Bend the right knee and place the right ankle on top of the left thigh a little above the knee (Fig. 188). Hold the balance for fifteen to thirty seconds, breathing normally. Then repeat to the other side.

The Tiptoe Posture limbers the legs and hips, tones the spine, abdomen, and nervous system, improves co-ordination and balance, and strengthens the ankle and knee joints.

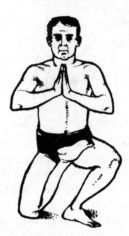

189

416. Horseface Posture: *Vatayanasana*

Vatayana means 'a horse'. The pose is said to resemble a horse's face.

Sit on the floor with the right leg folded on to the left thigh (half-lotus), the palms on the floor by the hips. Push the trunk up off the floor so that the right knee rests on the floor and the sole and heel of the left foot are flat on the floor with the heel near the right knee. Keep the back erect and hold the palms together in front of the chest (Fig. 189). Hold the pose for at least fifteen seconds, breathing deeply. Then repeat to the other side.

An alternative method of attaining the pose, requiring greater co-ordination and balance, is to lower yourself into it from the standing Tree Posture (No. 163, Fig. 66).

The Horseface Posture takes stiffness from the hips, limbers and firms the legs, tones the nervous system, and improves balance and concentration.

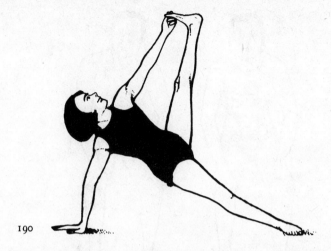

190

417. Inclined Big Toe Posture: *Utthita Padangusthasana*
Sit on the floor, with the legs extended together, and shift the bodyweight on to the right hip and leg. Keeping the head, trunk, and
legs stiffly in line, like an inclined board, support the body on the
right palm and straight right arm and the right foot. The left palm
rests on the left hip and the left leg and foot on the right leg and
foot. Bend the left knee and grasp the left big toe with the left hand.
Straighten the left leg and left arm, pulling the left leg to as near
vertical as you can (Fig. 190). Stay steadily in the pose for ten to
twenty seconds, breathing freely. Repeat to the other side, balancing
on the left arm and left foot.
    The Inclined Big Toe Posture strengthens, firms, and tones the
arms, back, and legs, makes the hip joints more supple, tones the
nervous system, and improves co-ordination, balance, and concentration.

MUSCULAR LOCKS (*BANDHAS*)

418. Recti Isolation:*Nauli*
Success in this muscle control, which comes more easily to men than
to women, depends on full mastery of the Abdominal Uplift
(*Uddiyana*, No. 162, Fig. 65). After a thorough exhalation the relaxed abdominal wall draws back into the thoracic cavity, creating

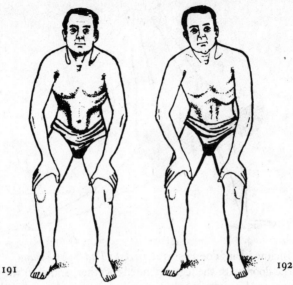

191   192

a deep hollow. Out of this hollow, with practice, you can bring forward the rectus abdominis muscles, both recti centrally (Fig. 191), or one singly to one side if you have more subtle control (Fig. 192). The peak of Yogic muscle control is to isolate left-both-right, and then across the abdomen again, in the opposite direction, right-both-left, achieving a wave-like motion that massages the organs of the abdominal cavity, burns up fat on the muscular wall, assists digestion, stimulates peristaltic activity in the intestines, and improves pelvic health. Its use in Yogic hygiene, in taking a natural enema while squatting in water, does not concern us here, but was discussed in *Yoga of Breathing*.

Leaning forward slightly and pressing the hands on the thighs, or on a chair-back, table-top, or other firm surface, assists the control. Standing before a mirror also aids mastery. Breathing is suspended during the control, so do not sustain an isolation or cycle for longer than ten seconds. Let go, take a few breaths, and then repeat. A cycle of five isolations or 'waves' may be performed to one exhalation.

VII Group B Postures: Programme Planning

Follow the rules and guidelines given at the end of the Group A postures. Warm-ups are optional. Precede and end the main programme with a few minutes of relaxation. Between two and five postures should be selected from each of the following sections:

All-body stretches: Nos 163-5, 168-71, 173-82, 192-3, 220, 255-7, 267-8, 279-85, 295-306.
Forward bends: Nos 183-8, 216-19, 221-33, 273.
Backward bends: Nos 194, 258, 263-8, 307-37.
Spinal twisting: Nos 170, 224, 233, 251-2, 262.
Sitting or kneeling: Nos 195-215.
Leg limbering: Nos 187-91,226, 234-43, 245-50, 253-4, 272-8, 294-300.
Abdominal squeezing and contracting: Nos 166-8, 170-2, 231-2, 234-44, 247-50, 259-61, 269-72, 279-93.
Balancing: Nos 375-417.
Inverted: Nos 338-74.
Abdominal muscle controls: Nos 162, 418.

VIII   Yoga Therapy

Laboratories in India have been investigating the therapeutic powers of the *asanas*, but much work remains to be done in this field. The postures should never be used as a substitute for medical treatment. The following table indicates the basic postures for which therapeutic claims have been made by eminent Yogins. They are thought to aid healing and to ward off the disorders named. When such basic poses as the Bow, Cobra, Shoulderstand, and so on, are mentioned, the whole series of that name should be understood in each case.

Disorder	*Posture*
Asthma	Abdominal Breathing, Bow, Corpse, Fish, Headstand, Locust, Lotus, Mountain, Shoulderstand.
Backache	Back-stretching, Big Toe, Bow, Bridge Cat, Cobra, Cowface, Fish, Headstand, Shooting Bow, Shoulderstand, Spinal Twist, Supine Thunderbolt, Wheel.
Bronchitis	Abdominal Breathing, Cobra, Fish, Locust, Lotus, Mountain, Shoulderstand.
Constipation	Abdominal Uplift, Back-stretching, Fish, Forward Bend, Head-Knee, Headstand, Knee Squeeze, Plough, Recti Isolation, Shooting Bow, Shoulderstand, Spinal Twist, Yoga Posture.
Diabetes	Back-stretching, Cobra, Corpse, Peacock Plough, Shoulderstand, Spinal Twist, Yoga Posture.

Gall bladder disorders	Bow, Cobra, Head-Knee, Noose, Peacock, Triangle.
Indigestion	Abdominal Uplift, Cobra, Corpse, Mountain, Peacock, Plough, Recti Isolation, Shoulderstand, Spinal Twist, standing stretch poses, Supine Thunderbolt, Yoga Posture.
Insomnia	Back-stretching, Cobra, Corpse, Locust, Mountain, Plough, Shoulderstand.
Kidney disorders	Bow, Cobra, Head–Knee, Locust, Noose, Shoulderstand, Spinal Twist.
Liver disorders	Boat, Noose.
Lumbago	Corpse, Locust, Plough, Spinal Twist, standing stretch poses.
Menopause disorders	Abdominal Uplift, Cat, Cobra, Corpse, Fish, Plough, Shoulderstand, sitting poses.
Menstrual disorders	Abdominal Uplift, Back-stretching, Cat, Cobra, Corpse, Fish, Forward Bend, Headstand, Plough, Recti Isolation, Shoulderstand, sitting poses.
Neurasthenia	Back-stretching, Corpse, Headstand, Hero's, meditation poses, Mountain, Warrior's, standing stretch poses.
Obesity	Abdominal Uplift, Back-stretching, Bow, Cobra, Forward Bend, Head–Knee, Plough, Spinal Twist.
Piles	Fish, Headstand, Plough, Shoulderstand.
Poor posture	Bow, Camel, Cobra, Cowface, Mountain, Palm Tree, Triangle.
Prolapse	Abdominal Uplift, Headstand, Shoulderstand.
Prostate disorders	Headstand, Shoulderstand, sitting and kneeling poses, Spinal Twist.
Reproductive organs	Back-stretching, Cobra, Headstand,

	Plough, Shoulderstand, Supine Thunderbolt.
Rheumatism	Back-stretching, Bow, Cowface, Head-Knee, Spinal Twist, Triangle.
Sciatica	Big Toe.
Sexual debility	Abdominal Breathing, Abdominal Uplift, Bow, Cat, Cobra, Dog Stretch, Foetus, Headstand, Hunkering, Plough, Recti Isolation, Shoulderstand, sitting and kneeling poses, Spinal Twist, Yoga Posture.
Tension	Abdominal Breathing, Abdominal Uplift, Back-stretching, Corpse, Forward Bend, Mountain, Shoulderstand, Slow-motion Exercises, Triangle.
Throat disorders	Lion.
Thyroid disorders	Bridge, Fish, Shoulderstand.
Varicose veins	Headstand, Shoulderstand, and all other inverted postures.
Wind pains	Abdominal Uplift, Knee Squeeze.

Volume III

Yoga of Meditation

I Why Meditate?

WHY MEDITATE?

The metaphysics, philosophy, and practices of Yoga have long fascinated a few Western scholars – but only in recent times have the practices been taken up with enthusiasm by many thousands of Europeans and Americans. In the great majority of cases, what they have taken up is an adaptation of Yogic disciplines to meet occidental needs, enhancing the quality of living. Most attention has been given to the postures (*asanas*), breath controls (*pranayama*), and relaxation exercises of Hatha Yoga, but a growing number of Westerners are now turning to the Yoga of Meditation for a variety of reasons, from its reasonable and valid use as a mental hygiene (all Yogic techniques are purificatory and promote tranquillity) to inner work towards Yoga's supreme goal of intuitive enlightenment. We should perhaps have written 'Goal', for the mystical experience sought is usually given a capitalization of its initial letter, whatever name it goes by – and there are many. The supreme goal of Yoga is the union ('Yoga' means 'union' or 'yoking') of the individual spirit with the universal spirit, the finding of one's essential nature (Self) beyond empirical ego, which has to be dissolved, and the seeing and experiencing of the ground of one's being. Thus such terms as Absolute, *Brahman*, God, Reality, Ultimate Reality, Cosmic Mind, Cosmic Consciousness, Universal Spirit, Over-soul, Over-self, Void, Buddha Nature, It, That – to name but a few – represent a goal for progress towards which body, breath, mind, and spirit are disciplined, refined, and perfected by psycho-physiological techniques, many of which provide great benefits for body and mind, in improved health, relaxation, tranquillity, and self-mastery, quite apart from the mystical end-goal for which they are a preparation.

MEDITATION AS MENTAL HYGIENE

Many levels of approach to Yogic meditation are possible. Readers may start out with one aim in mind, but switch to another level after a period of practice. One reason for meditating that is valid for every practitioner, whatever his viewpoint on Yoga's mystical frame of reference, is that meditation is a mental hygiene.

Such an approach is in no way unworthy of Yoga, for every discipline of Yoga has a purificatory nature. In this book's companion volume *Yoga of Breathing* we described techniques of posturing, breath regulation, relaxation, muscle and sexual controls, and hygienic practices, all of which traditionally serve the end of cleansing the organism. The psychological controls of Raja (Royal) Yoga are no less a purification than those of Hatha Yoga, but in Raja Yoga consciousness is worked upon directly, rather than indirectly through bloodstream, tissues, glands, and nervous system. Just as the techniques of the Yoga of Breathing cleanse the bloodstream, nerves, and body tissues, enhancing health and promoting poise and feelings of lightness, so do those of the Yoga of Meditation cleanse the mind, refine and clarify consciousness, lighten the spirit, and foster mental poise and equanimity. Meditation calms and tones the nervous system, relaxes, harmonizes psychic energies, recharges psychic batteries, and cultivates serenity.

HATHA YOGA AND RAJA YOGA

Some Raja Yogins dispense with the techniques of Hatha Yoga entirely, apart from the basic sitting postures for meditation, taking the view that if the state of consciousness is right, the body will be adequately cared for. This is an extreme view, though probably not without validity for the most advanced practitioners of Raja Yoga. The mainstream tradition sees the two approaches as inseparable, Hatha Yoga working on consciousness through bodily control and purification, and Raja Yoga working on the body through harmonizing the psychic energies and eliminating tensions and interference with the natural rhythm of nature.

Traditionally, Hatha Yoga is seen as a preparation for meditative Yoga. This is not to say that the former should be dropped in favour of the latter. Both should be practised, body influencing mind and mind influencing body to the heightened well-being of both. Swatmaram Swami, author of the *Hatha Yoga Pradipika* (which is translated 'a lamp [or light] on Hatha Yoga') says (**77**): 'There are many who are merely Hatha Yogins without the knowledge of Raja Yoga; I think them to be simple practitioners who do not get the fruit of their pains.' It may also be said that followers of the Yoga of Meditation are foolish if they aschew the aid of the exercises of the Yoga of Breathing.

THE QUIET MIND

Yoga meditation promotes psycho-physical poise and a quiet mind that protects against the stress of modern life, which destroys health and happiness, and is indeed a major killer in civilized society.

The newcomer to meditation receives a shock when he first sits down in a quiet place and turns his attention inwards. Our attention is normally turned outwards to cope with the challenges of the environment – but look within and you find that the mind is filled with the chatter of thought and the flashing of images; as rowdy as a cageful of mad monkeys, say some old Yoga texts. Yoga meditation sets out to reduce the clamour and the number of thoughts, to open up spaces between thoughts, to smooth out waves in the mind-stuff (*citta*).

Merely sitting still for a fifteen or twenty minute period each day – just sitting, letting thought flow and observing its flow – provides a mental hygiene of the kind we described. In fact, this is a meditative practice given pride of place by a leading school of Zen. But there are many other meditative methods, active and passive, to be described in the chapters to follow. The reader should experiment and select the method or methods best suited to his temperament, circumstances, and organism.

Meditation works upon the nervous system and the organism's physiological processes, and the results are extended beyond the duration of a daily session of contemplation to bring increased physical and psychical poise to life's daily activities. One experiences an inner sense of floating with the stream of life, with the Way or Course of Nature, which the Chinese call the Tao (pronounced 'dow').

William James, who made a still-unsurpassed study of the

psychology of religious experience early in this century, was impressed by the mental regeneration of a friend who had taken up Yoga practice, and wrote (132):

> The most venerable ascetic system, and the one whose results have the most voluminous experimental corrobation is undoubtedly the Yoga system in Hindustan.... The result claimed, and certainly in many cases accorded by impartial judges, is strength of character, personal power, unshakability of soul ... a very gifted European friend of mine who, by persistently carrying out for several months its methods of fasting from food and sleep, its exercises in breathing and thought-concentration, and its fantastic posture gymnastics, seems to have succeeded in waking up deeper and deeper levels of will and moral and intellectual power in himself, and to have escaped from a decidedly menacing brain-condition of the 'circular' type, from which he had suffered for years.... A profound modification has unquestionably occurred in the running of his mental machinery. The gearing has changed, and his will is available otherwise than it was.'

Laboratory investigation confirms scientifically the subjective experience of lowered blood pressure, relaxed muscles and mind; and EEG tests on meditators show that their brain waves exhibit a slow pattern distinct from that of ordinary waking, hypnosis, or sleep.

THE MYSTICAL DIMENSION

It is but a short step from harmony with Nature or the Tao to meditating for reasons that are religious, or at any rate mystical. So far we have given reasons for meditating that are apart from the metaphysical and spiritual dimension. The word 'Yoga' has a mystical meaning as the supreme goal, as well as one representing the practices used to realize the goal.

Today in the West there is a widespread yearning for psychic Wholeness and a 'religious' feeling (in its broadest sense) that is eclectic and has no place for the doctrinal rigidities and dead dogmas of institutionalized religion. 'How does one live with religious emotion in the twentieth century?' asks Monica Furlong, in *Contemplating Now* (123). 'The longing for meaning, for wholeness, and for what the French philosopher Hubert Benoit calls "inner work" is common to everybody, but no one any longer, is sure of what the "work" consists of.'

Well, the Yoga of Meditation is the oldest form of 'inner work' still alive and in use, and it is one which many thousands of occidentals are finding puts them in touch with the springs of spiritual life. To quote Miss Furlong again (123):

'Most people are not aware of such a call, yet they may feel the strongest attraction to make some sense of the 'God-feeling' within them, and be overwhelmed by feelings of sickness, sadness, depression and despair if they suppress it because they disagree with conventional kinds of religious belief, or are afraid that others will think them mad or odd. If it is true that 'this is a society that represses transcendence' then they will find it painful to begin with to admit to being driven by such an improper longing, but if they will get past this stage they will discover that most people have a very good idea what they are talking about and are suppressing similar longings and experiences of their own.

I believe that learning to admit transcendence may be one of the major undertakings of a man's life, perhaps the major undertaking, so that if it is ignored his personality may be stunted or destroyed. We are all contemplatives to a greater or lesser degree, and we all need, to the limit of our capacity, to admit the experience which we may, or may not, call God.'

Mystical experience transcends all religions and cultures, though each mystic tends to describe his experiences in the jargon of his particular religion and culture. But the sense of the unity of all things, the heart of the mystical experience, is not confined to followers of specific religions, and peak experiences of a spiritual nature can come unbidden to people who neither seek nor cultivate them.

Meditation offers the possibility of our opening up, as a flower to the sun, to the bright emotions of love and joy, even of ecstasy; of enriching immeasurably our relations with wives, husbands, children, parents, neighbours, and workmates – relationships based on I-Thou rather that I-It, in Martin Buber's well-known phrase.

GREATER SELF-MASTERY

Psychologists, neurologists, and doctors are now studying the psychological and physiological effects of Yoga practice and interpreting meditation in scientific language. Yoga, as an ever-developing living science, welcomes this investigation. Much to stimulate the intellect and imagination has resulted from such studies. There is the possibility, for example, that there are two distinct modes of consciousness, each related to one side of the brain. The left hemisphere controls language, verbal reasoning, and the time sense. The right hemisphere is responsible for intuition and 'spatial functions', including painting, sculpture, and dancing. Western culture, by this theory, has been left-hemisphere-orientated and Eastern culture has been right-hemisphere-orientated. This distinction will recur in a later chapter.

Laboratory tests have shown unusual patterns of brain wave production in meditators wired to EEG apparatus – waves distinct from those of the normal waking state, hypnosis, or sleep.

Meditators have demonstrated their ability to relax, to reduce their blood pressures, to slow down their heartbeats, to control, in fact, physiological functions thought to belong to the involuntary nervous system. This offers the possibility of regulating the health in ways not thought possible before. In addition to this, biofeedback equipment enables ordinary men and women to acquire control over physiological processes normally involuntary. After a short period of training in the use of the equipment, these subjects can display feats of self-mastery and conscious control over the involuntary nervous system of the kind demonstrated by exceptional Yogins.

MENTAL POWERS

The goal of acquiring exceptional mental powers (*siddhis*) is viewed with disfavour by respected Yoga masters, but it is a motivation for some people, and has been throughout Yoga's long history. Magic and the occult energies have always had a fascination for some sects of Indian Yoga and Taoist (Chinese) Yoga. Magic and the occult have also played a considerable role in Tantric Yoga, in particular that of Tibet.

That exceptional mental powers occur as a result of advanced Yoga meditation is claimed in all the major texts, including Patanjali's *Yoga Sutras*, but the main tradition holds that they are to be accepted lightly and not allowed to become distractions from the true goal of spiritual illumination.

WHAT IS MEDITATION?

At this point we should make clear what is meant by 'to meditate' in this work – and what 'to meditate' is not. It is neither to do what the dictionary defines as 'plan mentally, design', nor is it 'to muse, to think over', as is commonly assumed. There is a keen use of thought in Jnana Yoga, the way of the intellect, but most Yogas aim at a suspension of thought, a silencing of the mind's agitation.

Dictionary definitions of 'contemplation' bring us close to what is involved in oriental meditation. *The Concise Oxford Dictionary* defines 'contemplate' as 'gaze upon: view mentally'. The origins of the word are in the Latin *contemplum* or temple, an open space for observation. 'Contemplative' is defined as 'meditative, thoughtful; (of life in middle ages) given up to religious contemplation, opp. to active'. *Nuttall's Standard Dictionary* gives as one definition of contemplation, 'continued attention to a particular subject'.

Attention is the key. Meditation, as used in this book, is a general term applied to the methods of steadying, quieting, or opening the mind for purposes of altering states of consciousness. In the great religions its goal is a knowledge of the Absolute, personalized in Christianity and Islam, but impersonal in Vedantic Hinduism, Buddhism (a religion without a god), Zen, and Taoism. Esoteric and occult schools think more in terms of 'higher knowledge', 'heightened consciousness', or 'intuitive awareness'. The aim of meditation may also be, as shown above, at the less exalted (but valuable) level of relaxation and mental hygiene.

In terms of the Raja Yoga of Patanjali, meditation means sense withdrawal (*pratyahara*) and concentration (*dharana*), sustained into contemplation (*dhyana*), with the aim of triggering a super-conscious state (*samadhi*), which is one of intuitive realization of the identity of the individual soul or spirit and the cosmic soul or spirit.

MANY YOGAS

The inclusion here and there in this work of meditative practices from sources outside Hindu Yoga warrants an explanation. *All* techniques used to achieve some kind of heightened or higher consciousness or intuitive enlightenment may be considered as

Yogas. One can therefore talk of Hindu Yoga, Buddhist Yoga, Sufist Yoga, Taoist Yoga, and so on. There is even an Eskimo Yoga, using techniques corresponding with those of Indian Yoga. There are also Yogas that combine Eastern and Western methods of self-mastery, such as the inner work for 'the harmonious development of man' taught by George Gurdjieff and his successors.

Sufism (Islam's mystical wing) and Christianity were both influenced by Indian Yogic methods, and Buddhism's whole *raison d'etre* is the meditation (*dhyana*) of its founder, an Indian prince. Buddhist meditative methods are pure Yoga. Buddhism was carried from India to China, where developed the direct method of Ch'an (meaning 'meditation'), which took root in Japan as Zen (again meaning 'meditation'). Tibetan Buddhism has a large content of Tantric Yoga practice. Finally, it may be said that, wherever they are found in the world, contemplative practices essentially follow the techniques of Indian Yoga. They all utilize in some manner the beam of attention. Attention again and again is the key that unlocks the door to altered states of consciousness and Self-realization.

II   Yoga's Hindu and Mystical Setting

THE HISTORY OF YOGA

The practice of Yoga meditation has to be seen against the traditional backdrop of Hindu belief and culture. Though Yoga is not a
religion, it *is* a system of psycho-physiological techniques that
people can employ for spiritual unfoldment, and its history is linked
with that of Hinduism, into which it was incorporated by the
Brahmins, the priestly caste. And Yoga's whole *raison d'etre* is
mystical, its ultimate aim being the experiencing of the Reality
underlying all manifest forms. Therefore, to understand better
Yoga's goals, methods, and terminology, we should have some
acquaintance with its Hindu and mystical frame of reference.

Robert Linssen, the French Oriental scholar, says (144): 'Indian
thought largely emanates from a mixture of two currents: yoga,
established before the Vedic period, and Brahmanism, which
belongs to the period of the *Vedas*, the *Upanishads*, and the *Vedanta*.'
During the Mohenjo Daro excavations in the Indus basin, the John
Marshall expedition discovered intact ceramics about five thousand
years old on which were depicted Yogic meditative postures. Yoga
thus pre-dates the main Vedic currents of Indian thought, which
began about 1500-1000 BC with the *Rig Veda*, the *Sama Veda* and
the *Yajur Veda*, followed by the *Atharva Veda* about 1000-800 BC,
the *Brahmanas* about 800-600 BC, and the first *upanishads* about
800-500 BC. The six philosopical schools (*darshanas* or 'viewpoints')
developed about 200 BC-500 AD.

The different forms of Yoga have played a major part in forming
the spirit of modern India. Yoga is incorporated in Indian religion,
in vernacular literature, and in folk-lore. Professor Masson-
Oursel (144) calls Yoga a discipline of psycho-physiological behaviour
that is the permanent basis of Indian culture.

Yoga's mental disciplines are, to varying degrees, part of the meditative methods of Buddhism, Taoism, Ch'an, and Zen. The words 'Ch'an' and 'Zen' both mean 'meditation'. Yogic techniques are also found in Sufism, and they had some influence on Christian mysticism.

HINDUISM

Hinduism is in several respects a unique religion. Unlike Chrisianity, Buddhism, or Islam, it had no founder and is not centred on the personality, teachings, and historical activities of a founder figure. It grew gradually over a period of five thousand years, during which time it absorbed and assimilated several religions and cultural movements in India. Without embarrassment or discomfort, it contains a great gallimaufry of religious, metaphysical, and philosophical ideas.

K. M. Sen (165) says that it is

the recognition of 'many paths', each valid in itself but none alone complete, that gives to Hinduism its immense variety. The religious beliefs of different schools of Hindu thought vary and their religious practices also differ; there is in it monism, dualism, monotheism, polytheism, pantheism, and indeed Hinduism is a storehouse of all kinds of religious experiments.

For this reason Hinduism, throughout its long history, has been tolerant of all paths to spiritual truth, and has developed a remarkable capacity for absorbing disparate religious, metaphysical, and philosophical views. The multiplicity of viewpoints has been at the same time a strength and a weakness.

Hinduism is sometimes said to be a culture rather than a religion. K. M. Sen says that 'Hinduism is in fact a *dharma* rather than a religion in the restricted sense of the word.' *Dharma* is a difficult word to translate into English, for it has a cluster of meanings – 'way of life', 'civilization', and 'national consciousness' are three of them. Hinduism is a matter of conduct rather than of doctrinal belief. As Professor Radhakrishnan, in *The Hindu View of Life*, says (160): 'The theist and the atheist, the sceptic and the agnostic may all be Hindus if they accept the Hindu system of culture and life . . . what counts is conduct, not belief.'

'The attempt to translate it (Hinduism) into the verbal concepts and categorical structure of Western language leads to logical monstrosities,' writes Arthur Koestler, in *The Lotus and the Robot*, (139) Hinduism never had a St Paul or an Aquinas to tidy up its amorphous confusion. When the scholars get to work dissecting Hinduism, they end up with a multiplicity of parts labelled Vedism, Brahmanism, Saivism, Vaisnavism, and so on. But the Hindu, without straining, accepts all of the parts. He can incorporate the teachings of Buddha or Christ easily into his ideology – for he recognizes all paths to spiritual knowledge.

Hinduism is a national religion. The words 'Hindu' and 'India' share the same root – 'Indus.' Before the Islamic invasion, to be an Indian and to be a Hindu were one and the same thing. Hinduism is thought to have originated with the tribes of Aryans who migrated from Persia and the Eurasian steppes about 2000 BC., crossed the Hindu Kush, and settled in the valleys of the Indus and' the Ganges. Another wave of these nomads reached Syria and Egypt and founded the Hyskos empire about (1680-1580 BC). The Indo-European family of languages derives from the language the Aryans spoke, and includes most of the languages of Europe and a large part of south-west Asia. English and the other Germanic languages, the Romance languages derived from Latin, the Celtic, Greek, Slavonic, and Baltic languages all owe their origins to the speech of the Aryans. Sanskrit, the classical language of Hindu sacred literature and of Yogic philosophy, also derives from the Aryan language.

The polytheistic religion of the Aryans can be typified by the *Rig Veda*. Their gods personified the forces of nature: sun, fire, storm, and so on. They had both male and female deities. Their main method of worship was sacrifice in the open air. Some time between 800 and 500 BC Hindu polytheism gave way to monotheism.

Jainism and Buddhism emerged out of the complex Indian culture. Buddhism was strong for a time in India, reaching its peak during the third century BC. But Hinduism regained ascendancy and Buddhist masters and monks carried their religion to other lands. The meditative methods of Buddhism and Hinduism are closely related, and one leading school of Buddhism is called Yogacara. The Tantric Buddhism of Tibet, Nepal, and China incorporated many of the psycho-physiological techniques of Hindu Hatha Yoga. By the time of post-Buddhist Hinduism the main Yogas were all clearly established: Jnana, Karma, Bhakti, and so on.

THE HINDU GODS

The gods representing the single divine principle are numerous and of varying characters. The Hindu Trinity is composed of Siva, Vishnu, and the many-headed Brahma. Siva has a fierce character, needed to combat the demons; he is also a god of fertility, whose symbol is the phallus and whose symbolic animal is the bull. He is both a god of fertility and of destruction. The strongest Siva worship is found east of Benares. Vishnu has a milder character and is most worshipped west of Benares, where Bhakti (devotional) Hinduism is strong. He has many *avatars* or earthly incarnations, including the popular heroes Krishna and Prince Rama. Brahma, often confused with *Brahman* or Ultimate Reality, represents the divine power of creation. There are also Great Mother goddesses, such as the fearsome trio Durga, Kali, and Shakti.

CASTE

Since Vedic times each Hindu has been born into a caste, and each caste has had its rules and place in the Indian social system. The four main groupings are: i. *Brahmins:* the highest caste, the priests who alone could interpret the *vedas* and sacred writings. Today Brahmins are not always priests. ii. *Kshatriyas*: princes, warriors, and aristocrats. iii. *Vaisyas:* merchants, farmers, and professional people. iv. *Sudras:* servants and labourers.

The caste system may have originated before the Ayran invasion of the Indus Valley, but certainly the racial difference between the conquerors and the dark-skinned Dravidians contributed to its development. The fairer-skinned Aryans occupied the top castes, and the Indian labouring caste has tended to be dark-skinned. The Buddha was a Kshatriya by birth, but repudiated the caste system. There are many sub-castes. Each caste and sub-caste has its elaborate system of rules laying down which profession or employment a member should undertake, whom he should marry, what food he should eat, what clothing he should wear, what kind of house he should have, how it should be furnished, and so on.

It is to the credit of the drafters of the Indian constitution that there is no support in it for the caste system. It survives, but under mounting pressure. It remains strongest in south India. The complexity of modern urban living makes strict adherence to caste rules in cities impossible. Westerners are puzzled how caste has persisted, especially in the light of the lofty doctrine that the Self (*Atman*) of every man and woman is identical with the Over-self (*Brahman*).

STAGES OF LIFE (ASRAMAS)

Traditionally there are four stages or *asramas* laid down by the Brahmins for the life of the devout Hindu. They begin after childhood. i. The youthful period of discipline and education, during which the sacred writings are studied. ii. The period of the householder, the man occupied by his job, raising a family, and social responsibility. His duties should be performed in the spirit of Karma Yoga, and he may practise other Yogas. iii. The period of maturity, when his sons have grown up, married, and themselves become householders. Now he withdraws from family and social life, and takes instruction in spiritual development and Yoga at an *ashram*. iv. The final period, in which he becomes a wandering holy man, without property except for one robe, a staff, and a begging bowl. These aged mendicants are still a familiar sight in India.

The four-stage system has now been given a more modern look. For example, the Yoga schools (*ashrams*) are no longer crude huts with dried cow dung on the floor (as stipulated in some classic texts), but bright, clean, and attractive modern buildings in most cases.

The stages described above fit in with C. G. Jung's view that after middle age people develop a yearning, conscious or unconscious, for psychical Wholeness.

The final fourth stage of the devout Hindu's life is that of renunciation and non-attachment, in which he aims for *moksha* or *mukti* (Liberation). This concept is closely connected with two other Hindu ideas: *Karma* and Reincarnation.

KARMA

By the law of *karma* every human deed leaves a trace in the organism. We choose our actions and must be prepared to pay the price.

Each act shapes future action for good or ill. *Karma* should not be viewed as 'fate', as it popularly is in the West. A man takes responsibility for shaping his future life, or lives.

REINCARNATION

The concept of Rebirth is closely related to that of *karma*, for the *karmic* law of cause and effect extends through successive lives, according to Hindu belief, and hundreds, perhaps thousands, of lives may be needed to work off *karmic* impressions, a residue of which remain in even the enlightened man.

'Only in a long series of successive lives are the effects of our deeds and our actions undone,' writes Kovoor T· Behanan (6).

We live now because of our past *karma* and for the same reason we shall live again. Life is thus an expiation of the deeds of the previous existence and as long as it is accompanied by action and deeds the necessity for further expiation makes rebirth inevitable.

It is startling how a doctrine of rebirth like this, which can never be verified, has been accepted and believed as a solution for the riddle of existence. Cultured and illiterate alike find in it a just answer to the inequalities and sufferings of life. It inspires in its adherents a hope for the future coupled with submissive resignation in the face of present suffering. To say the least, the theory is, so far as the moral order is concerned, as logical as any other, which perhaps accounts for its acceptance. In its cardinal features the doctrine is found in the teachings of the ancient Greek philosopher, Pythagoras. Plato, too, believed in it.

MOKSHA (LIBERATION)

Moksha or *mukti* is release from *karma* and liberation from the cycle of rebirths. Buddhists use the term *nirvana* for this liberation. *Moksha* and *nirvana* sound negative states, and this view is reinforced by the use of the term 'Void'. But Hindus and Buddhists view them as fulfilments, as plentitudes, freedom, breaking of bonds, the opening of prison doors – fullness of being.

Moksha and *nirvana* are not annihilation, and we need not fear letting go our grip on the ego. All Yogas – Hindu, Buddhist, Sufist, and so on – share a common aim of dissolving the ego and realizing a higher Self. Swatmaram Swami, in the *Hatha Yoga Pradipika* ('a lamp [or light] on Hatha Yoga'), says (57): 'The Yogi in highest meditation is void within and void without like a pot in world space. He is also, like a pot in the ocean, full within and without.'

SACRED LITERATURE

Hinduism has no central founder figure: neither has it a supreme sacred book comparable in absolute authority with the Christian Bible or the Islamic Koran. However, certain works – principally the *Vedas*, the *upanishads*, and the *Bhagivad Gita* – are by Indian minds and hearts cherished as lofty expressions of Hindu wisdom. We have already pointed out how Hindusim accommodates a gallimaufry of concepts, many of which conflict. The same applies to Hindu sacred literature, in which conflicting ideas may be found within a single work.

Indian philosophy could be said to originate in the *vedas*, among the oldest of writings, though they are largely ritualistic, the main portion of each *veda* being taken up with the incantations (*mantras*) and hymns addressed to gods and goddesses, and the *Brahmanas*, written in prose, which deal with the rules and regulations for the performance of rites and sacrifices by the Brahmin priests. As appendages .to the *Brahmanas* there are the more philosophical *aranyakas*, whose closing passages are called *upanishads*, also known as *vedanta* (literally 'the end of the *veda*'). The word *veda* means 'knowledge' – compare the latin *videre*, 'to discern'. *Upanishad* derives from the root *sad*, which means 'to sit down'. *Upa* means 'near by', and *ni* means 'devotedly'. The whole word refers to the teachings received by the pupil sitting before a sage.

The *upanishads* educate and at the same time calm the spirit. Their monist thought, following on *vedic* polytheism, is poetical, lucid, and tranquil, But they not only criticize the earlier works to which they are appended – they mock them. The *upanishadic* sages were rebels who despised arid ritual and empty formulae. The *Chandogya Upanishad* contains a passage which compares the Brahmin priests to dogs marching in procession and chanting: '*Om!* Let us eat, *Om!* Let us drink, and so on!' OM (AUM) is the most sacred of all words to the Hindu.

The polytheism of the *Rig Veda* gave way to a search for unity within universal forms, and in the *upanishads*, with their teaching that *Atman* or Self equals *Brahman* or Cosmic Over-self, we find the purest Yogic philosophy. There are over two hundred *upanishads*, but ten or twelve are considered the most authoritative.

Few Westerners fail to appreciate, as poetry and as metaphysics, the beauty of the *upanishads*. The same may be said of the *Bhagavad Gita*, or 'Song of the Blessed Lord'. Both works have been translated several times into English and other European languages. The *Gita*, as it is popularly known, is part of the great epic called the *Mahabharata*. The Lord of the title is Krishna, a much-loved Indian deity, who in activities as an *avatar* or divine incarnation combines the qualities of a successful saint, warrior, poet, musician, and lover. The *Gita* takes the form of a discourse delivered by Krishna to Arjuna, the epic's hero, on the eve of a battle. Krishna instructs Arjuna in the way of duty and the ultimate goal of life. In doing so he expounds several Yogas.

The *Brahma Sutra*, written by Badarayana about the second century BC, sets out to explain the philosophy of the *upanishads*. The writer summarizes the views of earlier teachers, and refers to most of the leading systems of Indian thought. It is the third work in the threefold canon (*prasthanatraya*) on which the spiritual tradition of India is based (the first two works being the *upanishads* and the *Bhagavad Gita*).

BRAHMAN EQUALS ATMAN

One concept dominates the teaching of the *upanishads*, which express it again and again – the equation, *Brahman* equals *Atman*. The *Atman* is the Self, not the ego constructed principally by our parents, our teachers, and society. Yoga methods dissolve the empirical ego and permit the Self to be discovered. Self or *Atman* is then experienced as *Brahman*. *Brahman* is the divine principle 'in-forming' the universe, the essence and substratum of all things, all-pervading, the 'one without a second' (*ekamevadvitiyam*). *Brahman* is not God, if by God one means a personalized deity like the punishing and rewarding, wrathful and loving father-figure of Christianity; but the modern existentialist theologian's ground of being comes close to it. *Brahman* is the mystic One, and many labels are applied – though labelling the One is attempting the impossible.

'The most important step in the development of Indian philosophy was taken when the *Brahman*, the cosmic principle, and *Atman*, the psychic principle in man were looked upon as identical,' writes Kovoor T. Behanan (6). The identity of cosmic mind with our own pure consciousness is expressed in two sayings: 'that thou art' (*tat tvam asi*) and 'I am *Brahman*' (*aham Brahma asmi*). Dr Behanan says that this concept is 'a tacit assumption of mystics all over the world, irrespective of credal affiilations.' At this point Yoga becomes universal and transcends its Hindu setting. Mystics the world over believe in a unity behind the changing experiences and phenomena of life, and that this substratum is contacted and known by looking within.

'This idea [*Brahman equals Atman*] alone secures to the *Upanishads* an importance reaching far beyond their land and clime,' writes P. Deussen in *Outlines of Indian Philosophy* (116). He goes on, 'for whatever means of unveiling the secrets of Nature a future time may discover, this idea will be true for ever, from this mankind will never depart. If the mystery of Nature is to be solved, the key of it can be found only there where alone Nature allows us an interior view of the world, that is in ourselves.'

MAYA

What prevents us seeing that our essence and Cosmic Mind are one? The Indian philospher replies: '*maya* (illusion) and *avidya* (ignorance.)'

Yoga techniques, of which there are a variety, each with a different emphasis of approach – intellectual, devotional, psychical, physiological, and so on – cut aside the veil of illusion and disperse the fog of ignorance that prevents the clear perception and experience 'I am *Brahman*'. Indian teaching makes an analogy between the world seen as illusion (*maya*) and a coil of rope mistaken for a snake. Move closer and you see that what you took to be a dangerous snake is but a coil of rope. There is then nothing to do but relax and laugh. So, too, when the veils of illusion and ignorance are penetrated, one perceives one's real nature as 'the one without a second'. The enlightenment and awakening triggers joy and bliss, and we laugh because our real nature was there all the time, though we had failed to look in the right direction. But a glance that way would have been sufficient. As T'sen T'sang put it: 'A difference of a tenth of an inch and the Heaven and earth are set apart.'

THE MYSTICAL EXPERIENCE

We have just described the mystical experience, essentially the same for mystics of all nationalities, cultures, and religions, though dressed by them in the conceptual and verbal clothing of the culture and tradition to which they belong. Such description is always futile. The mystical experience of intuitive awareness and inner illumination transcends linear verbal thought. In it duality is overcome, subject and object fuse: there are no longer perceiver, perceived, and perceiving as separate entities – all three fuse together to become a unity that belongs to the cosmos itself.

William James, in his *Varieties of Religious Experience* (133), a work still unsurpassed in this field for its breadth and penetration, says:

This overcoming of the usual barriers between the individual and the Absolute is the great mystic achievement. In mystic states we become one with the Absolute and we become aware of our oneness. This is the everlasting and triumphant mystical tradition, hardly altered by differences of clime or creed. In Hindusim, in Neoplatoism, in Sufism, in Christian mysticism, in Whitmanism, we find the same recurring note, so that there is about mystical utterances an eternal unanimity which ought to make a critic stop and think.

III Yogic Philosophy

THE SIX SYSTEMS OF PHILOSOPHY

Yoga may be defined as mystical absorption. It is also a general name for the controls and techniques that perfect body, mind, and spirit so as to realize the mystical end-goal. Now we come to a third meaning. Yoga is one of the six systems of Indian philosophy (*darshanas*). *Darshana* means 'viewpoint' or 'vision', from the root *drs*, 'to see', 'to comprehend', 'to contemplate'.

The six schools of philosophy developed in the post-*upanishadic* period. For the theory behind its practice, Yoga borrows extensively from the Samkhya (or Sankhya) system, and the two names are often linked with a hyphen. The remaining four philosophies may also be paired, giving Samkha-Yoga, Mimansa-Vedanta, and Nyaya-Vaisesika.

Yoga differs from all the other systems in that it is not content, as they are, to expound metaphysical knowledge, but has devised and presented practical techniques whereby intellectual understanding can be reinforced by experiental knowing. Yoga says: 'Don't take our word for it Through psycho-physiological controls you can attain higher consciousness and experience on a level of Being the truth that will set you free.' This accounts for Yoga's great popularity and potency in Indian culture.

As all the Indian philosophies have the common aim of spiritual emancipation, it is thus possible for adherents of any school to borrow Yoga's practical techniques. This explains why leading Yoga masters may expound what is a predominantly Vedanta-Yoga teaching rather than the Samkhya-Yoga philosophy one might expect. But as all the systems have basically different approaches to metaphysical knowledge, in most respects they may be considered more complementary than contradictory.

Considering their age, these Indian philosophies are a remarkable achievement of human thought. Their texture is complex and dense. Count Hermann Keyserling, in writing his *Travel Diary of a Philosopher*, pointed out that Indian literature has more words for philosophical and religious thought than can be found in the Greek, Latin and German languages combined. We will here concisely outline the most important features of Yoga as a philosophy, particularly these most relevant to the practice of the Yoga of Meditation. Students of Yoga who wish to go deeper could not do better than start by reading the relevant chapters of Dr Behanan's *Yoga: A Scientific Evaluation*, which, though written in 1937, remains the clearest exposition for the general reader.

SAMKHYA YOGA

There is an old Indian saying: 'There is no knowledge equal to the Samkhya, and no power equal to the Yoga.' Samkhya is mainly a natural philosophy. Yoga takes from Samkhya its detailed account of the evolution of the known world and the nature of human consciousness. The leading Samkhya source text is Kapila's *Samkhya Sutras*, and the key work in the philosophy and practice of the Yoga of Meditation (Raja or Royal Yoga) is Patanjali's *Yoga Sutras*. *Sutras* are condensed statements – the word is usually translated as 'aphorisms'.

Richard von Garbe (124), a German oriental scholar, wrote that 'in Kapila's doctrine, for the first time in the history of the world, the complete independence and freedom of the human mind, its full confidence in its own powers, were exhibited.'

Samkhya and Yoga differ in two main respects. First, Samkhya is atheistical, but Yoga introduces – though awkwardly and weakly, it may be thought – a Supreme Being (*Isvara*), who stays aloof from human and worldly affairs, but acts as an inspiration. Second, Samkhya's approach to liberation is by way of metaphysical knowledge, intellectually accepted, whereas Yoga's approach is by way of psycho-physiological techniques and controls, though it uses Kapila's account of evolution, consciousness, the body-mind problem, and so on, as a theoretical support.

Samkhya explains the universe without seeing any need to introduce God. There is no anthropomorphized Creator. Kapila explained eternal evolution and dissolution in the universe in terms of *Purusha* (soul or spirit) and *prakriti* (basic substance), and the latter's evolutes. But Yoga, taking Samkhya's natural philosophy, added a Supreme Being, a liberated *Purusha*, who provides inspiration, but does not take an active role in human affairs. Thus God appears in Patanjali's *Sutras*, without fitting easily into the philosophical and metaphysical teaching of that work. Some scholars think that the appearance of *Isvara* in the *Sutras* was a later interpolation. Richard von Garbe says (124) of Patanjali's work: 'The passages which treat of God are unconnected with the other parts of the book – nay, even contradict the foundations of the system.'

VEDANTA

Most modern Yoga masters teach Yoga practice combined with the metaphysics of Vedanta: the '*Brahman equals Atman*' equation of the *upanishads*; the impersonal, all-pervading *Brahman* rather than a personal Creator, a concept which educated Indians find naive and unsophisticated. On this matter William James wrote (133):

> God as intimate soul and reason of the universe has always seemed to some people a more worthy conception than God as external creator. So conceived, he appeared to unify the world more perfectly, he made it less finite and mechanical, and in comparison with such a God an external creator seemed more like the product of a childish fancy. I have been told by Hindoos that the great obstacle to the spread of Christianity in their country is the puerility of our dogma of creation. It has not sweep and infinity enough to meet the requirements of even the illiterate natives of India.

Anta means 'end', and Vedanta is the knowledge found in the later *upanishadic* part of the *vedas* – *Brahman* as the one Reality. Samkhya-Yoga holds to the doctrine of the plurality of souls (*Purushas*), with *Isvara* (God) as a special *Purusha*. This clashes with the Vedanta *Brahman* concept, which is monist – *Brahman* is All, and each of us can say: 'I am *Brahman*.'

The best-known branch of Vedanta philosophy is Advaita Vedanta, founded by the brilliant Indian philosopher Sankaracharya, whose central tenet is non-duality.

Dr Behanan says (6) 'The vedanta has dominated the Hindu mind for so long that today most yogins have grafted the vedanta metaphysics to the yoga practice – *Brahman* alone is real. It is the adaptability of the system that makes yoga more a philosophy and a psychology than a religion.'

PURUSHA

We have Dr Behanan's assurance (6) that 'in its essential aspects the samkhya-yoga soul, called *purusha*, is not very different from the *Upanishadic Atman*.' However, the Samkhya Yoga doctrine of the plurality of souls (*Purushas*) marks a divergence from the monism of the *upanishads*, in which only *Brahman* is real.

Purusha is pure consciousness (*cit*), eternal, spaceless, passive, the Seer or Witness. It is the unchanging clear light against which the mind's thoughts and images becomes visible: not the images on the mental screen, but the projector's illumination. The relationship between *Buddhi* or Intelligence and *Purusha* is that the former reflects the latter.

Prakriti, the basic substance of the universe, serves *Purusha*. *Purusha* iniates cosmic evolution by coming into proximity with matter.

PRAKRITI

Dr Behanan (6) compares *upanishadic wisdom* with Samkhya *knowledge*. 'The wisdom of the *Upanishads* was, of course, the highest, but the *knowledge* of the samkhya had no equal because it was the boldest and most rational speculation in the field of natural philosophy.'

Samkhya means 'number'; it is the 'philosophy of number'. It probably received its name from its enumeration and classification of the twenty-five *tattwas* – the 'thatnesses' or categories of the known universe.

Samkhya Yoga teaches eternal alternating evolution and dissolution. Cosmic evolution is in the service of *Purusha* or Spirit, and proceeds from the subtle to the gross, from consciousness to gross atoms – the reverse of the customary direction of evolution as held by Western science.

The basis of all is *prakriti*, eternal and originally unmanifest.

Prakriti is often translated as 'Nature'. Dr Behanan (6) calls it 'primordial, undifferentiated matter' and Professor Wood (94) defines it as 'the basic substance or principle of the entire phenomenal or manifest world.'

The basic substance of things (*prakriti*) can be divided into three inherent qualities called *gunas*. These *tamas*, *rajas*, and *sattva* – or inertia, energy, and intelligence respectively. Alternative definitions of *sattva* are 'orderliness', 'purity', and 'illumination'. These three qualities or *gunas* combine to make up all the objects of Nature. They are both substance and energy. The predominance of a *guna* in a thing determined its essential nature.

Tamas represents mass, resistance, stability, solidity, and durability – though modern science tells us that all objects display ceaseless change – even the lamp-post that Dr Johnson kicked to disprove Bishop Berkeley's philosophical idealism. In the workings of the mind *tamas* is responsible for the stability of memory.

Rajas is the kinetic principle, responsible for the activity within the atom, and for change and motion everywhere in Nature. Within the mind it is responsible for the coming and going of thoughts and the ebb and flow of the emotions.

Sattva is the principle in Nature that makes for orderliness, that keeps the planets in their courses, designs the snow crystal's perfection, and regulates the involuntary functioning of the body. But *sattva* is found in its most characteristic element in the workings of consciousness. *Sattva* predominates in the 'mind-stuff', manifesting itself as intellect, will and feeling. It represents a pure and light quality, in contrast to the gross and heavy element in matter. But *sattva* is latent in heavy matter, just as *tamas* is latent in 'mind-stuff'. Energy (*rajas*) operates upon both *tanmas* and *sattva*.

STAGES OF COSMIC EVOLUTION

Prakriti's first evolute is *mahat*, *buddhi*, or Cosmic Consciousness, resulting from the three *gunas*, which were in dynamic equlibrium in primordial matter, being acted upon by *Purusha*. This is the plane of consciousness in which subject and object are fused, the goal for meditating minds in Yoga, Zen, Sufism, and other mystical traditions. *Buddhi* (intelligence) is passive at this stage.

In *mahat*, *sattva*, the basis of mental life, predominates. Thus, according to Samkhya-Yoga, the 'mind-stuff' originates immediately, reversing the customary scientific interpretation of evolution as a progression from inorganic to organic matter, and hence to whatever composes human consciousness. *Sattva*, being translucent, reflects spirit or *Purusha*. Dr Behanan provides an analogy (6) : 'A piece of rock and a crystal are both composed of atoms, but the latter can reflect the rays of the sun while the former cannot. *Sattva*, as against the other two *gunas*, has that something in its nature which, although different from *purusha*, makes the reflection of the latter possible.'

The next modification is *ahamkara*, the 'I' – sense. It is produced by energy (*rajas*). This should not be confused with pure consciousness, which is *Purusha*.

The process of evolution now takes on three aspects, each dominated by a separate *guna*. From the *sattvic* aspect develop the senses of sight, hearing, smell, taste, and touch. Samakahya-Yoga adds a sixth sense – mind or *manas* in its faculty of co-ordinating. The *rajas* aspect produces the motor organs – hands, feet, speech organs, excretory organs, and generative organs. The *tamas* aspect is responsible for the five potentials (*tanmatras*) of matter, corresponding to the cognitive senses listed above – light, sound, smell, taste, and touch. There is a further evolution from the *tanmatras* into the five gross atoms – earth, water, fire, air, and ether

The above make up twenty-four categories or 'thatnesses' (*tattwas*). *Purusha* brings their total to twenty-five. The diagram will help make the Samkhya-Yoga account of cosmic evolution more clear.

THE TWENTY-FIVE CATEGORIES (*TATTWAS*)

1. *Purusha*
2. *Prakriti*, Basic Substance
3. *Mahat*, *buddhi*, Cosmic Consciousness
4. *Ahamkara*, 'I' – Sense

The Six Senses	The Five Motor Organs	The Five Potentials (*tanmatras*)
5. sight	11. hands	16. light
6. hearing	12. feet	17. sound
7. smell	13. speech organs	18. smell
8. taste	14. excretory organs	19. taste
9. touch	15. generative organs	20. touch
10. *manas* (mind as co-ordinating faculty)		

The Five Atoms
21. earth
22. water
23. fire
24. air
25. ether

YOGA METAPHYSICS

Metaphysics seeks to grasp with the intellect 'the totality of things', which was Hegel's description of the Absolute. It was once a major concern of Western philosophy, but became uncertain when the Logical Positivists declared that statements that cannot be scientifically verified are without meaning, including talk of the Absolute or God. 'Is metaphysics possible?' then became the subject of the debate.

But Yogic and Western metaphysics differ in that the former does not rely on intellectual acceptance of a theory, but says something like this: 'Sit quietly, breathe evenly, silence your mind's chatter – and you will see into your inner nature and enter the plane of Being.'

In this work, with its practical approach, the metaphysical bases of Yoga provide only a backdrop to its practice. The reader is free to question the validity of the backdrop's design. But whatever his (or her) views on speculative Yogic metaphysics and philosophy, there can be no doubt that practical benefits accrue on many levels from the practice of Yoga. These were described earlier, in the chapter entitled 'Why Meditate?'

And few readers will fail to agree with Kovoor T. Behanan, when he concludes his 'scientific evaluation' of Yoga by saying (6): 'As far as the metaphysical tenets of yoga are concerned, they are an audacious and poetic leap in the dark – worthy enough to occupy a spacious hall in the "Mansions of Philosophy" that the human mind has spun in its irrestible desire to explain the warp and woof of the unknown.'

IV   Sitting for Meditation

SITTING FOR MEDITATION

This chapter is concerned with the pre-requirements for meditation, the two most important of which are a poised and stable sitting posture and the right attitude to take towards controlling the mind.

PLACE

The *Bhagavad Gita*, which calls itself a 'scripture of Yoga' and is the most translated work of world literature after the Bible, provides guidance in how to set about meditating. It says:

6.11. Having in a cleanly spot established a firm seat, neither too high nor too low, with cloth, skin and kusa grass thereon.

The room chosen for regular meditation should be clean and airy, and free from draughts and extremes of temperature, either hot or cold. The surroundings should be as pleasant and restful as possible for all the senses. Choose a place likely to be free from interruptions, either by people or the impingements of sense stimuli on the eyes, ears or skin. An outdoor place is sometimes suitable, but most meditators sit down to quieten the mind in bedrooms or other rooms in their homes.

A cushion will be a fully adequate substitute for the 'cloth, skin, and kusa grass' mentioned in the *Gita*. Place it on an even floor.

CLOTHING

Clothing should be light and comfortable. Remove the tie, collar, belt – anything which constricts or is likely to constrict. (No clothing at all should be worn when circumstances permit, but becoming chilled will not aid meditation.) Remove all objects from the pockets of trousers, shirts, and so on. Do not wear shoes or stockings.

CLEANLINESS

Bathe or sponge the whole body before sitting down to meditate; or wash the face and hands at least. Brush the teeth and rinse out the mouth with water. Empty the bladder, and the bowels too, if possible. Cleanliness and purification are an important part of Yoga practice.

EATING AND DRINKING

> 6,16. Yoga is not possible for him who eats too much, nor for him who does not eat at all, nor for him who is addicted to too much sleep, nor for him who is [ever] wakeful, O Arjuna.

The *Gita* here gives guidance for the eating and sleeping habits of a Yogi. A lesson can also be drawn in relation to sitting for meditation. If the stomach is full, respiration and circulation of the blood are impeded, and Yogins say that the movements of *pranic* energy currents are checked. Nor is an uncomfortably empty stomach desirable for a meditator, for it results in distracting sensations. Allow at least two hours to go by after a main meal before sitting down to meditate.

Overeating or undereating are alike detrimental to success in Yoga. A Yogic rule is that one should finish a meal feeling that a little more could have been taken. An old text put it like this: 'Half [the stomach] for food and condiments, the third [quarter] for water and the fourth should be reserved for free motion of air.'

SLEEP

Sleeping too much or too little is detrimental to the lucidity and alertness of mind required for meditation. Though by meditating in the Yogic manner one recharges mental batteries and touches deep levels of energy, the practice should not be used to refresh a fatigued mind. Meditation requires a clear and alert mind; a tired mind will be unable to sustain one-pointedness.

MODERATION

The Yogin is enjoined to show common sense and moderation in his habits of eating, drinking, sleeping, and daily exercise. Self-mortification and grim asceticism are not supported by the *Gita* or any of the main textual authorities.

6, 17. To him whose food and recreation are moderate, whose exertion in actions is moderate, whose sleep and waking are moderate, to him accrues Yoga which is destructive of pain.

POSTURE FOR MEDITATION

6, 13. Holding erect and still the body, head, and neck, firm, gazing on the tip of his nose, without looking around.

Descriptions of the possible Yogic postures or *asanas* for meditation are given in *Yoga of Posture*. The most famous posture for meditation is the Lotus Posture, sometimes called the Buddha Pose. However, it is a difficult pose for the average Westerner, and may take many months to master. Much easier poses can be used. The essential factors are to sit keeping the back upright and to have the head and neck poised in line with the spine. Beginners may for a time utilize a wall or chair-back to provide support for the spine. In the main traditional postures the legs are crossed in some manner. The easiest Yoga posture is Easy Posture (*Sukhasana*) in which the legs are crossed tailor's fashion and the knees are kept as low as is comfortable. But if this proves difficult to sustain you can always sit on a straight-backed chair in the Egyptial Posture.

EGYPTIAN POSTURE

This way of sitting on a straight-backed chair resembles a pose often depicted in Egyptian sculpture. The feet and knees are kept together, and the soles of the feet are flat on the floor. The palm of the right hand rests flat on the top of the right thigh a little above the

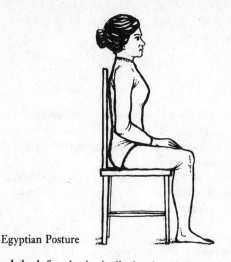

Egyptian Posture

knee, and the left palm is similarly placed above the left knee.

Maharishi Mahesh Yogi, the most successful *guru* in the West, does not insist on the cross-legged posture for his Transcendental Meditation, and says that sitting on a chair can be satisfactory so long as the back is kept erect. However, the unmatchable compactness and stability of the cross-legged Yogic postures will be apparent to anyone who takes the trouble to master at least one of them. The Easy Posture is not difficult, as its name reveals.

Lying on the back is not considered a suitable position for meditation because it causes drowsiness and dullness of mind. We shall see later that the mind should be in a normal state of wakefulness for meditation – neither dull nor very active.

EASY POSTURE (*SUSKHASANA*)

Sit on a cushion on the floor, cross the ankles, and lower the knees towards the floor as far as is comfortable. Keep the head, neck, and backbone in upright line. Rest the palm of the right hand on the right knee and the palm of the left hand on the left knee. Sometimes cross the right ankle over the left, and sometimes cross the left ankle over the right.

The knees will lower further as the weeks go by. When they rest easily on the floor it is time to move on to the Perfect Posture.

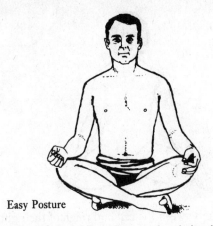

Easy Posture

Become accustomed to the Easy Posture by sitting in it while watching television, listening to records, feeding the baby, and so on. Remember that the body has to be forgotten in the tuning within of meditation; by practising sitting cross-legged at other times you can make the sitting posture comfortable and unobtrusive to the mind during meditation.

When Patanjali listed *asanas* or postures as the third of his eight limbs (*angas*) of Yoga, he was not primarily concerned with the numerous postures for good health that are found in Hatha Yoga, but with steady sitting postures for meditation. The most important thing is that the head, neck, and spine should be held poised easily in upright line. These essentials for sitting in meditation are aided by the practice of the Yoga of Posture, whose exercises and muscle controls strengthen the spine and back muscles, improve posture, and develop suppleness in the leg and hip joints.

PERFECT POSTURE (*SIDDHASANA*)

Siddha means 'adept'. This pose is so named because it is a favourite of 'perfected' Yogins. The right leg is bent at the knee, and by grasping the ankle, the right heel is pulled in against the pernieum, which is the soft flesh between the genitals and anus. The left leg is then folded and pulled back so that the left heel is against the pubic bone and the outer edge of the left foot, with the soles upturned, is

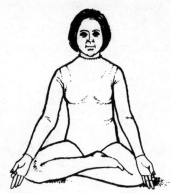

Perfect Posture

inserted in the fold between the calf and thigh of the right leg. Both knees are kept down on the floor. Place the right palm on the right knee and the left palm on the left knee, or clasp the hands loosely in the lap. Keep head, neck, and backbone in a straight vertical line. Sometimes reverse the roles of the legs so that the left heel is tucked in against the perineum and the right foot is pushed into the fold between the thigh and calf of the left leg.

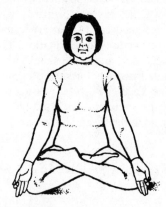

Lotus Posture

LOTUS POSTURE (*PADMASANA*)

In this famous pose, which occidentals find difficult, both feet are upturned on the thighs, right foot on left thigh, left foot on right thigh, each as high up the thigh as possible. Draw the feet up by pulling on the ankles. Here again the knees must be down firmly on the floor; if one is raised the pose will be unstable and lopsided. The hand positions may be as given for Perfect Posture – that is, on the knees or clasped limply in the lap.

Preparatory exercises for both Perfect and Lotus positions were given in *Yoga of Posture*.

It is important to use for meditation a posture which is firm and in which the body is at ease. An old Chinese Buddhist text says: 'If the body is at ease, the Tao will prosper.'

Before leaving this section on posture for meditation, it is necessary to explain that when the *Gita* instructs the Yogin to gaze 'on the tip of his nose' this should not be done other than momentarily. Sankaracharya says (164): 'He is to gaze *as it were* on the tip of his nose. Here we have to understand the words "as it were": for the Lord [Krishna] means to prescribe, not the very act of "gazing on the tip of his nose", but the fixing of the eye-sight within (by withdrawing it from external objects); and this, of course, depends on the steadiness of mind.'

If the gaze is directed to the front of the nose the attention is drawn in and integrated. The eyes should then be closed and the gaze released. The brief focusing of the gaze has helped sense-withdrawal (*pratyahara*) and instantly induced a concentrated state of mind. Some texts instruct that the attention should focus on the navel or a little below it, which 'nails down' rising thoughts. The space between the eyebrows is another much-favoured spot for directing and fixing the attention.

BREATHING

Breathe quietly, through the nostrils, not the mouth. During meditation the breathing rate will slow down and establish an even rhythm between inhalation and exhalation. The breath controls described in detail in *Yoga of Breathing* will aid in calming the nervous system and stimulating the physiological processes that aid meditation.

Breath control (*pranayama*) is the fourth of Patanjali's eight limbs of Yoga. The Yoga system uniquely utilizes the influence of breathing on mental states: fast and jerky breathing excites the mind, but slow, smooth, and rhythmic breathing calms it.

RIGHT ATTITUDES

6, 12. Making the mind one-pointed, with the actions of the mind and the senses controlled, let him, seated there on the seat practise Yoga for the purification of the self.

'A normal state of mind is needed for starting meditation,' says Maharishi Mahesh Yogi (146).

The mind should neither be dull nor very active. When it is dull, tending to sleepiness, it loses the capacity for experience. When it is very active, it remains in the field of gross experience, and, as it were, refuses to enter into the field of subtle experience, just as someone very active on the surface of the water does not sink.

One-pointedness of mind is the practical aim of the Yoga of Meditation. The attention rests steadily on one object until the knower, the known, and knowing become one in Enlightenment.

6, 10. Let the Yogin try constantly to keep the mind steady, remaining in seclusion, alone, with the mind and body controlled, free from desire, and having no possessions.

In these three lines from the *Gita* the conditions for successful Yoga meditation are concisely presented.

Quietness, privacy, and a secluded place in or outside of the home are needed for practice. The likelihood of disturbance should be reduced to a minimum. The abrupt ringing of a telephone bell in the room in which you meditate can have an unpleasantly jarring effect on the nervous system, so stay well away from telephones, or leave the receiver off the hook. 'During meditation the mind engages itself in the deeper levels of the thought-process', says Maharishi Mahesh Yogi (146): 'if it is disturbed and suddenly made to come out into the gross levels of sensory perception, it will experience a great contrast between the subtle and the gross fields of perception. This sudden contrast will damage the mind's serenity and will upset the nervous system.'

Meditation should be practised alone, as the presence of one or more other persons in the room will prove a distraction and prevent relaxation. One is all too conscious of their proximity and breathing presence.

The body should be stable and without movement, the spine kept upright and the head and neck in line with it. Suitable postures were described earlier in this chapter.

The mind has to be quietened and then kept steady. Such control is virtually effortless in correct performance. Concentration, after its initial gentle impulse, like a singer launching a soft head note, sustains itself and becomes free-flowing in the higher contemplative stages. One should not be trying to do this or that during meditation, for each intention is a distraction and a cause of tension and strain.

Professor Wood says (94):

Before you meditate you choose your subject or object of meditation, and there is then an act of will in which you tell your mind to keep to that subject and not to wander away from it.

This concentration on the chosen subject then goes by itself, and you need not think of it. If you have decided to walk in a certain direction the legs go on walking; you need not think of this act of will at every stage. An act of will goes on operating until another act of will changes it. Similarly, the act of concentration is still there while the meditation is going on, though it has been forgotten – 'subconscious' or 'unconscious' is the new word for this, though really it is now a habit, an act of the mind lapsed into inert form or motion.

'Free from desire' Maharishi Mahesh Yogi translates as 'expecting nothing'. A longing for Self-knowledge is necessary for the fully-committed Yogin, but no expectations should be entertained when he sits down to meditate. To expect any particular psychological or spiritual experience during meditation is certain either to block its attainment or to produce results that are ego-projections and not truly of the Self. The expectations are based on the known, which is the conditioned past; whereas Self-realization is a timeless and unconditioned experience, transcendent, on another plane of consciousness, hence totally new.

'Having no possessions,' says the *Gita*. Interpretations of this vary from the literal way of renunciation of the *sannyasi* to the state of going into meditation empty-handed, that is, without mental baggage, objects of thought or emotions that have to be grasped or recorded by consciousness.

During the stage of sense-withdrawal (*pratyahara*) one 'gives up' the external sense objects or possessions to turn the attention inward and sink down to subtler layers of consciousness. The meditating Yogin has also to be free from the tensions created by the tug-of-war between polar opposites and the interplay of the three *gunas*. Thus, the *Bhagavad Gita* states:

2, 45. The Vedas treat of the triad of the *gunas*. Be, O Arjuna, free from the triad of the *gunas*, free from pairs, free from acquisition and preservation, ever remaining in the *Sattva*]Goodness], and self-possessed.

But the major possession the Yogin must release is the ego, which dissolves during meditation.

COMING OUT OF MEDITATION

Instruction in this is omitted in many manuals, but it is important for the health of the nervous system that the meditator should return gradually from the subtle to gross levels of activity. A Chinese Buddhist text cited by Charles Luk (145) puts it:

Entry and exit should be both orderly for then
The states of coarse and fine do not impair each other.
This is like a horse that's tamed
At your will to stay or go.

At the conclusion of meditation, sit quietly for a few minutes before opening the eyes. Blink the eyes a few times as though releasing energy from them and clearing them. Unfold the legs and stretch them out straight along the floor. Stretch the legs away from the body for a few seconds, at the same time stretching both arms straight up from the shoulders so that the fingertips reach up towards the ceiling. Lower the arms. Take two or three deep abdominal breaths while sitting on the floor. Massage the legs with the hands for about a minute. Then stand up. Never jump up immediately meditation has ended.

HOW LONG SHOULD MEDITATION LAST?

It has been found that sessions of meditation lasting twenty to thirty minutes once or twice a day are most effective.

V   Patanjali's Royal (Raja) Yoga

THE YOGA SUTRAS

'In (the) basic literature of Yoga, the *Yoga-Sutras* of Patanjali stand
out as the most authoritative and useful book,' says I. K. Taimini
(89), one of the best modern commentators on this work. 'In its 196
Sutras the author has condensed the essential philosophy and
technique of Yoga in a manner which is a marvel of condensed and
systematic exposition.'

Patanjali divides his famous work into four sections. Section 1
answers the question 'What is Yoga?', and since the goal of mind-
stilling by Raja Yoga is the higher state of consciousness called
samadhi, this section is called *Samadhi Pada*. *Pada* means 'part of
a book'.

The first part of Section 2 investigates the causes of suffering
(*klesa*), and the second part describes the external practices (*bahir-
anga*) of Raja Yoga. The *sadhaka* (seeker or aspirant) is here shown
how to make a start with practice (*sadhana*) whereby he can achieve
his goals. Section 2 is called *Sadhana Pada*.

The first part of Section 3 deals with the internal practices
(*antaranga*) leading the aspirant to *samadhi*. The second part
describes the psychic powers (*siddhis*) that may be acquired. The
section is called *Vibhuti Pada*. *Vibhuti* means 'divine power'.

Section 4 deals with the philosophy and metaphysics of Yoga and
the nature of mind and consciousness. The practical aim behind the
theory is emancipation or spiritual freedom (*kaivalya*). Hence this
final section is called *Kaivalya Pada*.

THE *SUTRA* METHOD OF EXPOSITION

Indian philosophical works employ the *sutra* method of exposition –

terse, close-knit, packed so densely with meaning that a commentary on each *sutra* is necessary.

Sutra means 'thread'. The English word 'suture' and its Latin root *sutura* are linked etymologically with the Sanskrit *sutra*. The condensed statements are strung together to outline a philosophy. *Sutra* has the secondary meaning 'aphorism'. 'Just as a thread binds together a number of beads in a rosary, in the same way the under-lying continuity of idea binds together in outlining the essential aspects of a subject,' says Mr Taimini (89).

The most important characteristics of this method are utmost con-densation consistent with clear exposition of all essential aspects and continuity of the underlying theme in spite of the apparent discontin-uity of the ideas presented. The latter characteristic is worth noting because the effort to discover the hidden 'thread' of reasoning beneath the apparently unconnected ideas very often provides the clue to the meaning of many *Sutras*. It should be remembered that this method of exposition was prevalent at a time when printing was unknown and most of the important treatises had to be memorised by the student. Hence the necessity of condensation to the utmost limit. Nothing essential was, of course, left out, but everything with which the student was expected to be familiar or which he could easily infer from the context was ruthlessly cut out.

This makes for difficulty for the modern student of Yoga con-fronted by the printed text: the meaning has to be mined from the dense prose. Fortunately, commentaries are usually available. To quote Mr Taimini again (89):

We have to remember that in a treatise like the *Yoga-Sutras*, behind many a word there is a whole pattern of thought of which the word is a mere symbol. To understand the true significance of the *Sutras* we must be thoroughly familiar with these patterns. . . . Luckily for the earnest student, Yoga has always been a living Science in the East and it has had an unbroken succession of living experts who continually verify by their own experiments and experiences the basic truths of this Science. This has helped not only to keep the traditions of Yogic culture alive and pure, but to maintain the meanings of the technical words used in this Science in a fairly exact and clearly defined form.

In India the seeker has through the centuries been able to receive explanations of Patanjali's condensed exposition of the Royal Path from the mouths of the 'living experts'. Today we can obtain the necessary clarification from the printed word. Many distinguished exponents of the Yoga of Meditation have translated the *Sutras* into English and provided commentaries. Without such expansions and elucidations of the highly-contracted aphorisms we would have little chance of getting at the real meaning of the text. A difficulty is that there are no exact English equivalents for many of the Sanksrit terms; translators go as near as they can, and often cannot do other than retain the use of the original Sanskrit word.

We are using here the translation of Manilal Nabhubhai Dvivedi (22), still one of the clearest. Quotation marks are used to denote quotations from his explanatory notes, based on the famous commentary of Vyasa and others. His translation I have changed in one brief but important respect. For his 'contemplation – absorption – trance' I substitute 'concentration – contemplation – *samadhi*', the terms I have used throughout this book for the final three stages of meditation.

SECTION 1 OF THE *YOGA SUTRAS*:
STILLING THE MIND

1, 1. Now, an exposition of Yoga [is to be made].

Here, in the very first *sutra*, it is clear that Patanjali is not the originator of Yoga, which goes back many centuries before Patanjali's birth. But Patanjali is about to expound its teaching and methods. The 'Father of Yoga', as Patanjali is called, is its first systematizer. Little is known of him, and his identity is disputed by scholars. He is thought to have lived and written the *Yoga Sutras* in the third and second centuries BC.

1,2. Yoga is the suppression of the transformations of the thinking principle.

Or it could be called checking the mind's modifications. Here Raja Yoga is summed up in only a few words. Its aim and practice is stilling the mind. The Sanskrit original has only four words: *Yogas citta-vritti-nirodha*. *Citta* is the mind-stuff, *vritti* (literally 'whirlpool') the mind's movement, and *nirodhah* means 'restraint'.

This Yoga is achieved by meditation that it is not thinking about something, but the quietening of thought, reducing the waves until the surface of the mind is calm and pellucid so that the white light of pure consciousness (*Purusha*) can shine in all its clarity. Dvivedi says, 'It should be distinctly borne in mind that the thinking prin-

ciple is not the *Atman*, the *Purusha*, who is the source of all consciousness and knowledge. The suppression of the transformations
of the thinking principle does not, therefore, mean that the Yogin
is enjoined to become nil, which certainly is impossible.'

Citta manifests itself when consciousness is acted upon by matter.
Its modifications can be reduced to one, as in *sabija samadhi* or
samadhi 'with seed'. But the ultimate aim is to inhibit all transformations, in *nirbija samadhi*. The *jivatma* or individual soul then
frees itself from its entanglement in matter (*prakriti*), the substance
of the manifest world, and finds itself joined with *paramatma* or
universal soul.

1,3. Then the seer abides in himself.

'When all the *vrittis* or transformations of the thinking principle
are suppressed, there remains only the never-changing eternal seer,
Purusha, in perfect *sattva* [purity], being only the perceiver. The
ultimate fact of consciousness is itself and nothing else. This un-
alloyed bliss is the proper state of the highest Yoga called *Nirbija
Samadhi*,' says Dvivedi.

The third *sutra* tells us what happens when the mind's movements
are inhibited. The Seer is *drashta* or *drashtri*, the Witness or Looker.
The meditator knows his essential nature. This, in short, is Self-
realization. We are talking about the Self that is beyond the empirical
ego; the latter is the public and private self mainly constructed by
parents and society. The pure Self, our essential nature, is there all
the time waiting to be uncovered. There is a profound mystery here.
For we have already reached our goal if we but knew it. The Yogi
works through Time to reach a goal which is the discovery that at the
core of his being he was on the plane of the Timeless all along.

1, 4. But otherwise [he] becomes assimilated with transformations.

We should endeavour not to be caught up in the mind's agitation
and movement, which prevents us knowing our real nature. The
Buddhists call it 'Buddha nature' or 'Buddha mind', because it was
this the Buddha uncovered when he meditated beneath a *bodhi* tree.

1, 5. The transformations are five fold, and painful or not-painful.

Even the pleasurable states of mind are disruptive. The discerning
Yogin notes that desire for pleasure holds the seeds of pain. The next
sutra lists the five transformations of the mind.

1, 6. [They are] right knowledge, wrong knowledge, fancy, sleep and
memory.

The following five *sutras* describe these transformations:

1, 7. Right knowledge [is] direct cognition or inference or testimony.

1, 8. Wrong knowledge is false conception of a thing whose real form does not correspond to that conception.

'A post mistaken for a man,' says Dvivedi. Or a coiled rope mistaken for a snake.

1, 9. Fancy is the notion called into being by mere words, having nothing to answer to it in reality.

1, 10. That transformation which has nothing for its basis is sleep.

Sleep is a transformation, but *samadhi* is 'pure cessation of all transformations'.

1, 11. Memory is the not-allowing a thing cognised to escape.

1, 12. Its suppression is secured by application and non-attachment.

'Its' refers to transformations of the thinking principle. Non-attachment is called *vairagya*. Application means meditation. 'That which attracts the mind and makes it assume various forms as passions, emotions, sensations, etc., is nothing but *raga*, attachment; and *vairagya*, therefore, is . . . the absence of all attachment,' says Dvivedi.

1, 13. Application is the effort towards the state.

Dvivedi comments that ' *Sthiti* or "state" is that state in which the thinking principle, as it were, stands, unmoved and unmodified, like the jet of a lamp in a place not exposed to the wind. The steady, sustained effort to attain this *Sthiti* is called application.'

1, 14. It becomes a position of firmness, being practised for a long time, without intermission, and with perfect devotion.

The point is that the mind comes at an advanced stage to a position in which, though apparently performing the ordinary functions of life, it is really at rest.'

1, 15. The consciousness of having mastered [every desire] in the case of one who does not thirst for objects perceptible or scriptural, is non-attachment.

Dvivedi comments that 'it is only when the mind reaches this condition of freedom from attachment, that true knowledge begins to dawn upon it, as right reflection in a mirror cleared of dirt.' Non-attachment should not be equated (though it often is) with feelings of indifference or coldness.

1, 16. That is the highest, wherein, from being the *Purusha*, there is entire cessation of any, the least, desire for the *Gunas*.

Purusha and the *gunas* were dealt with in an earlier chapter. *Purusha* is pure consciousness, spirit, or soul. The *gunas* are the three inherent qualities of *Prakriti*, which is primordial matter. They are *tamas* or inertia, *rajas* or activity, and *sattva*, which may be translated as rhythm, orderliness, or purity. 'This kind of *vairagya* is called *para* or the highest, as distinguished from the former which is only *apara* or lower,' says the commentary.

SECTION 1 OF THE *YOGA SUTRAS*: *SAMADHI*

Patanjali now goes on to describe *samadhi*, the goal of meditation. The practical work of stilling the mind to trigger this superconscious state is left until Sections 2 and 3. *Samadhi* is higher consciousness, the final stage of meditation. It has itself several stages or qualities, progressively finer. In Yogic meditation the attention drops like a pebble towards the sea- or river-bed of consciousness. A better simile, perhaps, would be produced by reversing the movement: a cork released from the sea- or river-bed and floating upwards to break the surface and meet air and sun.

In dealing with the stages of *samadhi* we are on very subtle psychological territory in which the distinction is made (1, 17 and 1, 18) between *samprajnata samadhi* and *asamprajnata samadhi*.

1, 17. Conscious [*samprajnata samadhi*] is that which is attended by argumentation, deliberation, joy, and the sense of being.

'Though the mind is free from transformations, still it is conscious of that which it identifies itself with, and hence this *Samadhi* is called conscious (*Samprajnata*),' says the commentary.

1, 18 The other is that which consists only of *Samskaras*, being brought on by the practice of the cause of complete suspension.

This is *asamprajnata samadhi*. The prefix *a* means 'not'. *Samskaras* are mental impressions traced by past experiences. *Pra* means 'higher', and *jna* means 'knowledge'. *Prajna* is variously translated as 'intelligence', 'wisdom', 'consciousness', and 'higher consciousness'.

I.K. Taimini says that *Prajna* is 'the higher consciousness working through the mind in all its stages'. He makes a distinction between the *samprajnata samadhi* and *asamprajnata samadhi* and the *sabjia samadhi* and *nirbija saamdhi* (*samadhi* 'with seed' and 'without seed', respectively) described by Patanjali towards the end of Section 1. Other commentators use the two sets of terms interchangeably. The difference for Mr Taimini is that he sees the first pair as alternating stages, and the final pair as the culmination of a process which he likens to an aeroplane passing in and out of cloud and finally emerging from the last cloud in the sky into clear air and light, which is consciousness of *Purusha*. This is achieved by breaking through progressively subtler vehicles and planes of consciousness. 'The recession of consciousness towards its center is thus not a steady and uninterrupted sinking into greater and greater depths but consists in this alternate outward and inward movement of consciousness at each barrier separating two planes,' (89) he says.

In the Transcendental Meditation taught by Maharishi Mahesh Yogi progress is made similarly by a succession of 'drops' into consciousness, which the Maharishi calls (146) 'turning the attention inwards towards the subtler levels of a thought until the mind transcends the experience of the subtlest state of the thought and arrives at the source of the thought'.

Dr Behanan (6) defines *samprajnata samadhi* as 'the stage of trance-contemplation in which the subject is conscious of the object of concentration,' and *asamprajnata samadhi* as 'the stage of trance- contemplation in which the subject is not conscious of the object of concentration.' Professor Wood describes the former as 'the kind of *samadhi* which has an objective *bhumi*' (ground or object of meditation and the latter as 'the superior kind of *samadhi*, in which the contemplation has no objective ground.'

Conscious (*samprajnata samadhi*) can be divided into four stages: *savitarka*, *nirvitarka*, *savicara*, and *nirvicara*. Here, Dr Behanan (6) gives the clearest account.

Since *samadhi* is the last of the right stages and the goal towards which all efforts are directed, it is important to understand the nature of the yogin's experiences in this condition. Even here several grades are said to exist and the one quality which characterizes them all is the relative or total loss of subject-object awareness. That state in which the mind is one with the object (*artha*), together with the concept (*jnana*) and the name (*sabda*), called *savitarka*, is the lowest kind of *samadhi*. The object remains gross because it is identified with concept and name. In short, the associations formed in our waking life still persist.

The next stage of *samadhi*, *nirvitarka*, is a grade higher than the above, in that the associations of name and concept are dropped off. The object is just the object without predicate relations. In the *savicara prajna*, the grossness of the object is no longer felt; its place is taken by the subtle constituents of matter (*tanmatras*). Perception, if one may call it such, is determinate because the *tanmatras* are subject to time, space and casuality. In the fourth kind of *samadhi*, *nirvicara*, the *tanmatras* are finally dispossessed of the conceptual notions of time, etc.

These four stages are also called conscious-*samadhi* (*samprajnata-samadhi*), because there is, though only vaguely, a union between the subject and the object; the object is, so to say, still there. The *buddhi* continues to function as long as the object remains and the feeling of personality, accompanied by deliberation (*vitarka*), reflection (*vicara*), and joy (*ananda*), persists.

But the yogin's aim is to surpass the *citta* stage entirely: This condition is reached in the *superconscious-samadhi* (*asamprajnata-samadhi*), *Prakriti* (nature), through *citta*, does not bind the *purusha* any more, the sense of personality and the resultant joy are no longer experienced. The ultimate truth dawns on the yogin and the *purusha* abides in itself.

The stages of *samadhi*, which should not be identified with the unconsciousness of dreamless sleep or coma, are described by Patanjali later in Section 1:

1, 41. In the case of one the transformations of whose mind have been annihilated, there is entire identity with, and complete absorption in, the cogniser, the cognition, and the cognised, like a transparent jewel.

Meditator, the object, and the process of contemplation have fused.

1, 42. The argumentative condition [of the concentrated mind] is that which is mixed with thoughts of word, meaning and understanding.

The commentary says: ' This and the following *Sutra* refer to the *Sthula* or gross division of *Samprajnara Samadhi*. . . . When the mind apprehends a word and meditates upon its meaning and form, as also upon the understanding of either . . . it is called *Savitarka Samadhi* we are still holding in mind the name (*sabda*) and the normal conceptual associations.'

1, 43. Non-argumentative is that in which the meaning alone is present as if quite unlike itself, or memory being dissolved.

This is *nirvitarka samadhi*, the next grade up, in which word and understanding have been dropped.

1, 44. By these, the deliberative and non-deliberative having reference to the subtle elements are also explained.

The 'subtle elements' are the *tanmatras*.

1, 45. The province of the subtle ends with the indissoluble.

1, 46. These constitute seeded-meditation.

'Inasmuch as there is consciousness in this kind of *Samadhi* it is called seeded, for there is the seed which, on waking, may grow into various distractions from the condition of *Samadhi*'.

1, 47. The purity of the non-deliberative being reached, internal contentment follows.

'The last stage of *Samadhi* develops a sense of complete intellectuality, or complete absorption in the soul. . . . This is called *Adhyatmaprasada*. The qualities of *rajas* and *tamas* being entirely annihilated, so to speak, and *sattva* alone remaining . . . it is possible to experience the bliss consequent upon true recognition of the *Purusha*,' says the commentary.

1, 48. The intellect is there truth-bearing.

1, 49. Its subject is different from that of revelation and inference, for it refers to particulars.

1, 50. The impression thereof stands in the way of other impressions.

Dvivedi comments: 'We know that the last truth impressed on the mind is none other than blissful cognition of the *Purusha*. The mind ceases to transform itself into anything besides this impression.'

1, 51. The prevention of that even, leads to the prevention of all, and thus to meditation without seed.

Even the impression of having uncovered the *Purusha* is a seed (*bijas*). When even this fades away, *samadhi* with seed (*sabija*) gives way to *samadhi* without seed (*nirbija*), in which there is only pure consciousness'

Swami Vivekananda (171) describes the two stages with characteristic eloquence:

You remember that our goal is to perceive the Soul itself. We cannot perceive the Soul because it has got mingled up with nature, with the mind, with the body. The ignorant man thinks his body is the Soul. The learned man thinks his mind is the Soul; but both of them are mistaken. What makes the Soul get mingled up with all this? Different waves in the *Citta* rise and cover the Soul; we only see a little reflection of the Soul through these waves. So, if the wave is one of anger, we see the Soul as angry; 'I am angry,' one says. If it is one of love, we see ourselves reflected in that wave, and say we are loving. If that wave is one of weakness, and the Soul is reflected in it, we think we are weak. These various ideas come from these impressions, these *Samskaras* covering the Soul. The real nature of the Soul is not perceived as long as there is one single wave in the lake of the *Citta*; this real nature will never be perceived until all the waves have subsided; so, first, Patanjali teaches us the meaning of these waves; secondly, the best way to repress them; and thirdly, how to make one wave so strong as to suppress all other waves, fire eating fire as it were. When only one remains, it will be easy to suppress that also; and when that is gone, this *samadhi* or concentration is called seedless. It leaves nothing, and the Soul is manifested just as It is, in Its own glory.

Soul is of course *Purusha*. Later (in his *Raja Yoga*) (171) Vivekananda says:

in this first state of *samadhi* (*samadhi* with seed) the modifications of the mind have been controlled, but not perfectly, because if they were, there would be no modification. If there is a modification which impels the mind to rush out through the senses, and the Yogi tries to control it, that very control itself will be a modification. One wave will be checked by another wave, so it will not be real *samadhi*, in which all the waves subside, as control itself will be a wave. Yet this lower *samadhi* is very much nearer to the higher *samadhi* than when the mind comes bubbling out.

A similar distinction is made in Zen Buddhism, where you have the stages of 'present-heart' (*ushin*) and no-heart' (*mushin*), heart here meaning consciousness. As an old Zen poem puts it: 'Being mindful of not-thinking is thinking nevertheless. O that I were now beyond thinking and non-thinking.' This sums up the difficulty and the final stage of Yogic meditation when concentration sustained into contemplation moves beyond thinking and non-thinking into *samadhi*.

SECTIONS 2 AND 3 OF THE *YOGA SUTRAS*
THE EIGHT LIMBS OF YOGA

Having described the goal of Yoga meditation in Section 1, Patanjali turns in Section 2 to the disciplines that bring it about. He describes eight limbs (*angas*) making up the eightfold path of Raja Yoga. Raja means 'king'. The stages of this Royal Way are:

i.   Abstinences (*yamas*)
ii.   Observances (*niyamas*)
iii.   Postures (*asanas*)
iv.   Breath control (*pranayama*)
v   Sense withdrawal (*pratyahara*)
vi   Concentration (*dharana*)
vii.   Contemplation (*dhyana*)
viii.   Self-realization (*samadhi*)

The first two limbs are rules of conduct, ethical disciplines that ensure the Yogin is approaching the serious business of Self-realization in a suitable frame of mind. On an ethical plane they provide the purification that is essential preparatory training in Yoga.

There is a sense, however, in which Patanjali is here putting effect before cause and the cart, as it were, before the horse. Yogic morality reaches its full flowering in the Self-realized person. The same thing is true of the Eastern 'ways of liberation' in general. In Zen Buddhism, for instance, Christians are perplexed to find little or nothing in the way of ethical do's and don'ts. This is because the Zen masters know that the Zen experience, attained through meditation and other disciplines, will transform the personality of the aspirant, who will then, naturally, as a fully-realized human being, become compassionate, loving, calm, joyous, honest, truthful, and so on. Patanjali, too, was probably aware of the difficulties of being ethical by an effort of will on a lower plane of consciousness than the advanced Yogin can achieve, but felt that the attempt would do some good in creating a right attitude in the neophyte and in refining thought and emotion to some extent.

Stages 3 to 8 follow in natural order. One sits steadily in a Yogic posture (*asana*) of meditation which holds the back erect. One breathes quietly and evenly (*pranayama*). One withdraws the senses from their external objects and turns the attention inwards (*pratya-hara*). An object of concentration is then held steadily by the mind (*dharana*), sustained into the free-flowing attention that is contemplation (*dhyana*). The final stage of Self-realization (*samadhi*) was dealt with in the last section; in this we will examine the preceding seven limbs.

The Five Abstinences (*Yamas*)

2, 30. Forbearance consists in abstaining from killing, falsehood, theft, incontinence, and greediness.

These five moral qualities go much deeper than just not-doing, and can be expressed as positives instead of negatives: non-violence, truthfulness, non-stealing, continence, and non-covetousness.

Non-violence (*ahimsa*) is not just avoiding killing, violence, and injury, but means also a positive compassion for all sentient creatures. It means avoiding anger and violent thoughts, and being gentle of mind. Where there is violence there is usually fear behind it. The practices of Yoga make for non-fear (*abhaya*) and for non-anger (*akrodha*).

Non-violence was the favourite precept of Mahatma Gandhi, who said of it:

> *Ahimsa* is not merely a negative state of harmlessness but it is a positive state of love, of doing good even to the evil-doer. But it does not mean meek submission to the will of the evil-doer: it means the putting of one's whole soul against his will. Working under this law of our being, it is possible for a single individual to defy the whole might of an unjust empire, to save his honour, his religion, his soul, and lay the foundation for that empire's fall or its regeneration.

In Indian folk-lore many stories are told of wild animals becoming gentle in the presence of a Yogi. Patanjali says: 'Near him in whom non-violence has fully taken root, all beings renounce enmity.'

Truthfulness (*satya*) has a deeper meaning than not telling lies. It means that our attitude to others should be marked by sincerity, integrity, and authenticity, to use a term loved by existentialists. There is also the deeper dimension expressed in the saying: 'Truth is God, God is Truth.'

Non-stealing (*asteya*) extends beyond physical objects to the psychological sphere – taking undeserved credit, for example.

Continence (*brahmacharya*) refers at one level to the austerity expected of the Hindu undertaking advanced Yoga practice. His *guru* commands chastity because of respect for the sexual energies which can be harnessed for spiritual ends. Sensual excitement would waste energy and distract the mind from its concentration and goals. Chastity is not, however, expected of the married 'householder Yogin', but continence would apply in a wider dimension of non-attachment to sensual pleasures – which does not mean trying not to enjoy a walk in pleasant surroundings or a cool drink on a hot day, but an attitude of not clinging to pleasures and not craving for their repetition. Think of a mirror, which receives but does not grasp.

Non-possessiveness (*aparigraha*) means not the absence of all possessions, but not clinging to them or craving unnecessary things. At the same time the Yogin is expected to reduce his possessions to a reasonable simplicity. This rule counters the Western mania for accumulating wealth and possessions, both seen as marks of prestige and identified with success in life. The Yogin has a very different concept of what constitutes the main goals of life.

The Five Observances (*Niyamas*)

2, 32. Observances consist in purity, contentment, mortification, study, and resignation to *Isvara.*

I prefer 'austerity' to 'mortification' in translating the third observance.

Purity (*saucha*) means both bodily and moral purification. Purification is much in evidence in Yogic practice. The breath controls, postures, hygienic processes, and dietary rules described in *Yoga of Breathing* all contribute to psychophysical purity, whereby body and mind are prepared for the progressive refinement of consciousness that is the Yoga of Meditation. Yogins are instructed to change the quality of their body cells by eating *sattvic* foods, and *sattva* is the *guna* which predominates in pure consciousness. Internal (ethical) purity is obtained by obeying the abstinences and observances.

Contentment (*santosha*) is cultivation of calmness and equanimity of mind. In this the immobile postures (*asanas*) and smooth, rhythmic breath controls (*pranayama*) are helpful. All the Yogic disciplines foster contentment and those qualities of character that so impressed William James in persons who had been practising Yoga for some time. Peace of mind comes, the Yoga masters say, when body and mind are kept pure. Yogins should be cheerful and uncomplaining – *tush*, the root from which *santosha* comes, means 'to be pleased'.

Austerity (*tapas*) refers to strength of character and to resolute pursuit of Yoga's goal of union of Self (*Atman*) and *Brahman*. The word *tapas* means purification by burning, which is often mistaken as self-mortification. This observance sometimes leads to fasting, a meagre diet, and other forms of asceticism. A moderate austerity trains the will and develops body and mind for the highest Yogic practice, but the *Bhagavad Gita* and the most respected Yoga masters warn against excessive asceticism and self-mortification.

In discourse 17, 5–6 of the *Gita* Lord Krishna says: 'Those men who practise terrific austerities (*ghara tapas*) . . . weakening all the elements in the body – fools they are – and Me who dwell in the body within; know thou these to be of demoniac resolves.'

Study (*svadhyaya*) includes reading the *upanishads*, the *Bhagavad Gita*, and the most highly-regarded literature of Yoga, and deep reflection on what is read. It also includes self-study, the stripping away of the 'not-I' selves described in the chapter on Jnana Yoga.

Resignation to *Isvara* (*Isvara Pranidhana*) is resignation to God, *Brahman*, That, It, Tao, or whatever title you wish to give the

Absolute. Nature, if you wish, which we are *of* and not just *in*. The observance can be taken as advice to let go, to stop clinging to the ego – a source of frustration, dissatisfaction, and tension – and to trust in the Self that is at the centre of wholeness of being. The ego thinks it is in charge and has an inflated concept of its own importance. Modern psychology has revealed to us the great regions of the psyche below the surface of consciousness, and C. G. Jung used the term Self over and above the ego for the organizer and integrator of the total psyche, of which the conscious part in which the ego operates is but a small part.

Isvara, the Supreme Being, is probably a later interpolation into Patanjali's *Yoga Sutras*, in which he sits uneasily as a model *Purusha*, an inspiration, and a recipient of devotion. The ego is melted by the fire of devotion (Bhakti Yoga), just as in Jnana Yoga it is whittled away by the well-honed intellect and in Raja Yoga dissolved by stilling the mind's agitation and modifications. In Christian language *Isvara pranidhana* is 'Not my will but Thy Will be done', 'Love God and do what you like', and losing your soul to find it. In Taoist language it is floating with the flow of life and Nature, the Tao.

The differing functions of the two aspects of Yogic ethical training are cogently summed up by I. K. Taimini (89) : 'The practices included in *Yama* are, in a general way, moral and prohibitive while those in *Niyama* are disciplinal and constructive. The former aim at laying the ethical foundation of the Yogic life and latter at organizing the life of the *Sadhaka* for the highly strenuous Yogic discipline which is to follow.'

Postures (*Asanas*)

2, 46. Posture is that which is steady and easy.

The *asanas* in Raja Yoga are the seated meditative postures, whereas in Hatha Yoga the whole organism receives attention from a wide range of posturing, improving suppleness and flexibility, toning the nervous system and the glands, purifying the bloodstream and firming and strengthening the muscles, in a system unrivalled in its completeness and effectiveness for these purposes. In *Yoga of Posture* over four hundred *asanas* are described.

Patanjali has here in mind only a few of the most stable sitting postures. The aim is to keep the body steady and the back straight, the chin held level and the head poised easily in line with the spine. This stage was described earlier in the chapter entitled 'Sitting for Meditation'.

The aim of meditative posture is not to focus attention on the body, but, on the contrary, to enable the meditator to forget about the body and to give his total attention to quietening the mind. Hence Patanjali continues:

2, 47. By mild effort and meditation on the endless.

To make sense, this *sutra* has to be joined with 2, 46. Thus: 'By poised effort and meditation on the infinite posture is steady and easy.'

Patanjali goes on to say that by mastering posture the Yogin is made free from assaults from the pairs of opposites. These are both bodily and mental: heat and cold is an example of the former, and joy and sorrow of the latter.

Breath Control (*Pranayama*)

2, 49. This being [accomplished], *pranayama* [follows] – the cutting off of the course of inspiration and expiration [of the breath].

This should not be taken literally. Suspension of breathing (*kumbhaka*) is a part of *pranayama*, as discussed and described in the large section given to Yogic breath regulation in *Yoga of Breathing*, and of the arousal of *kundalini* energy, but as far as meditation is concerned what is required is reducing the breathing to such smoothness and quietness that it is made as unobtrusive as the immobile and 'invisible' body.

Another feature prominent in Hatha Yoga thinking should also be pointed out. *Prana* is the life force, considered to be potent in the air we breathe. It is also the connecting link between matter and mind. I. K. Taimini (89) writes: '*Prana*, which exists on all the planes of manifestation, is the connecting link between matter and energy on the one hand and consciousness and mind on the other. Consciousness expressing itself through the mind cannot come into touch with matter and function through it without the intermediate presence of *Prana*.' Swami Vivekananda, a much earlier interpreter of Yoga to the West, put it (171): 'In this body of ours the breath motion is the "silken thread"; by laying hold of and learning to control it we grasp the pack thread of the nerve currents, and from these the stout twine of our thoughts, and lastly the rope of *Prana*, controlling which we reach freedom.'

Pranayama prepares the mind for meditation. It conduces to calming the mind-stuff (*citta*). The word itself indicates that it is restraint (*yama*) of *prana*, the life-force. Negative and positive *pranic* currents in the body are equalized and channelled in Hatha Yoga practice. Patanjali says that *pranayama* produces two positive results:

2, 52. Thence is destroyed the covering of light.

This does not mean that *Purusha* is uncovered – otherwise what need would there be for the remaining four stages? It is a reference to the '*tattvic lights*', the luminosity of the energy channels of the subtle body (*see* the chapter on Kundalini Yoga). That *Purusha* is not referred to is revealed by the following *sutra :*

2, 53. The mind becomes fit for concentration.

Pranayama, in common with the preceding stages, prepares the mind for concentration (*dharana*), contemplation (*dhyana*), and Self-realization (*samadhi*), which are the internal meditative techniques whereby the light of *Purusha* really is uncovered.

But first there is the initial process of turning inwards, called *pratyahara*.

Sense Withdrawal (*Pratyahara*)

2, 54. Sense-withdrawal is, as it were, the imitating by the senses of the thinking principle, by withdrawing themselves from their objects.

2, 55. There follows the greatest mastery over the senses.

Vivekananda (171) is clearer here: '2, 54. When the senses have withdrawn from their objects and transmuted themselves into the modes of consciousness, this is called "the Withdrawal", *Pratyahara*.' And the *Vishnu Purana* expands this a little: 'The adept in yoga gives himself up to "Withdrawal" and stops the traffic of the senses with their objects which are word, sight, etc., to which they invariably attached. He then makes his senses work for his Consciousness and the ever-agitated senses are controlled. No yogi can achieve the aim of yoga without controlling the senses.'

Two groups of sense-distractions have already been removed – those resulting from poor posture and from uneven breathing. We did this by making the body posture stable and at ease, and by regulating the breathing so that it flows smoothly and rhythmically.

Pratyahara is the initial process of turning the attention inwards, of inhibiting the reception of the bombardment by a myriad sense impressions to which we are at every moment subjected. This withdrawal of attention from external objects affects all the senses. Unless an object before one is being used for visual attention, the eyes should be closed. The sense responses of the skin, ears, nose, and tongue should also be closed down, as though by turning down the volume of a radio – though the analogy applies to only one sense, whereas all the senses should be shutting down to some degree in *pratyahara*. The sensations of sight, touch, hearing, smell, and taste are quelled. This requires practice, but as the days go by you will become more proficient in shutting out the external world.

A considerable amount of inhibition of external stimuli goes on automatically – otherwise our nervous systems would be so overloaded that they would collapse and suffer a total shut-down. A kind of inbuilt filtering valve has evolved which lets through to consciousness only those sense stimuli that are of interest and value to us. The function of the filtering valve is to preserve the individual and the human species as a whole. However, though this filtering goes on continually, unless you have already had experience of meditation in the Eastern style you will find it strange at first to withdraw into yourself as completely as you do in *Pratyahara*.

Now one problem immediately faced in Yoga meditation is that when we turn the attention inwards, having drawn it back from what is going on externally, we discover the unaccustomed world of what is going on *internally* – strange internal movements to do with physiological processes, little tensions and itchings, gurgles in the stomach, and so on. And, strangest of all, we find that our heads seem filled with unruly thoughts – some old Yoga texts refer to a cage full of excited monkeys. We have to learn to reduce and quieten these turbulent thoughts, which parade through the mind, dispute, and play, quite without invitation. Fortunately, we have the aid of a powerful technique in this work of stilling the mind's turbulence. It is Yogic concentration or *dharana*.

Concentration (*Dharana*)
Patanjali ends Section 2 of the *Yoga Sutras* with sense-withdrawal (*pratyahara*), and opens Section 3, called *Vibhuti Pada* (*vibhuti* means 'divine power'), with concentration (dharana). In fact, the first three *sutras* of Section 3 summarize concisely the nature of the final three stages of meditation in Raja Yoga.

3, 1. Concentration is the fixing of the mind on something.

It is best if the object selected for concentration is something fixed and unchanging – or at least appears to be, for science tells us that everything is in a state of movement and change. It may be a rose, a candle flame, the space between the eyebrows, a piece of broken glass, a tree on the horizon, or one of a million or more other objects. It may be a diagram drawn for the purpose of meditation (a *yantra*); or, if we employ the ears instead of the eyes to focus attention, it may be a voiced word or phrase held to have special meaning in this respect (a *mantra*), which may be spoken inwardly rather than aloud. It is possible for other senses – touch, for example – to provide the means whereby the field of consciousness can be narrowed. One can also narrow thought to a single thought.

In early training a small fixed object a few feet away, on which the gaze can rest, makes a good focus for concentration. After a few weeks, the eyes can be closed and the object held before the minds' eye.

Whatever the object chosen, the beam of attention should finally be held unwavering. If the mind wanders from its limited field of attention, it should be gently brought back, coaxed rather than dragged.

An analogy may be made with the spotlight which picks out, for the audience's attention, the movements of performers on a theatre stage. The stage is the area of the spotlight's beam of attention, and over this limited range it is free to roam.

We must keep the beam of our attention within a small area. Eventually the quality of the flow of attention changes and concentration gives way to a higher stage – contemplation (*dhyana*).

Contemplation (*Dhyana*)

3, 2. The unity of the mind with it is contemplation

'It' is the object of concentration. 'Absorption or *dhyana* is the entire fixing of the mind on the object thought of, to the extent of making it one with it. In fact the mind should, at the time, be conscious only of itself and the object,' says Drivedi.

Now the spotlight has stopped its slight movement up and down and from side to side and fixes unwavering on one point. If one sits immobile, quietly breathing, retracts the senses, and concentrates the mind on a restricted field, eventually the attention may be held steady without distraction or interruption. This is the stage of contemplation or *dhyana*, the penultimate of Patanjali's eight limbs of Yoga. A state of mental poise is sustained in an effortless flow. Now the meditator is close to breaking through to a new mode of consciousness. There is a change of quality from gross to subtle.

Self-realization (*samadhi*)

3, 3. The same, when conscious only of the object, as if unconscious of itself, is *samadhi*.

That is, the first stage of *samadhi*: consciousness, with seed. In the advanced stage of *samadhi* without seed, the meditator, the thing meditated upon, and the process of meditation are merged and become one, and consciousness is fully integrated.

3, 4. The three together constitute *Samyama*.

Samyama is the name given to the final three stages of meditation – *dharana*, *dhyana*, and *samadhi* – when practised successively with one and the same object.

3, 7. The three are more intimate than the others.

The internal stages of concentration, contemplation, and Self-realization are more intimate than the external stages that go before.

3, 8. Even it is foreign to the unconscious.

Even *samyama* is preparatory to seedless *samadhi*.

YOGIC METHODS OF MEDITATION

The techniques of Yoga meditation are more varied than those of the other esoteric psychologies. They may incorporate difficult and possibly dangerous psycho-physiological controls, as in Kundalini Yoga. They may require mastery over breath and muscle, as in Hatha Yoga. They may harness the energy of the libido, utilizing sex either directly or indirectly as a way to mystical experience, as in Tantric Yoga. They may be powerfully imaginative, as in Tibetan Yoga. They may make use of the vibratory power of human speech, as in Mantra Yoga, or the magico-occult power of design and form, as in Yantra Yoga. When the power of analytical reason is used to cut away layer upon layer of 'not-I' material that has accrued from parental and social conditioning to uncover the pure naked Self, then that is Jnana Yoga. There is concentration of the heart, of devotion, in Bhakti Yoga, and of action, work, and service in Karma Yoga. Patanjali's Raja Yoga, the 'Royal Way', emphasizes 'one-pointing' the mind and stilling thought. Some techniques are given in other chapters, and a few helpful concentrative methods will be described here.

Claudio Naranjo, in his study of contemplative exercises among the traditional disciplines (156), distinguishes between two types of meditation: 'concentrative' and 'opening-up'. The 'opening-up'

method is mostly found in use in Buddhist schools. Yoga mainly
utilizes concentrative exercises, and Patanjali's famous treatise, as
we have seen, teaches that awareness is to be focused on a fixed
point and the mind made steady. This is called concentration or
dharana.

VI   Techniques of Concentrative Meditation

CONCENTRATION (*DHARANA*)

Concentration (*dharana*) is the only one of the last three stages of Patanjali's Raja Yoga that comes under any measure of conscious control, and that, as was explained in describing the right attitude for meditation in the chapter on sitting for meditation, need only extend to the initial impulse that focuses the attention on the chosen spot. We may compare this with the impulses with which a great singer launches a note, which is then sustained and supported by the stream of breath and the diaphragm and some other body muscles. Or, to use different anologies, we may think of the skater's glide over the ice or the divers' leap from the springboard. The deeper stages of contemplation and Self- realization come to us by a kind of grace, provided the right quality of attention has been put into flow. They are not something that can be performed or willed. Start thinking 'I will do this' or 'I will do that' and you are right back where you started from, with thought, a buzzing active mind.

Concentration is preceded by sense-withdrawal (*pratyahara*). As a tortoise might withdraw its head into its shell, so you pull in the attention from external sense objects. Internal sounds and sensations take the place of external stimuli – such unfamiliar stimuli as itchings, tinglings, audible gurglings, the thump-thump of the beating heart, the passage of air in the nostrils and trachea. From these stimuli, too, you should withdraw.

The technique of *pratyahara* is as well known to the Christian mystic as to the Hindu Yogin. This is how Meister Eckhart (128) describes it:

The best and utmost of attainment in this life is to remain still and let

God act and speak in thee. When the powers have all been withdrawn from their bodily forms and functions, then is this word spoken. Thus he says: 'In the midst of the silence the secret word was spoken to me.' The more completely thou art able to in-draw thy faculties and to forget those things and their images which thou hast taken in, the more, that is to say, thou forgettest the creature, the nearer thou art to this and the more susceptible thou art to it.

Here the soul is scattered abroad among her powers and dissipated in the act of each: the power of seeing is in the eye, the power of hearing in the ear, the power of tasting in the tongue, and her powers are accordingly enfeebled in their interior work, scattered forces being imperfect. It follows that for her interior work to be effective, she must call in all her powers, recollecting them out of external things to one interior act.

To achieve the interior act one must assemble all one's powers as it were into one corner of one's soul, where, secreted from images and forms, one is able to work. In this silence, this quiet, the Word is heard.

In concentrative meditation the attention is fixed on one thing. If the beam chases after a sound or a thought, bring it back gently to rest on the meditation-object. When unbidden thoughts appear, check the kind of chain reaction, based on association, that could lead to several minutes of involuntary reverie. It can be appreciated that concentrative meditation is valuable training on a practical level, bringing a steady flow of attention to bear on work and life's activities in general. The mental faculty of concentration strengthens with practice. 'Genius is concentration,' Schiller said.

Dharana is restricting the attention to one point. It is concentration without tension. No clenching of fists, no biting of the lower lip, no knitting of the brow. The meditating Yogi should give the appearance of relaved serenity. Yet he is giving all of himself to concentrative meditation – a whole person wholly attending. There is no thought of results. We have already discussed the right attitude to take for meditation in the preceding chapter.

In popular usage concentration means applying discursive reasoning to a chosen subject, excluding all irrelevant thoughts and painstakingly working with relevant thoughts. The field of attention becomes a small circle, but within that circle thought is busily engaged. Yogic concentration (*dharana*) is a very different matter, for it reduces a stream of thought to one thought, the object of attention, and there holds it unwavering. The object of attention is unimportant, and may be the most trivial of things. It is not that the single thought-track in the mind-stuff (*citta*) is so important that all other thoughts must be kept away, but that the method of holding a single percept in the mind is being used to still thought entirely. When sustained effortlessly, like a great singer's soft head-note floating on the breath, that single furrow across the mind's calm fades away like the grin on the face of the Cheshire cat in *Alice in Wonderland*. At a press conference in London I heard Maharishi Mahesh Yogi describe the technique as 'using a thorn to remove a thorn from one's flesh.'

Some writers on Yoga give preliminary exercises in which the meditator thinks about all aspects of the meditation object until he has exhausted all possible lines of thought about it. He then goes on to hold the mind steady. Thinking about and around a subject is the common Western concept of concentration – we do quite enough of it, and my view is that even the beginner should go direct to holding the attention steady, which is *dharana* proper.

Dr Kovoor T. Behanan, who undertook training in India with a famous teacher in order to make a scientific evaluation of Yoga, says (6):

Another road open to the yogin to achieve his special goal is that of concentration, where attention is focused on a point. If a flower is chosen as the object of concentration, there is no consideration of its size, weight, or any other qualities whatsoever; it is mentally reduced to a point and kept before the mind as a mere idea. Any thought about the qualities or relations of objects only leads to a perpetual succession of ideas and this is precisely what the yogin wants to avoid. However barren this kind of focusing of the attention may seem, yogins claim that one-pointed concentration is dynamic enough to reach deeper levels of consciousness.'

STEADY GAZE MEDITATION

Trataka or gazing steadily at an object is one of the six purifying processes of Hatha Yoga, having the purpose of 'clearing the vision'. As a cleansing exercise the gaze is prolonged, without staring, but also without blinking, until the eyes begin to water. The eyes do not move and the gaze remains fixed on one point. Clairvoyance is one of the psychic powers said to result from the practice. Here, however, we are concerned with fixed gazing as a technique of of meditation and not as a hygiene for the eyes – though such meditation can be looked upon as a hygiene for the mind.

In visual concentrative meditation one should not gaze until the eyes water or become sore. Blink naturally when necessary, and as soon as the eyes tire close them and hold the image of the concent-ration-object before the mind's eye. Later you will have the ability to produce it at will by visualization.

A small object is preferable to a large one, though a small part of a larger object may be selected and, of course, large objects become small objects to the gaze when they are at a distance. A leaf on a tree may be the focus of attention, or the tree itself if it is on a distant horizon. Out of doors, the concentration-object may be a tulip or a daisy, a stone, a pebble, a clod, a piece of broken bottle – anything on on which the gaze can be fixed. Indoors, it may be an apple, a rose in a vase, the vase itself, a cross, a crust of bread, or a leaf on a bush in the garden visible beyond the window of the room you are meditating in. A picture may provide numerous points of interest, one of which should be selected. Hindus sometimes concentrate on a picture of a revered *guru*, saint, or diety. When gazing at a portrait, it is custom-ary to focus the gaze on the space between the eyebrows or on the person depicted. A steady candle flame in a darkened room is some-times suggested, both for *trataka* and for concentrative meditation. It is an apt choice, for four reasons. First, in the *Gita* we find:

6,19 'As a lamp in a sheltered spot does not flicker', — this has been thought, as the simile of a Yogin of subdued thought, practising Yoga in the Self.

Second, light is associated with mystical enlightenment. Third, the eyes are drawn to a bright point. Fourth, the bright image is easily retained as an after-image when the eyes are closed.

For some or all of the reasons just given, bright objects – a silver coin, the glint of sunlight on water or rock – have a strong appeal for many meditators. The seventeenth-century Christian mystic Jacob Boehme achieved enlightenment on gazing upon his cobbler's crystal as it reflected bright sunlight.

But points on which to focus the gaze are for all practical purposes limitless – and (again for practical purposes) the concentration-object can be as mundane as an old bath plug or a rusty can. However, it is understandable that for regular use meditators often select a religous symbol or an object that has either intrinsic beauty or associations with tranquillity.

There are obvious advantages in focusing on an object that is available at any time: hence the frequent mention in classic texts of tip of the nose, the space between the eyebrows (for the inner gaze), and the navel. However, in commenting on verse 13 of discourse 6 of the *Bhagavad Gita* in the chapter on sitting for meditation, it was pointed out that the tip of the nose should provide only a momentary location for the gaze. A prolonged gaze on the nose or between the eyes with the inner gaze could strain the eye muscles. If any body part or process is to be taken as the focus of concentrative meditation, far and away the best choice is breathing – a technique of meditation to be described later in this chapter.

Ideally, any external object chosen for steady gaze meditation should be on a level with the eyes. An object placed a little below eye level will not tire the eyes, but one placed above eye level, so that the eyes have to turn up, will cause fatigue.

Sit firmly in one of the meditative postures, head, neck, and backbone in vertical line, motionless, breathing slowly and smoothly, looking steadily at the concentration-object. 'Cease from thine own activity, fix thine eye upon one point,' instructed Jacob Boehme, in one of his *Dialogues*. 'Gather in all thy thoughts and by faith press into the Centre.' Do not stare: look *through* the eyes rather than *from* them. The eyes should not be widely opened, as in a stare, or they will soon tire. Blink when necessary, or the eyes will become dry and painful. Frederick Spiegelberg, in *Spiritual Practices of India*, (167) says that the meditator should gaze 'in a calm, relaxed manner, somewhat as though he were looking at his face in a mirror.'

In early practice the attention will slip away and unbidden thoughts will intrude and attempt to set up the chain reaction called reverie. Each time you become aware of having lost concentration, bring the torch beam of attention back to its task and produce again the soft impulse that sustains concentration for a while. You should look and feel serene. Poised in body and mind, simply *look*. When concentration is effortlessly sustained, subtler and deeper levels of mind will be known. And if you are concentrating upon, say, an apple or a rose, you will get to know it – its 'appleness' or 'roseness', what the Zen Buddhists call its 'suchness' – as you have never known it before.

AN EXPERIMENT IN VISUAL CONCENTRATION

In steady gaze meditation after a time the object concentrated upon becomes more vivid and luminous. Being held in the light of attention without interference from concepts and associations that normally operate in perception of this object, and without reflection, the perception strikes with a clarity and freshness such as one is likely to find in young children. Children do not have this freshness of vision for long: soon a mesh of categories acts upon every perception of known objcets. As the result of a study of eidetic imagery in children, H.Werner states (173):

The image ... gradually changes in functional character. It becomes essentially subject to the exigencies of abstract thought. Once the image changes in function and becomes an instrument in reflective thought, its structure will also change. It is only through such structural change that the image can serve as an instrument of expression in abstract mental activity. This is why, of necessity, the sensuousness, fullness of detail, the colour and vivacity of the image must fade.

Arthur J. Deikman (115),who has written several interesting papers on the nature of human consciousness and the modes of consciousness observed in mystical experience, sees mystic phenomena as' a consequence of a deautomatization of the psychological structures that organize, limit, select, and interpret perceptual stimuli'. He carried out experiments in which subjects gazed steadily upon a blue vase, meditating in the Patanjali manner, though nothing so exotic or mystical was mentioned to the subjects. They were told (114):

The purpose of the sessions is to learn about concentration. Your aim is to concentrate on the blue vase. By concentration I do not mean analyzing the different parts of the vase, or thinking a series of thoughts about the vase, or associating ideas to the vase; but rather, trying to see the vase as it exists in itself, without any connections to other things. Exclude all other thoughts or feelings or sounds or body sensations. Do not let them distract you, but keep them out so that you can concentrate all your attention, all your awareness on the vase itself. Let the perception of the vase fill your entire mind.

The instructions were, as we have seen, to use the blue vase as an object of Yogic concentration, though the subjects were not aware of this.

Each session of concentration lasted half an hour, and there were forty or more sessions spread over several months. The subjects' perceptions of the vase changed in directions similar to those reported by meditating Yogins – the vase became 'luminous', 'more vivid', 'I really began to feel, you know, almost as though the blue and I were perhaps merging or that the vase and I were. It was as though everything were sort of merging.'

Mr Deikman sees these changes as being a ' "deautomatization", an undoing of the usual ways of perceiving and thinking due to the special way that attention was being used.' He also sees these changes in consciousness as the working of a receptive mode, which research indicates is related to the right hemisphere of the brain; the contrasting acting mode (which predominates in the West) is related to the left hemisphere of the brain.

This experiment did not, of course, prove or disprove any of the metaphysical claims of the great religions, but it did give support to the changes in consciousness described by Patanjali and Raja Yogins.

A STABLE IMAGE EXPERIMENT

In another experiment which could throw light on steady gaze meditation, a group of physiological psychologists devised a method of keeping a visual image stable on the retina by use of a tiny projector mounted on a contact lens which the subject wears. The image from the projector falls constantly on the retina. Now normally our eyes keep on the move. The larger movements are called saccades, but there are tiny movements even when we try to hold the gaze motionless on some object. These tiny movements are called optical nystagmus.

The interesting thing about these experiments is that when the subjects looked at a stabilized image the image vanished. There was no visual experience whatever. A similar effect occurs when a subject gazes upon a completely clear visual field, a *ganzfeld*, such as a white-washed surface or the two halves of a table-tennis ball placed over the eyes. After about twenty minutes some subjects report a 'blank-out', a total disappearance of the sense of vision for a short period. Such a period is marked by a burst of alpha activity in the brain as recorded by an electroencephalogram (EEG). Similar alpha rhythms were recorded in the stabilized image experiment using a projector.

High alpha activity has been recorded in meditating Yogins and Zen monks.

Professor Robert E. Ornstein, in his book *The Psychology of Consciousness* (158), has pointed out the similarity of the 'blank out' experience to that of mystics who have taken meditation as far as the experience of 'void', 'white light', 'cloud of unknowing', and so on. He thinks the two experiences have 'essential similarities and are produced through quite similar procedures.' He also says:

> One consequence of the way our central nervous system is structured seems to be that, if awareness is restricted to one unchanging source of stimulation, a 'turning off' of consciousness of the external world follows. The common instructions for concentrative meditation all underscore this; one is advised to be constantly aware of the object of meditation and nothing else, to continuously recycle the same input over and over.

VISUALIZATION MEDITATION

> The Raja Yoga – By this knowledge the modifications of the mind are suspended, however active they may be: therefore, let the Yogi untiringly and unselfishly try to obtain this knowledge. When the modifications of the thinking principle are suspended, then one certainly becomes a Yogi: then is known the Indivisible, pure Gnosis.
>
> Let him contemplate on his own reflection in the sky as beyond the Cosmic Egg.... Through that let him think on the Great Void unceasingly. The Great Void, whose beginning is void, whose middle is void, whose end is void, has the brilliancy of tens of millions of suns, and the coolness of tens of millions of moons. By contemplating continually on this, one obtains success.

The above description of Contemplation of the Great Void, taken from the *Siva Samhita* (91), is one of the plainer examples of visualization meditation, which in Tantric and Tibetan Yoga can become elaborate and colourful fantasies. But however intricate the visualization, in the end the mind becomes still and clear and knows the white light of pure consciousness (*Purusha* or *Atman*).

A mental image of a flower, a tree, or a deity may be held in mind for a time, and then gradually dismantled, piece by piece, until only a clear light remains. Here is an example of this method, as described in *The Tibetan Book of the Dead* (121):

Whosoever thy tutelary deity may be, meditate upon the form for much time – as being apparent, yet non-existent in reality, like a form produced by a magician. . . . Then let the vision of the tutelary deity melt away from the extemities, until nothing at all remaineth visible of it; and put thyself in the state of the Clearness and the Voidness – which thou canst not conceive as something – and abide in that state for a little while. Again meditate upon the tutelary deity; again meditate upon the Clear Light; do this alternately. Afterwards allow thine own intellect to melt away gradually, beginning from the extremities.

Most of the visualization contemplations are much more complex than the two examples already given. However, there is a movement from complexity to clearness and voidness as contemplation moves from gross to luminous and subtle stages.

GROSS, LUMINOUS, AND SUBTLE CONTEMPLATION

A revered *guru*, god, or goddess is conjured up in gross contemplation (*sthula dhyana*). The appearance of the figure and the setting can be detailed and colourful. The *Gheranda Samitha* (90) gives two examples:

[Having closed the eyes] let him contemplate that there is a sea of nectar in the region of his heart: that in the midst of that sea an island of precious stones, the very sand of which is pulverized diamonds and rubies. That on all sides of it, Kadamba trees, laden with sweet flowers; that, next to those trees, like a rampart, a row of flowering trees, such as malati, mallika, jati, kesara, campaka, parijata and padma, and that the fragrance of these flowers is spread all round, in every quarter. In the middle of this garden, let the Yogin imagine that there stands a beautiful Kalpa tree, having four branches, representing the four *Vedas*, and that it is full of flowers and fruits. Beetles are humming there and cuckoos singing. Beneath that tree let him imagine a rich platform of precious gems, and on that a costly throne inlaid with jewels, and that on that throne sits his particular Deity as taught to him by his *Guru*. Let him contemplate on the appropriate form, ornaments and vehicle of that Deity. The constant contemplation of such a form is *Sthula Dhyana*.

Another Process: Let the Yogin imagine that in the pericarp of the great thousand-petalled Lotus [Brain] there is a smaller lotus having twelve petals. Its colour is white, highly luminous, having twelve bija letters, named ha, sa, ksa, ma, la, va, ra, ym, ha, sa, kha, phrem. In the pericarp of this smaller lotus there are three lines forming a triangle, a, ka, tha; having three angles called ha, la, ksa: and in the middle of this triangle, there is the *Pranava Om*. Then let him contemplate that there are two swans, and a pair of wooden sandals. There let him contemplate his *Guru Deva*, having two arms and three eyes, and dressed in pure white, anointed with white sandal-paste, wearing garlands of white flowers; to the left of whom stands *Sakti* of blood-red colour. By thus contemplating the *Guru*, the *Sthula Dhyana* is attained.

In contrast, luminous contemplation (*jyotir* or *tao dhyana*) is inner gazing upon the formless *Brahman*, the all-pervading cosmic spirit, manifesting itself as a mass of clear light. *Brahman* is contemplated again, as invisible cosmic energy, in subtle contemplation (*suksma dhyana*).

Though such heightened and developed powers of visualization in the service of contemplation may fascinate us, they cannot be said to belong to our practical approach to Yoga meditation, capable of quickly producing results on all the levels of approach described in the chapter entitled 'Why Meditate?' But, the techniques of meditation described in the rest of this chapter are accessible to all readers.

THOUGHT OBSERVATION AND REDUCTION

Vivekananda wrote (171):
From our childhood upwards we have been taught only to pay attention to things external, but never to things internal, hence most of us have nearly lost the faculty of observing the internal mechanism. To turn the mind, as it were, inside, stop it from going outside, and then to concentrate all its powers, and throw them upon the mind itself, in order that it may know its own nature, analyse itself – is very hard work. Yet that is the only way to anything which will be a scientific approach to the subject.

To sit motionless, eyes closed, and look within the mind is not the simple matter that it first appears. The necessary awareness takes practice, and the difficulty lies not so much in doing as in having to be a mere passive spectator who must not interfere. It comes as a shock for the beginner to find what an unruly place his mind is: nevertheless, in this exercise, the role expected is that of a detached observer. In time the mind will become calmer and the number of thoughts active in it become less.

The method was described by Charles Baudouin in his book *Suggestion and Auto-suggestion* (107):

Seat yourself for a while and allow your thoughts to take their own course freely. It [the mind] behaves like a frisky monkey. Let the monkey jump about; wait and take note. Your thoughts will entertain ugly ideas, so ugly that you will be surprised. But day by day, these errings will become less numerous and less extensive. During the first months you will have a thousand thoughts; then you will have no more than seven hundred; and the number will progressively diminish.

The image of an excitable monkey is one frequently used in Yogic literature in describing the mind. As you observe the parade of thoughts, note how they link by association – your personal associations based on conditioning, memory, and experience. It is essential to observe with detachment, to become a dispassionate spectator. Do not comment upon the thoughts; do not make judgments; do not show surprise, anger, dismay, sorrow, or any other emotion. Just observe the stream of thought with passive awareness.

After a time the number of thoughts will decrease. You will then be able to concentrate on single thoughts, to watch them rise, cross the mind, and go. Later on gaps will appear between thoughts, as though between beads on a thread. The space between the thoughts is more important than the thoughts themselves, which are unimportant in this exercise. The intervals between thoughts reveal pure awareness, the golden thread on which the beads of thought are strung. There, momentarily, one tastes the pure Self. That taste, however brief, is worth infinitely more than any number of words. 'He who tastes not, knows not,' said the Sufist Rumi.

BREATHING MEDITATION

Professor Ornstein, in *The Psychology of Consciousness* (158), tells how some American friends of his

made a hopeful journey to India. Attracted by the repute of a certain famous *guru* (teacher) they hitchhiked across country, found a very inexpensive trans-Atlantic flight, and then travelled overland, with great difficulty, all the way to the Himalayas in the Indian subcontinent.

Finally, after walking for days and days, they reached the *ashram* (a sort of 'religious living association') of the *guru*. After allowing them some time to calm down, the *guru* saw them. Their hopes were high: perhaps they would receive a mysterious 'secret initiation' or maybe even a genuine 'magic word'. When they had outlined their trek, their difficulties, their expectations, and their hopes, the *guru* instructed them: 'Sit, facing the wall, and count your breaths. This is all.'

The technique of breathing meditation is well known in Yoga, Zen, and other schools of Buddhism, and has been mentioned many times in manuals on these disciplines. The seekers expected something more esoteric. In fact, the *guru's* 'This is all' was quite a lot. There is much that can be said for breathing meditation, especially for beginners, which most Westerners are.

Breathing meditation is accessible to all meditators and effective as a mental hygiene and for touching deep levels of energy and consciousness. Respiration provides an unchanging stimulus for Yogic concentrative meditation, is with us minute after minute throughout life, and accompanies us everywhere. Further: breath has close associations with the life-force (*prana*), and with subtle energy currents in the body, and consciousness itself. *Prana*, Yoga holds, is the connecting link between matter and mind. It is worth noting, also, that *Atman*, the Self to be realized, originally meant 'breath'. The German word *Atem* ('breath') has the same root as the Sanskrit *Atman*.

Some Yogins use the heartbeat as a focus for attention, but not all can acquire the knack of listening in to their heartbeats, nor do all find it the most suitable of concentration-objects, in spite of its being the pulse of life. The slower pace of breathing (slower than the beating heart) and its calming effect on the mind makes it an ideal process for contemplation. Within a few minutes of our seating ourselves motionless in poised posture, breathing slows down and becomes smoother. We can become conscious of our breathing instantly at any time and in any place, and fasten our attention on it quickly and easily. If we surrender to the respiratory rise and fall, inhalation and exhalation, we have the sensation not so much of breathing as of being breathed; and in an instant we are brought, in a way nothing else can do so effectively, close to our essential being.

Normally we only become aware of our breathing when we are agitated or excited, or have just made a strenuous physical effort;

but in breathing meditation we follow the slow smooth motions of calm breathing.

You can choose a point on which to fix the attention – either the point in the nose where incoming air first strikes or a point a little below the navel. This point in the belly is much favoured by Japanese Zen meditators, who stress its importance as the body's centre of gravity, and also the need for breathing deep into the belly. By fixing the attention there, thought is said to be 'nailed down'.

Breathe through the nostrils, unless they are so badly blocked that you are forced to breathe through your mouth. The meditative postures with head, neck and backbone in upright line favour deep healthful breathing. Readers who have already put into use the *pranayama* exercises given in *Yoga of Breathing* will have no problems here. As instructed there, breathe deeply into the adbomen; the diaphragm moves down and the ribs expand. The reverse process occurs during exhalation: the abdomen draws back and flattens, the diaphragm rises, and the thorax draws in. This deep diaphragmatic and abdominal breathing is beneficial to health, and the habit should be cultivated at *all* times. It relaxes and calms the mind, thus assisting meditation.

Once meditation commences the breathing should be left to itself without conscious regulation. Though one should breathe correctly, in the healthy, Yogic manner, during meditation, filling the lungs fully is not part of it. The motionless silence of sitting meditation requires only a small supply of oxygen. During meditation respiration will become slower, smoother, more rhythmic and, all meditation being a change from the gross to the subtle, finer. A text in Chinese Yoga says (145): 'The breath seems to have vanished in spite of the presence of the respiratory organs which seem to be useless; the practiser thus feels as if his breath comes in and out through the pores all over his body. This is the highest attainment in the art of breathing.'

Beginners should for a month or so count each breath they take, either on each inspiration or each expiration, from one to ten, and then go back to one. Counting beyond ten produces mounting mental effort and as the score increases the competitive element may intrude, which would mar the relaxed quality of meditation. Attention should be focused on one of the two places mentioned earlier: the point in the nostrils against which the incoming air is first felt to strike, or a place in the belly a little below the navel.

After a month of counting breaths, drop the counting. When the attention wanders to some distracting sound or sensation, or thoughts enter the mind, return once more to concentration on your breathing. Show no impatience. Return again and again. Eventually the number of interruptions of concentration will become much fewer – and one day, perhaps, there will be not meditator and his breathing, but a transcending of the subject-object dichotomy in the tranquillity of pure Being. It may only last a moment or so at first, but the experience is likely to be repeated subsequently in longer periods of peaceful union.

THE WITNESS

In this Yoga technique you observe any daily activity as though you were a detached and dispassionate spectator of yourself. This applies not only to your physical actions, but also to your states of mind. Detached, without passing judgments or commenting, be calmly aware of life's daily activities, whatever they may be: in the home, at work, in play, in social life, driving a car, emptying the bladder, eating a sandwich – there is no need to select activities, for whatever is being done *now* is the object of contemplative awareness. We learn a great deal about ourselves from self-observation, and the awareness leads to beneficial changes in the personality in the direction of greater equanimity, sensitivity, and alertness. We learn, too, the importance of the here and now, and to live more in the present.

The Buddhists call it 'mindfulness'. A Buddhist monk may be told to walk, and be mindful of every step. Walking becomes meditation. We have already seen that breathing can become meditation. Tibetan Yoga Masters instruct their pupils to make meditation exercises of their occupations: whether it be street cleaning, shoemaking, making pottery, clerking, serving in a shop, or whatever, every movement may be performed with contemplative awareness. Making a meditation exercise of everyday activities is common to many Buddhist schools. Asked 'What is Zen?', a Zen Master replied: 'When you are hungry eat, when you are tired sleep.' And Zen monks are said to receive sudden enlightenment (*satori*) on seeing a Master eat rice or perform some other everyday act.

Krishnamurti makes much of self-observation in his books and lectures, calling the mental attitude choiceless or passive awareness. Another name for it is bare attention. In the system of 'harmonious development' taught by George Gurdjieff it is known as self-remembering. Gurdjieff studied and worked with the Sufis and most of his exercises were of Sufic origin. Sufism uses the shell of Islam for its home, rather in the manner of the hermit crab, but claims to be the essence of all religions. Its methods have affinities with those of Yoga and other Eastern esoteric psychologies. It is customary in most of these systems to combine concentrative meditation in short sitting sessions once or twice a day with this more 'open' form of contemplation during everyday activity. Alternating contraction and expansion, one might say.

The Karma Yogin, who follows principally the path of service and action (*karma*), makes everyday activity a sacrament, an act of devotion to the divine principle. He fully attends to each action. The most commonplace activities of life are thus given a rich dimension through contemplative awareness.

VII   Mantra Yoga

JAPA

Patanjali includes *japa* among a Yogin's observances. *Japa* is repetition of a letter, syllable, word, phrase, sentence, or sound considered to possess magical, occult, spiritual, or mystical potency, and called a *mantra*. It may be voiced aloud or thought inwardly. The latter technique has been made popular in the streamlined method taught by the *guru* Maharishi Mahesh Yogi under the name Transcendental Meditation. We will devote a separate chapter to TM, as it is known for short, and here discuss traditional methods.

Mantras are incantatory and mystical sounds. They provide a form of concentrative meditation. The voiced *mantra* should be repeated in a voice that is alive and resonant. The mystical aim is to utilize the power of sound vibrations to influence modalities of consciousness. A *mantra* may be repeated hundreds, even thousands of times.

As a Yoga method, *japa* has the virtue of simplicity, but can easily degenerate into arid, mechanical, and empty repetition. At its profoundest Mantra Yoga explores the influence of sound vibrations in a universe which science tells us is made up of vibrations. It is known that sound vibrations can destroy buildings and make peop!e ill. That they can also have healing power is shown by the many successful experiments with music therapy.

LISTENING TO INTERNAL SOUNDS

Nada or listening to internal sounds is one of the practices of Mantra Yoga. The Yogin sits in a meditative posture and seals his right ear with his right thumb and his left ear with his left thumb, his eyes with his index fingers, his nostrils with his middle fingers, and his lips with the remaining four fingers.

The *Siva Samhita* (91) describes the variety of internal sounds that the Yogin should concentrate upon:

From practising this gradually, the Yogi begins to hear the mystic sounds [*nadas*]. The first sound is like the hum of the honey-intoxicated bee, next that of a flute, then of a harp; after this, by the gradual practice of Yoga, the destroyer of the darkness of the world, he hears the sounds of ringing bells; then sounds like roar of thunder. When one fixes his full attention on this sound, being free from fear, he gets absorption [*Samadhi*].

MUSIC

The Mantric Yogin is said to hear the sound of the cosmos, the music of the spheres, and in advanced meditation a single universal tone. The poet Schlegel wrote: 'Through all the tones there sounds, throughout the colourful earth, a gentle tone, sustained, for him who listens secretly.' Schumann used these lines to preface his *Fantasia in C Major*.

It is widely acknowledged that great music can communicate states of consciousness from composer to listener, in a language beyond words and so close to Being. When composing one of his symphonies, Gustav Mahler felt not so much that all his deepest questions had been answered as that there were no longer any questions to be asked. Hazrat Inayet Khan, a Sufi, says: 'Music is behind life and rules life: from music springs all life. The whole of creation exists in rhythm.'

POETRY

The incantatory element in Mantra Yoga is important. It should be recalled that it has made a considerable contribution to English and European poetry. Poetry differs from prose in having something of the quality of music, an incantatory element, and the words in good poetry say more than they mean in the narrower sense. In most national literatures, verse has preceded prose and has accompanied song and dance. Geoffrey Ashe, in a chapter on poetry in *The Art of Writing Made Simple* (103), says:

Why this prevalence of rhythm? To answer the question is to identify the first word which we can supply to poetic language in general. It is *incantatory*. If that term conveys a hint of primitive magic, I cannot help it. The hint is justified. In fact the great themes of ancient poetry, the myths, may well have arisen out of earlier magic rituals. But however that may be, the incantatory quality is present in all true poems.

Poetry is the nearest language comes to expressing mystical experience. In England, for several centuries, the mystical tradition has been sustained more by poetry than by the Church. The philosopher Martin Heidegger suggests that poetry can lead us to Being. If so, it is a kind of Yoga.

OM (*AUM*)

Mantra Yoga belongs to the long history of man's striving to find the word whose utterance unlocks the door to Absolute Knowledge. Franz Kafka (135) summed up the search in a diary entry dated 18 October 1921:

It is entirely conceivable that life's splendour forever lies in wait about each one of us in all its fullness, but veiled from view, deep down, invisible, far off. It *is* there, though not hostile, not reluctant, not deaf. If you summon it by the right word, by its right name it will come. This is the essence of magic, which does not create, but summons.

In Mantra Yoga magical or mystical potency has been ascribed to certain words, the most powerful of which is held to be OM. 'In the beginning was the Word.' To the Hindu that word is OM. It is the *pranava*, the 'word of glory', representing the Absolute.

This most famous of *mantras* is composed of three letters, AUM, which becomes OM on being voiced. The AU sound is pronounced as in the English 'house'. The AU sound begins at the back of the throat and comes forward to the front of the face, which singers call 'the mask'. The lips are closed for the M sound, which is usually sustained half as long again as the preceding AU sound.

The three letters AUM represent the aspects of *Brahman* or the Absolute found in the Hindu Trinity: Creator, Destroyer, and Preserver.

André van Lysebeth, a leading European teacher of Hatha Yoga, says (52) that the sounding of OM and other *mantric* vocables gives a vibro-massage to various glands and vital organs in the thoracic cavavity and the abdomen, stimulates deeper breathing, and tones the nervous system. But it is the influence on consciousness that concerns us in the Yoga of Meditation. The *Mundaka Upanishad* says: 'OM is the bow, the individual self is the arrow, the spirit is the target. One should then become one with it like the arrow that has penetrated the target.'

SOME OTHER MANTRAS

The *mantras* of Indian Yoga are usually Sanskrit letters, syllables, words, or sentences. *Mantras* other than OM are often preceded by it. The well-known OM MANI PADME HUM means 'OM, the jewel in the lotus.' In OM TAT SAT, TAT or 'That' refers to *Brahman*, and SAT is pure being. Two other well-known *mantras* are SOHAM, meaning 'He is I', and HANSAH, meaning 'I am He'.

As we shall see in the chapter on Bhakti Yoga, the Krishna Consciousness Movement have as the lynch-pin of their practice the *mahamantra* (great *mantra*): HARE KRISHNA, HARE KRISHNA, KRISHNA KRISHNA, HARE HARE, HARE RAMA, HARE RAMA, RAMA RAMA, HARE HARE. This is chanted again and again (*japa*).

KINDS OF *JAPA*

Japa can be performed in a variety of ways. If we look at Tantric practice we find the following kinds and methods:

  i. Daily (*nitya*). Morning and evening as instructed by a *guru*.
  ii Circumstantial (*naimittika*). For festival days and special occasions.
  iii For desired results (*kamya*). With special attainments in mind.
  iv Forbidden (*nishiddha*). Forbidden are the mixing of *mantras*, those from an unqualified instructor, those voiced incorrectly or without knowledge of their meaning.
  v Penance (*prayaschitta japa*).
  vi. Unmoving (*achala*). Immobile, firmly seated.
  vii Moving (*chala*). While standing, sitting, lying, walking

about, or performing any activity. Repetition is inward; the lips do not move.

viii   Voiced (*vachika*). Repeated aloud.

ix   Whispered (*upanshu*). Only the practitioner hears the *mantra*.

x   Bee (*bhramara*). The sound 'Ah' is produced low in the throat and sustained as long as is comfortable to a breath. A rapid inhalation is then made and the bee-sound repeated, and so on. It is sometimes called 'beetle-droning'.

xi   Mental (*manasa*). Alain Danielou(14)calls this 'the very soul of *japa*. The *mantra* is not uttered aloud at all, but remains revolving in the mind. The eyes are closed. Meditation on the meaning of the *mantra* predominates over all other thoughts.'

xii   Uninterrupted (*akhanda*). For those who have renounced the world. Continued for hours.

xiii   Non-uttered (*a-japa*). The meaning of the *mantra* is held in the mind and absorbed.

xiv   Circumambulatory (*pradakshina*). While walking in a temple or a garden.

MANTRAS IN OTHER TRADITIONS

The *mantra* method is not exclusive to Yoga. Concentrating and stilling the mind by repetition of words or sounds is found in other mystical traditions.

The priests of ancient Egypt saw the utterance of certain words in ritualistic moments as a way to open up consciousness to cosmic energies. The name of God or divinity is widely used for *japa* in other traditions. The Sufists perform *dhikr*, which means both 'repetition' and 'remembrance'. There is a tradition in the Pure Land Buddhism sect of Japan that if you can recite the *nembutsu* or name of Buddha once in the correct meaningful way, with the whole of your being, that is enough to produce enlightenment. Chanting *mantras* is the main method of another Japanese Buddhist sect, the Shingon-shu (Shingon means *mantra*). That the early Christians utilized a form of *japa* for concentrative meditation is clear from the contents of the *Philokalia*, a collection of writings by the Christian Fathers (first millenium), first published in Venice in 1782. The

'Prayer of the Heart' has remained a part of the Greek Orthodox tradition: 'Lord Jesus Christ, son of God have mercy upon me.' St John Climacus wrote: 'If many words are used in prayer, all sorts of distracting pictures hover in the mind but worship is lost. If little is said or only a single word pronounced, the mind remains concentrated.'

Transcendental Meditation, the method of deep relaxation and going to the source of thought taught by Maharishi Mahesh Yogi, is a streamlined presentation of one of the varieties of Mantra Yoga, silent repetition of a word. The Maharishi has made it the most wisely practised Yoga meditation in the West.

VIII The Transcendental Meditation of Maharishi Mahesh Yogi

MAHARISHI MAHESH YOGI

Maharishi Mahesh Yogi, the most widely known present-day *guru*, was born on 18 October 1911 in Uttar Kashi, son of an income tax official. He took a degree in physics at Allahabad University, worked for a time in a factory, and then in the early 1940s became a pupil of Swami Brahmananda Saraswati, with whom he stayed thirteen years. After his teacher's death he went into seclusion for two years, during which he developed his method of Transcendental Meditation, a streamlined form of Mantra Yoga suited to the needs of active people. In 1959 he took the method to America and Europe. The publicity attendant on temporary associations with stars of the entertainments industry made the tiny, chuckling *guru* a household name in the western world. TM as it is known for short, has steadily gained adherents in many countries. Persons who enrol at a TM centre are not asked to alter their way of life, though it is believed that the influence of meditation will produce changes. Persons of all religions or none are welcomed, TM being a technique and not a religion or a philosophy. As a Hindu, Maharishi Mahesh Yogi believes in the law of *karma*, reincarnation, and other concepts given little support in the Western world; but non-Hindu meditators are not asked to renounce their own religious viewpoints, nor, for that matter, their worldly pleasures.

THE METHOD

The technique of Transcendental Meditation could hardly be simpler.

One mentally repeats a word while sitting still. The lips and tongue should not move. A Yoga sitting posture is not expected if the meditator does not find it comfortable. The eyes are closed and the attention is turned inwards. No mental force should be used: each time the mind is found to have wandered, the *mantra* is reintroduced.

At his or her initiation, each person who enrols for TM is given a Sanskrit word as a personal *mantra*. It is claimed that there is a specific word to suit the nervous system of each applicant. This, and a certain amount of mumbo-jumbo at the initiation, savours of an occultism out of step with the customary straightforward and commonsense presentation of the method. No real evidence has been offered in support of the claim, and some scepticism on this is expressed even within the organization. My view is that the choice of word is not of great importance either in Mantra Yoga or in TM – its *use* is what counts, leading the meditator to deep relaxation. It is necessary only that the word should be easily pronounced (Westerners report difficulty in this respect with some of the words given for TM) and that it should have no unpleasant or tension-producing associations. A meaningless word, which the Maharishi prefers, avoids distracting the attention with associated thoughts.

The Maharishi also insists that the method, simple though it is, cannot be taught by book instruction, and that meditators need to check progress with his personally-trained instructors.

He stresses the importance (as we did earlier in this book) of not thinking about or expecting results – that way, he says, the attention is undivided and the meditator will not 'fall victim to auto-suggestion and only imagine that experience.'

EFFORTLESS MEDITATION?

The Maharishi denies that the mind is controlled in Transcendental Meditation, and says that the mind moves naturally towards a field of greater happiness, which he calls bliss consciousness. This statement has led some of his followers to say that TM is not Yoga and that no Yogic concentration is involved. The Maharishi has certainly simplified and streamlined a technique of Yoga, and he has himself said many times that TM is his version of Yoga meditation. His teaching that asceticism, austerity, strong will-power, and iron discipline are not needed and that the natural movements of the mind can be harnessed is timely, and welcomed by the majority of people today. However, I think one should be cautious about saying that no control and no concentration are involved in it, and that it is not a form of concentrative Yogic meditation. The Maharishi has developed a particularly easeful method of meditation, but it seems to me to be clearly within the mainstream Yogic tradition.

The Maharishi's instruction to repeat a *mantra* mentally, and to go back to it when the attention is found to have wandered from it, is familiar in all forms of concentrative Yoga meditation. Occasionally the writers of Yoga texts may employ metaphors that seem to imply a degree of iron control of the mind, but what is actually required is not concentration in the common Western sense of the word, as we made clear earlier in describing the right attitude to Yoga meditation. *All* Yoga meditation should be comfortable. Whatever the method used, to become aware that the attention has wandered is usually enough to switch it automatically back to its position. For example, the method of breathing meditation described earlier in this book can be just as easeful and gentle as Transcendental Meditation. It can be combined with use of the silent *mantra*, which is mentally repeated either on each inhalation or on each exhalation.

There is, moreover, a whole class of meditation which Claudio Naranjo calls 'opening-up', in contrast to the other main class of 'concentrative', meditation. The opening-up methods include the Zen meditation of 'just sitting' (*shikan-taza*), favoured by the Soto school, in which there is no object, not even a silent *mantra*, for the mind to fix on. Yet even here a meditative poise of mind, which is surely a kind of attention or concentration, is required. Zen Master Yasutani Roshi describes it thus: (175) 'Now, in *shikan-taza* the mind must be unhurried yet at the same firmly planted or massively composed, like Mount Fuji, let us say. But it also must be alert, stretched, like a taut bowstring. So *shikan-taza* is a heightened state of *concentrated* awareness wherein one is neither tense nor hurried, and certainly never slack.' (The italics are mine.)

The Maharishi appeared to concede that concentration, of however natural a kind, was involved in TM in reply to a question I heard put to him at a press conference in London's Festival Hall in 1974. Asked whether the repetition of a *mantra* was not a form of concentration, the *guru* skilfully replied, with one of his famous chuckles, that in this TM was 'using a thorn to remove a thorn from the flesh'. Using a thorn nevertheless.

That there is more to this than just semantic confusion is clear from a few words (118) spoken by the Maharishi in a television discussion which was transmitted by the British Broadcasting Corporation on 5 July 1964: 'We, in meditation, don't make an effort. We allow the mind to get into these more effortless [*sic*] states, because in experiencing the subtlest state of thought, effort is less and less, and less, and less, and then no effort, absolutely no effort.'

So only the deeper stages of meditation are effortless. The dive may be effortless, but only after one has walked to the end of the springboard and made the jump in the correct manner. In TM the silent *mantra* provides the springboard. Similarly, Patanjali's *dharana* gives way to *dhyana*, which flows effortlessly into *samadhi* – what the Maharishi calls bliss consciousness.

TM LABORATORY-TESTED

Laboratory research into Transcendental Meditation reveals that during meditation the following physiological changes occur:

i   Heartbeat and breathing rates slow down.
ii   Oxygen consumption and metabolicnate falls by twenty per cent.
iii The blood lactate level drops. This level goes up with stress and fatigue.
iv   Skin resistance to electric current increase fourfold, a sign of relaxation.
v   EEG readings of brain wave patterns shown increased alpha activity – again a sign of relaxation.

These findings, in subjects who had been meditating between one month and nine years, show that TM induces deep relaxation even though the meditator is neither asleep nor in a hypnotic trance.

For the claim that TM releases 'creative intelligence' there has not been any reliable evidence.

THE SOURCE OF THOUGHT

The Maharishi equates the mentally 'sounded' *mantra* with thought,

which is 'the subtle state of speech' and 'a subtle form of sound'.
He likens the rise of a thought to surface consciousness to a bubble
that rises to the surface of the ocean. In his *Science of Being* (147) he
says:

> A thought starts from the deepest level of consciousness and rises
> through the whole depth of the ocean of mind until it finally appears as a
> conscious thought at the surface. Thus we find that every thought stirs
> the whole range of the depth of consciousness but is consciously
> appreciated only when it reaches the conscious level; all its earlier
> stages of development are not appreciated.

By repeatedly diving down during meditation – compare this
with the analogy of a pilot flying in and out of clouds used in
discussing Raja Yoga – thought can be known at all the points of its
journey to the surface of consciousness. At its subtlest level thought
is transcended.

> When the conscious mind transcends the subtlest level of thought, it
> transcends the subtlest state of relative experience and arrives at the
> transcendental Being, the state of pure consciousness or self-awareness.
> This is how, in a systematic manner, the conscious mind is led, step
> by step, to the direct experience of transcendental absolute Being.

The Maharishi says that Being cannot be experienced through
any of the senses, which are in the relative field. Sensory perception
is transcended in 'a state of consciousness in which the experiencer
no longer experiences'. This comes about for reasons we made clear
in discussing Patanjali's Raja Yoga: knower, known, and knowing
become one.

LEVELS OF CONSCIOUSNESS

One does not have to read the writings of Maharishi Mahesh Yogi
long to discover that he is teaching, in his own way, the *upanishadic*
creed of finding the Self and knowing it to be one with *Brahman*.

He says that by meditating one reaches a state of consciousness
beyond the well-known states of dreamless sleep, dreaming sleep,
and wakefulness. This fourth state he calls Transcendental Consciousness. Its physiological concomitant is deep relaxation. Beyond
this stage are three more.

The fifth stage is Cosmic Consciousness, in which Transcendental
Consciousness is carried into everyday activity. In Cosmic Con-

sciousness, one acts, but is aware that the Self is untouched by action. The Maharishi says that Cosmic Consciousness can be achieved through meditation alone, and by the ordinary man without his becoming a recluse or undergoing harsh disciplines.

It is more difficult to reach the final two stages. In God Consciousness the Self and activity are united. The final stage is called Union. In it one 'looks out on the world with the eyes of God'.

DR HERBERT BENSON AND THE 'RELAXATION RESPONSE'

The manuscript of this book was already going to press when I read with great interest Dr Herbert Benson's *The Relaxation Response* (William Morrow, New York, 1976). Here was laboratory-tested confirmation of views I expressed earlier in this chapter.

In 1968 Dr Benson and colleagues at the Harvard Medical School studied the physiological changes during meditation of volunteer practitioners of Transcendental Meditation. The findings were those mentioned above – a marked decrease in the body's oxygen consumption (hypometabolism), the production of Alpha waves in the brain, and so on. Dr Benson's findings are much quoted by the 'sellers' of TM, as one might expect. But they do not mention Dr Benson's subsequent studies and findings, which he described in *The Relaxation Response*.

Dr Benson says that the physiological changes seen in meditators using the TM technique are duplicated by other techniques of meditation, as long as four basic factors are present: (1) A quiet environment; (2) A mental device that provides a constant stimulus; (3) A passive attitude that does not worry about distracting thoughts; (4) a comfortable position.

Dr Benson himself teaches the simple technique of combining silent repetition of a word with awareness of breathing – the combination suggested earlier in this chapter and which I have used effectively for several years. His patients sit comfortably, close their eyes, become aware of their breathing, and mentally repeat the word 'One' on each exhalation.

Dr Benson's own words should be quoted: 'It is important to remember that there is not a single method that is unique in eliciting the Relaxation Response. For example, Transcendental Meditation is one of the many techniques that incorporate these [four] components. However, we believe it is not necessary to use the specific method and specific *secret*, personal sound taught by Transcendental Meditation. *Tests at the Thorndike Memorial Laboratory of Harvard have shown that a similar technique used with any sound or phrase or prayer or mantra brings forth the same physiologic changes noted during Transcendental Meditation . . .* In other words using the basic necessary components, any one of the age-old or the newly derived techiques produces the same physiologic results regardless of the mental device used.' (*The Relaxation Response*, pp 113-4).

Dr Benson's investigations lead him to believe that 'the passive attitude is perhaps the most important element in eliciting the Relaxation Response'. This would explain the effectiveness of Transcendental Meditation – for Maharishi Mahesh Yogi attaches supreme importance to effortlessness – the passive attitude – in his simple, streamlined technique.

IX   Yantra Yoga

FORM-SYMBOLS

At the same time that the sound symbol (*mantra*) is being repeated (*japa*), a form or design symbol (*yantra*) may be gazed upon. It may also be a single means of concentrative contemplation. *Yantras* represent in the visual field what *mantras* represent in the aural. They are diagrams drawn for the purpose of finding the centre of one's being or Self-realization. As art works to be gazed upon they range from the simple to the colourful and elaborate. *Yantra* meditation is practised mainly by the Yogins of Tantric Hinduism and Tantric Buddhism.

The Yogin sits in a meditative posture and concentrates on the form-symbol with his gaze, holding the mind steady and opening to the deep meaning of the symbol. Some forms of *yantra* meditation include a psychic journey before the mind becomes silent. Some Yogins close their eyes and visualize the *yantra*, holding it firmly in the mind.

MANDALAS

The most notable and elaborate *yantras* are the *mandalas* in which the designer includes concentric circles, sometimes within a square. *Mandala* is a Hindu word meaning 'circle', and a circle is the most important oriental symbol for unity and wholeness. It is the symbol of the Self. Its artistic representation is an object of contemplation whereby the state of consciousness it objectifies is evoked in the beholder.

Forms of the *mandala* in Christian symbolism are the nimbus and the rose window; the central symbol (*yantra*) of Christianity is the cross, however. In Zen painting the circle represents enlightenment and human perfection. Circles called 'sun wheels' appear in rock engravings that date back to the Neolithic age, before the invention of the wheel. *Mandala* construction (of a simple kind) and meditation is even found among the Eskimos. Peter Freuchen, in his *Book of the Eskimos* (122) tells how an Eskimo will sit before a large stone and with a small sharp stone start carving a circle upon the large stone. He will continue the circular movement for hours, sometimes days, until he passes into a trance.

Professor Eliade (119), an eminent authority on religious symbols, here describes the function of the *mandala* in both its external and its interiorized form:

The term itself means 'a circle'; the translations from the Tibetan sometimes render it by 'centre' and sometimes by 'that which surrounds'. In fact a *mandala* represents a whole series of circles, concentric or otherwise, inscribed within a square; and in this diagram, drawn on the ground by means of coloured threads or coloured rice powder, the various divinities of the Tantric pantheon are arranged in order. The *mandala* thus represents an *imago mundi* and at the same time a symbolic pantheon. The initiation of the neophyte consists, among other things, in his entering into the different zones and gaining access to the different levels of the *mandala*. This rite of penetration may be regarded as equivalent to the well-known rite of walking round a temple (*pradakshina*), or of the progressive elevation, terrace by terrace, up to the 'pure lands' at the highest levels of the temple. On the other hand, the placing of the neophyte in a *mandala* may be likened to the initiation by entry into a labyrinth: certain *mandalas* have, moreover, a clearly labyrinthine character. The function of the *mandala* may be considered at least two fold, as is that of the labyrinth. On the one hand, penetration into a *mandala* drawn on the ground is equivalent to an initiation ritual; and, on the other hand, the *mandala* 'protects' the neophyte against every harmful force from without, and at the same time helps him to concentrate, to find his own 'centre'.

But every Indian temple, seen from above, is a *mandala*. Any Indian temple is, like a *mandala*, a microcosm and at the same time a pantheon. Why, then, need one construct a *mandala* – why did they want a new 'Centre of the World'? Simply because, for certain devotees, who felt in need of a more authentic and a deeper religious experience, the traditional ritual had become fossilised: the construction of a fire altar or the ascent of the terraces of a temple no longer enabled them to rediscover their 'centre'. Unlike archaic man or the man of Vedic times, the Tantric devotee had need of a *personal experience* to reactivate certain primordial symbols in his consciousness. That is why, moreover, some Tantric schools rejected the external *mandala*, and had recourse to interiorised *mandalas*. These could be of two kinds: first, a purely mental construction, which acted as a 'support' for meditation, or, alternatively, an identification of the *mandala* in his own body. In the former case the yogi places himself mentally within the *mandala*, and thereby performs an act of concentration and, at the same time, of 'defence' against distraction and temptation. The *mandala* 'concentrates'; it preserves one from dispersion, from distraction. The discovery of the *mandala* in his own body indicates a desire to identify his 'mystical body' with a microcosm.

The *mandala* concentrates and integrates the mind of the meditator; he makes a psychic journey, entering the *mandala*, and passing to its centre so that the centre of his Being and that of the *mandala* coincide.

The psycho-analyst C. G. Jung made the discovery that some mentally-ill patients, when given a box or paints or crayons, will draw *mandala* shapes without being aware of their significance. He found *mandala* depiction most frequent in patients moving towards psychic wholeness, a process he termed Individuation. The circle motif also appeared in the dreams of such patients.

The Ganapati Yantra

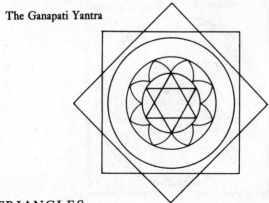

TRIANGLES

Triangles surrounded by concentric circles appear frequently in

Hindu *yantras*. The triangles usually interpenetrate, some pointing down and some pointing up. A triangle pointing up represents Siva, the male cosmic principle, and one pointing down represents Shakti, the female cosmic principle. A central point (*bindi*) represents *Brahman*, the Absolute. The word *bindu* has a number of meanings and shades of meaning. It is a dot or period, vitalizing a consonant when placed above it; it is seed; it is semen; it is Void or Emptiness.

Aniela Jaffe, in her contribution to the book *Man and his Symbols* (131), writes:

> But a great many of the eastern meditation figures are purely geo-metrical in design; these are called *yantras*. Aside from the circle, a very common *yantra* motif is formed by two interpenetrating triangles, one point-upward, the other point-downward. Traditionally, this shape symbolizes the union of Shiva and Shakti, the male and female divinities, a subject that also appears in sculpture in countless varia-ations. In terms of psychological symbolism, it expresses the union of opposites – the union of the personal, temporal world of the ego with the non-personal, timeless world of the non-ego. Ultimately, this union is the fulfilment and goal of all religions: it is the union of the soul with God. The two interpenetrating triangles have a symbolic meaning similar to that of the more common circular *mandala*. They represent the wholeness of the psyche or Self, of which consciousness is just as much a part of the unconscious.

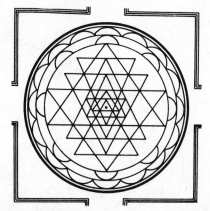

The Mandala
of the Srichakra

The mandala of the *srichakra* has nine basic triangles that represent 'nine fundamental natures' or 'nine wombs' whereby 'duality evolves from unity', corresponding to the nine elements of which we are composed: skin, blood, flesh, fat and bones, known as the 'five damsels of Siva', plus the 'four *srikantha*' (*srikantha* is another name for Siva), which are marrow, seed, vital energy and individual soul (*jiva*).

The *srichakra* is another name for the *sahasnana chaktra*, 'the lotus of a thousand petals', the highest of the *chakras* or energy centres of the subtle body, located at the tip of the head. This *mandala* thus represents the successful ascent of latent force, called *kundalini* or serpent power, to the *srichakra*. This movement is achieved through intense concentrative meditation (*mantra* and *yantra*) and advanced breath controls. This branch of Yoga, hazardous unless under the personal direction of a reliable *guru*, is called Laya or Kundalini Yoga.

X   Kundalini (Serpent Power) Yoga

Nothing that has been written in either the classic or the modern literature of Yoga gives us an opening to fit *kundalini* into our practical approach. All accounts agree that intensive and even hazardous discipline for many years is required by this Yoga path, which can be traced back to the Indus Valley civilization which ended about 3000 BC, and probably was known before that.

The method is a combination of concentrative meditation, which utlizes *mantras* and *yantras*, breath controls, and muscular contractions (*mudras*) and locks (*bandhas*). Some of the *mudras* and *bandhas* were described in *Yoga of Breathing*, but they were given there for the purpose of enhancing sexual health and fitness. Breathing exercises (*pranayama*), also described in *Yoga of Breathing* are considered an essential preliminary to attempting to arouse the body's latent power as they purify the channels (*nadis*) through the energy flows. As the methods of awakening *kundalini* are complex and not without danger, and require expert supervision, they will not be described here. However, we will concisely indicate the salient concepts of Kundalini Yoga, also called Laya (Latent Power) Yoga.

These are:
  i *Kundalini* or serpent power is an energy latent in the body, said to be coiled at the base of the spine.
  ii The *chakras* or vital centres represent stages in the ascent of the power.
  iii The *sushumna* is the channel which carries the *kundalini* force.
  iv Bliss consciousness (*samadhi*) is triggered when *kundalini* has travelled via the *sushumna* and through the vital centres to the highest *chakra*, the *sahasrara*, the 'thousand-petalled lotus' at the crown of the head.

SERPENT POWER

The concept of a key universal energy that can be activated in the body and controlled by meditation is found in a number of esoteric traditions. Life-energy theories have a long history in India, China, Japan, Korea, and Hawaii. In Yoga the universal force has aspects as Shakti, the female creative power, and as *prana*, which has also a meaning as 'breath'. The latent force within the body is called *kundalini*, or serpent power. Yogins always refer to *kundalini* as 'she'.

According to Yogic tradition, *kundalini* is a concentration of Cosmic Life Energy or *prana-Shakti*, dormant at the base of the spine and symbolically represented as a serpent, coiled three and a half times, closing with her mouth the entrance to the fine channel (*sushumna*) leading upwards through the spinal cord to the crown of the head, where Siva awaits, triggering *samadhi*. The ascending force passes through several key centres, called *chakras*, of which by main tradition there are seven.

WILHELM REICH

Kundalini force is referred to variously by writers as electro-magnetic energy, psychic force, and so on – but its nature remains a mystery.

Supporters of the orgone energy theory of the Austrian psycho-analyst and natural scientist Wilhelm Reich point out the similarities between Reich's concept of cosmic energy and the Yogic *prana*, and between his theory of bodily 'rings' and the *chakras*. Some neo-Reichians shy off the term 'orgone', but common to all Reichian therapists is his idea of a flow of energy in the body which if blocked causes illness.

For an account of Reich's theories on vital energies see W. Edward Mann's *Orgone, Reich and Eros*. There Professor Mann says (148): 'Indian thinking, both Hindu and yoga, on the body, its energy basis and potentials, is very similar to Reich's. Already some young Reichians are attempting to integrate the two approaches; given the interest of many Western youth in Oriental concepts and philosophy, we can expect interesting developments from such combinations.'

CHAKRAS

The *chakras*, literally 'wheels', are said to be vortices of *pranic* energy, each associated with special powers that can be awakened by concentrative meditation. However, there are three approaches to interpreting these vital centres. The first equates them with nerve plexuses, glands, or actual centres, in the body. Such equations are only partly successful. A second view is that the *chakras* belong to a subtle or astral body, the *sukshma sharira*. The third idea is that the *chakras* are symbols indicating points for concentrative meditation. The first and second approaches have been those most frequently promulgated. Indries Shah indicates that the Sufis take the third view in relation to *lataif,* which has similarities to the *chakra* system (166): 'In Yoga, the *chakras* or *padmas* are conceived as physically located centres in the body, linked by invisible nerves or channels. Yogis generally do not know that these centres are merely concentration points, convenient formulations whose activation is part of a theoretical working hypothesis.'

The most recent attempt to show *kundalini* as a biological phenomenon is by Gopi Krishna, whose Research Foundation for *Kundalini* has branches in Europe and North America.

The symbology of the *chakras* is complex and highly imaginative. In most cases a *chakra* has its seed sound-symbol (*bija-mantra*), its form symbol (*yantra*), its colour, its presiding god and goddess, and so on. The lower five *chakras* correspond to the five elements. The coiled serpent sleeps in the lowest *chakra* (*muladhara*).

Buddhist Tantrists recognize only four *chakras*, the first at the navel, and the fourth in the head. Some ancient statues depict the Buddha with a swelling on the top of the head indicating the activated brain *chakra* (*usnisa-kamala*).

The seven *chakras* of Kundalini Yoga, with their main symbols and associations, are as follows:

Root Centre (*Muladhara Chakra*)
Location: base of the spine, between the anus and the genitals. Form-symbol: lotus with four petals. Sound symbol: *lam.* Colour: yellow. Element: earth. Presiding god: Brahma the Creator. Goddess: Dakini.

Pelvic Centre (*Swadhistana Chakra*)

Location: at the genitals. Form-symbol: lotus with six petals. Sound symbol: *vam*. Colour: white. Element: water. Presiding god: Vishnu. Goddess: Rakini.

Solar Plexus Centre (*Manipura Chakra*)

Location: at the solar plexus. Form-symbol: lotus with ten petals. Sound symbol: *ram*. Colour: red. Element: fire. Presiding god: Rudra. Goddess: Lakini.

Heart Centre (*Anahata Chakra*)

Location: at the heart. Form-symbol: lotus with twelve petals. Sound-symbol: *yam*. Colour: blue. Element: air. Presiding god: Isha. Goddess: Kakini.

Throat Centre (*Vishuddha Chakra*)

Location: at the throat. Form-symbol: lotus with sixteen petals. Sound-symbol: *ham*. Colour: white. Element: ether. Presiding god: Sadashiva. Goddess: Sakini.

Brow Centre (*Ajna Chakra*)

Location: between the eyebrows, the 'third eye'. Form-symbol: lotus with two petals. Sound-symbols: OM (AUM). Colour: snow white. Presiding goddess: Hakini.

Crown of the Head Centre (*Sahasrara Chakra*)

Location: at the cerebrum. Form-symbol: lotus with a thousand petals. Presiding god: Siva. This is the centre of Self-realization (*samadhi*).

The rich and colourful symbolism of the *chakras* goes far beyond the concise summary given above.

THE *SUSHUMNA*

The *sushumna* is the fine channel which carries *kundalini* energy. Taking the two main views, it is either physically located as the vagus or pneumogastric, the tenth cranial nerve, or is considered to be part of the invisible network of channels of the astral body. The former view is argued in detail by Dr Vansant Rele in *The Mysteri-*

ous Kundalini (**69**); he also states the case for the *chakras* being nerve plexuses. On either side of the astral tube or *sushumna* run two other tubes called *ida* and *pingala*, which carry nerve currents up and down the body.

SELF-REALIZATION

Throughout its long history Kundalini Yoga has been practised by persons seeking magical and occult powers. The writers of Tantric texts in their enthusiasms have exaggerated such powers, and also are guilty of oversimplyfing the means to success. A single *mantra* or *mudra* is credited with the power to raise *kundalini* to 'the thousand-petalled lotus' in the cerebrum. The result is *samadhi*, the realization of the true Self beyond the ego that is the goal of all the Yogas.

The process of raising *kundalini* from *chakra* to *chakra* can take hours of psycho-physical control and concentrative meditation, and it may take decades of regular practice before the brow centre is reached, if it ever is. According to the jacket blurb of the British edition of his *Secret of Yoga* (**43**), Gopi Krishna, after seventeen years of meditation, 'unexpectedly experienced the awakening of *kundalini*, and subsequent severe ordeals which few have survived.' And Swami Vishnudevananda (**92**) says that only a few famous Yogins have taken serpent power to the crown of the head. As things now stand, *kundalini* is not the easiest of paths to the Self.

XI   Yoga of Action (Karma)

WISDOM IN ACTION

Karma Yoga is called 'the Yoga of Action' (*karma* means 'action'), but it must be understood that a special quality of action is intended, one far removed from the 'go-getting' so admired in the Western world. This special quality at its purest is called actionless action (*naishkarmya karma*), and results from non-attachment (*vairagya*). In the *Bhagavad Gita*, in which the most inspired instruction in 'the way of action' is to be found, the need for non-attachment is stressed again and again, but this is only really complete when the individual has found and lives in his Self (*Purusha* or *Atman*), which is untouched by action and is over and above it as pure Being.

By the universal law of *karma*, good actions beget good results and likewise evil action produce evil results. Intentions count as actions, and one does not suffer for unintentional evil actions. Thoughts, good or bad, normally tend to be acted out in some way, and may become habits. Hence the saying: 'We sow a thought, we reap an act. We sow an act and reap a habit. We sow a habit and reap a judgment.' The law of *karma* is at work in our dealings with wife, children, parents, relations, colleagues in work, and so on. The Hindu believes he has future lives – a great many of them if need be – to build up *karmic* credit to effect release from the round of rebirths. Few people in the Western world believe in reincarnation, but we can all see how to some extent our thoughts, actions, and habits build up a store of future misfortune or future good for us in this one life we are sure of.

Despite a relationship with the law of *karma*, Karma Yoga does not make much of good and bad deeds, in the sense of listing them and reiterating warnings against 'sin' or 'wickedness'. The emphasis is on non-attachment, and action performed with full attention in the here and now and in a spirit of care and compassion – love guided by wisdom.

Karma Yoga is wisdom in work and action. The Karma Yogin's actions are marked by poise of body, mind, and spirit. In this the other main Yogas can make their contribution: Hatha Yoga for better posture, balance, and relaxation; Raja Yoga for equanimity and control of mind: Jnana Yoga for knowledge of Self; and Bhakti Yoga to impart a feeling tone of love and worship to all life's activities, even the humblest. Karma Yogins reinforce wisdom in work and action with set periods of meditation for mental hygiene and deeper insight, but there is a sense in which meditation and contemplation are possible at any moment. Each action, when performed with right attention, becomes contemplative. A similar approach is found in Buddhism: Zen Buddhists talk of 'every moment Zen' (Zen means 'meditation'). A Zen Master, asked 'What is Zen?' replied: 'When you are hungry eat, when you are tired sleep.'

In Karma Yoga, love and duty having become one, duties become sources of happiness. The dustman who performs his work with mindfulness is the equal of the surgeon performing a delicate operation in the same spirit, and superior in Yogic terms if the latter works only with thought of the money he will receive. Right attitude is all-important.

Karma Yoga is seen at its finest in a life of service. Mahatma Gandhi exemplified the spirit of Karma Yoga; Albert Schweitzer could also be mentioned in this connection.

Karma Yoga means service and work without clinging to the fruits of action. This is a difficult concept for Westerners to grasp. More often than not it leads to a rich return in efficiency, effectiveness, and productivity. A poised detachment from work, accompanied by steady application, is a sure technique for consistent and skilled results.

GITA YOGAS

Karma Yogins turn to the *Bhagavad Gita* for inspirational instruction in the Way of Action. This great work, which calls itself a Yoga scripture, is not without appeal for Westerners: over a hundred translations have been made into English and other European languages. The chapter headings reveal that the *Gita's* range of instruction is not so much Yoga as Yogas – Samkhya Yoga, Karma Yoga, Jnana Yoga, Sannyasa Yoga, Dhyana Yoga, Vijnana Yoga, Abhyasa Yoga, Bhakti Yoga. There is also mention in the text of Buddhi Yoga and Atman Yoga. The nature of these Yogas can be summarized as follows:

Samkhya Yoga – Yoga of Science (literally 'number')
Karma Yoga – Yoga of Action
Jnana Yoga – Yoga of Self-knowledge
Sannyasa Yoga – Yoga of Renunciation
Dhyana Yoga – Yoga of Meditation
Vijnana Yoga – Yoga of Comprehension
Abhyasa Yoga – Yoga of Steady Effort
Bhakti Yoga – Yoga of Devotion
Buddhi Yoga – Yoga of Wisdom
Atman Yoga – Yoga of Self

There is considerable overlapping of the Yogas, so that it is virtually impossible to practice any one of the above Yogas without practising several of the others. Things become less confused if we reduce the Yogas to three that between them absorb all the others. These are Karma Yoga, Jnana Yoga, and Bhakti Yoga.

Lord Krishna's instruction to Arjuna in the discourses of the *Gita* overlaps with that given by Patanjali in his *Yoga Sutras*. In both works one finds the key sequence of internal Yoga – concentration (*dharana*), contemplation (*dhyana*), and Self-realization (*samadhi*). The insights gained by meditation are to be carried into everyday action. The Yogin established in wisdom goes about his duties with actionless action, a paradoxical and difficult concept also taught in Taoism and Zen, in which it is called non-action (*wu-wei*).

NON-ATTACHMENT

Non-attachment (*vairagya*) is the key to practising Karma Yoga. It is often misinterpreted by Westerners as apathy, indifference, or coldness: it is true that the writers of the old Yoga texts, by their use of forceful simile and metaphor, often give that impression.

In the second discourse of the *Gita*, Lord Krishna instructs:

2, 47. Thy concern is with action alone, never with results. Let not the fruit of action be thy motive, nor let thy attachment be for inaction.

2, 48. Steadfast in devotion do thy works, O Dhanamjaya, casting off attachment, being the same in success and failure. Evenness is called Yoga. . . .

2, 51. For men of wisdom cast off the fruit of action; possessed of knowledge [and] released from the bond of birth, they go to the place where there is no evil.

Krishna and Arjuna hold their conversation on a battlefield, shortly before the start of the battle. Arjuna is told by the god that he is committed to action in the relative world; he cannot do otherwise. However, the young warrior must act while aware of the Self within that is untouched by action. And he must act without thought of result. Which is not the same thing as not having any aims, not caring, or not accepting the result when it comes.

Maharishi Mahesh Yogi (146) comments on Discourse 2, verse 47: This does not mean that Arjuna is not to fight for the sake of winning the battle; it does not mean that the action should be done without caring for its result. That would be hypocrisy.

It is the anticipated fruit of an action that induces a man to act. It is desire for a result that makes him begin to act and enables him to persist in the process of action. The Lord wishes to show that the result of the action will be greater if the doer puts all his attention and energy into the action itself, if he does not allow his attention and energy to be distracted by thinking of results. The result will be according to the action, there is no doubt about that. . . .

The teaching of non-anticipation of the fruit of action has an even deeper, cosmic significance in that it is supported by the very process of evolution. If a man is held by the fruit of action, then his sole concern is centred on the horizontal plane of life. Seeing nothing higher than the action and its fruit, he loses sight of the Divine, which pervades the action and is the almighty power at its basis leading it to ultimate fulfilment. He thus loses contact with the vertical plane of life, on which the process of evolution is based.

Thus it is clear that the lord's teaching on the one hand supports activity and on the other upholds evolution and freedom.

Non-attachment means not clinging to objects, emotions, images, ideas. One cannot avoid action, one cannot avoid things; but it is possible to act without having an attitude of possessiveness. The Sanskrit word *niryogakshema* is used in the *Gita* to convey the state of being 'independent of possessions' – which does not mean not having any at all (though Yogins generally make do with very little) but carries the meaning that (147) 'in this state one is not required to think of gaining what one does not have or of preserving what one has.'

We are speaking now of a kind of streamlined living that finds delight in the most important things, which are also seen to be the simplest things. In this way one acts free from bondage to things. So many people are held captive by their possessions, though they think it is the other way round.

In Discourse 3 Lord Krishna teaches Arjuna that every action should be performed as an act of devotion, as a sacrifice (*yajna*). With clear vision, obtained by Yoga, it will be obvious where one's duty lies and one acts accordingly. The man with knowledge of the Self (*Atman* or *Purusha*) is capable of actionless action (*naishkarmya karma*). He acts because one cannot live in the relative world without acting, but he is not the slave of things – whether material objects, emotions, or thought. Having an attitude of non-grasping and non-anticipating, he is free to give his total attention to what he is doing in the manner which the Buddhists call mindfulness, which is the total man totally attending. Thus pruning a rose bush, buttoning a coat, typing a manuscript, boiling an egg, ironing a shirt, and any of the multiplicity of crafts, arts, trades, and professions becomes a form of contemplation and at the same time a form of worship.

'The place where there is no evil,' referred to in the *Gita* 2, 51, is the state of spiritual freedom (*Moksha*). The highest non-attachment is found in the liberated Yogin.

THE *GITA'S* TEACHING OF KARMA YOGA

The key passages in the *Bhagavad Gita* giving guidance on Karma Yoga occur in the third discourse. The following verses were translated into English by A. Mahadeva Sastri. The commentary given within quotation marks is that by the philosopher Sankaracharya, whose name is spelt in several other ways – *acharya* means 'religious teacher'. He is thought to have lived between 510 and 478 BC, though some scholars place him later.

3, 3. In this world a two fold path was taught by Me at first, O sinless one: that of the *Samkyhas* by devotion to knowledge, and that of the Yogins by devotion to action.

The understanding gained by Jnana Yoga, the Yoga of Knowledge, and by contacting pure consciousness by meditation, can be

carried into everyday action and action itself can be a form of
contemplation in the way described earlier. It is understandable
that the path of Karma Yoga should be deemed suitable for people
caught up in family, social, and commercial life. Karma is the Yoga
of the market place, but the Self-realized Yogin is untouched by its
clamour and its profusion of sense stimuli and objects of consciousness.

3, 4. Not by abstaining from action does man win actionlessness, nor
by mere renunciation does he attain perfection.

'By abstaining from action man cannot attain to actionlessness
(*naishkarmya*), freedom from activity, i.e. devotion in the path of
knowledge, the condition of the actionles: Self.' *Naishkaryma* can
also be translated as 'non-action' or 'actionless action'. One acts, but
in the knowledge that the Self is not touched.

3, 5. None, verily, even for an instant, ever remains doing no action;
for every one is driven helpless to action by the energies born of nature.

'The energies (*gunas*) are three, *Sattva*, *Rajas* and *Tamas*. "Every
one" means every living being that is ignorant [*ajna*], who knows not
[the Self]; for, it is said of a wise man that he is one "who is
unshaken by the energies" (14, 23).' 14, 23 reads: 'He who, seated
as a neutral, is not moved by *gunas;* who, thinking that *gunas* act,
is firm and moves not.'

3, 6. He who, restraining the organs of action, sits thinking in his mind
of the objects of the senses, self-deluded, he is said to be one of false
conduct.

In a word, a hypocrite. The organs of action are the hand, the
foot, and so on. Stopping physical action while indulging in mental
activity of the kind mentioned would be hypocritical.

3, 7. But whoso, restraining the senses by mind, O Arjuna, engages in
Karma Yoga, unattached, with organs of action, he is esteemed.

The hypocrite of 3,6 is here contrasted with the Karma Yogin
who performs actionless action, with the senses controlled. Verse 42
of discourse 3 says: 'They say that the senses are superior; superior
to the senses is mind; superior to mind is reason; one who is even
superior to reason is He.' 'He' is the Self (*Atman*).

3, 8. Do thou perform [thy] bounden duty; for, action is superior to
inaction. And even the maintenance of the body would not be possible
for thee by inaction.

3, 9. Except in the case of action for Sacrifice's sake, this world is action-bound. Action for the sake therefore, do thou, O son of Kunti, perform, free from attachment.

Maharishi Mahesh Yogi says that sacrifice (*yaghya*) should be given a broader meaning than religious ceremony, making it an action which aids evolution in the direction of higher consciousness. Worthwhile acts can also be viewed as devotional 'offerings'.

3, 19. Therefore, without attachment, constantly perform the action which should be done; for, performing action without attachment, man reaches the Supreme. . . .

3, 27. Actions are wrought in all cases by the energies of Nature. He whose mind is deluded by egoism thinks 'I am the doer'.

He who 'by egoism identifying the aggregate of the body and the senses with the Self, i.e., who ascribes to himself all the attributes of the body and the senses and thus thoroughly identifies himself with them – he, by nescience, sees actions in himself: as regards every action, he thinks "I am the doer".'

We have learned earlier that it is the three *gunas* that act and not the Self. The ego keeps thinking 'I' do this, 'I' do that. The ego bolsters its need for power by saying it acts, when lucid thought reveals that Nature (the interacting *gunas*) is responsible. Consider the meaning of saying 'I am hungry', 'I am angry', and so on. And ask yourself whether you breathe or are breathed.

3, 28. But he who knows the truth, O mighty-armed, about the divisions of the energies and [their] functions, is not attached, thinking that the energies act upon the energies.

'He who is versed in the classification of the energies [*gunas*] and their respective functions holds that the energies as sense-organs move amid the energies as sense-objects, but not the Self. Thus holding, he forms no attachments for actions '.

3, 30. Renouncing all actions in Me, with thy thought resting on the Self, being free from hope, free from selfishness, devoid of fever, do thou fight.

'Fever' here can mean anguish, grief, or delusion. Maharishi Mahesh Yogi translates (146): 'Surrendering all actions to Me by maintaining your consciousness in the Self, freed from longing and the sense of "mine", fight, delivered from the fever [of delusion].' To 'maintain your consciousness in the Self' while engaged in action requires an ability to retain the state of higher consciousness even in the market place and not just during the dive within in meditation. The Maharishi says:

Maintenance of transcendental Self-consciousness along with activity in the waking state of consciousness requires co-existence of the two states of consciousness. The ability of man's nervous system, which is the physical machinery through which consciousness expresses itself, has to be developed to express these two states simultaneously. This is brought about by regularly interrupting the constant activity of the waking state of consciousness with periods of silence in transcendental consciousness. When, through this practice, the nervous system has been permanently conditioned to maintain these two states together, then the consciousness remains always centred in the Self. The Lord explains that this centering of consciousness in the Self is the way of 'surrendering all actions to Me.'

'All this is threaded on me,' says the *Gita*, 7, 7. We are one with the divine principle. Awareness of this on a plane of universal consciousness is the aim of all the Yogas. The Karma Yogin realizes it through selfless service, acting without thought for the fruits of action, non-grasping and non-clinging, his action a form of renunciation, devotion, and worship.

XII   Yoga of Devotion: Bhakti

BHAKTI PRACTICE

Bhakti is the Way or Yoga of Devotion. Here again we have a form of meditation. Acts of devotion or adoration – in Hinduism, usually directed to chosen deities, Krishna being a favourite – should be performed in the meditative or contemplative manner: that is, the whole person wholly attending. For the Hindu, sincere devotion produces good *karmas*, and the Bhakti way merges naturally with that of Karma, the Yoga of Selfless Action. Devotion should be without egoism or expectation of rewards – petitioning God with prayers in the Christian manner is not customary. Bhakti thus fulfils the major purpose of all the esoteric Eastern psychologies, which is to dissolve the ego and to find the Self. Purification is an important feature of all Yoga practice. Here it is consciousness that is purified, the steady flame of Bhakti love burning up such spiritual impurities as hatred, anger, greed, pride, and other destructive emotions.

Bhakti makes a strong appeal to the Indian masses – it has always been their favourite Yoga. It requires simplicity of heart and a steady flow of devotion. It does not require education or a well-honed intellect; though, in the way that Yoga paths overlap, the intellectual approach does not exclude the worshipful: the two may work in harness.

But when not tempered by detachment and intellectual objectivity Bhakti adoration can pass into hysteria and possession. It then becomes the equivalent of the most emotional of the Christian sects: snake-handling, speaking with tongues, and the like occur. A report (18) on Bhakti worship and celebration in Bengal Vaishnaism lists the following behaviour observed as a result of arousing intense love of Krishna: '*nrtya* [dancing], *viluthita* [rolling on the ground], *gits* (singing), *krosana* [loud crying], *tanu-motana* [twisting of the body], *hujkara* [shouting], *jrmbha* [yawning], *svasa-bhuman* [profusion of sighs], *lokanapeksita* [disregard of popular opinion], *lalasrava* [foaming at the mouth], *atta-hasa* [loud laughter], *ghurna* [giddiness], *hikka* [hiccup].'

If adoration is steady it finds its own forms. Bhakti practice is an opening-up to the heart's will and direction. Worship takes different forms in different cultures. The Hindu expresses devotion in singing hymns of praise, in dancing, and in repeating (*japa*) *mantras*.

BHAKTI HYMNS

Bhakti songs of praise are often of lyric beauty, and are not without resemblances to Christian hymns.

The taming and steadying of the senses that is an important part of Yogic meditation is found in the following seventeenth-century Bhakti hymn by Tukaram (**108**):

THOUGH *HE* SLAY ME

Now I submit me to thy will,
Whether thou save or whether kill;
Keep thou near or send me hence,
Or plunge me in the war of sense.

Thee in my ignorance I sought,
Of true devotion knowing nought.
Little could I, a dullard, know,
Myself the lowest of the low.

My mind I cannot steadfast hold;
My senses wander uncontrolled.
Ah, I have sought and sought for peace.
In vain, for me there's no release.

Now bring I thee a faith complete
And lay my life before thy feet.
Do thou, O God, what seemeth best;
In thee, in thee alone is rest.

In thee I trust, and, hapless wight,
Cling to thy skirts with all my might.
My strength is spent, I, Tuka, say;
Now upon thee this task I lay.

Mahatma Gandhi was said to have a special affection for the
following Vaishnavite hymn (18):

He is the true Vaishnava who knows and feels another's woes as his own.
Ever ready to serve, he never boasts.
He bows to everyone, and despises no one, keeping his thought, word,
and deed pure.
Blessed is the mother of such an one. He reverences every woman as
his mother.
He keeps an equal mind and does not stain his lips with falsehood; nor
does he touch another's wealth.
No bonds of attachment can hold him.
Ever in tune with Ramanama, his body possessed in itself all places
of pilgrimage.
Free from greed and deceit, passion and anger, this is the true Vaishnava.

MANTRAS

Bhakti employs concentrative meditation in repetition (*japa*) of
mantras. 'The principle of *bhakti* is that the things we love and
dwell upon we become,' says Ernest Wood (94).

Hence the *mantras* of the gods and goddesses, whose powers and virtues are effective, as they are names. That is why people sing hymns, and
why in Indian villages there is constantly the singing of songs with the
repetitions of names or praises (*bhajans*) which are set to pleasing music
relating the sound to the thought and to that extent forming a mental
home or habitat where the mind can rest in an upward-turned condition.

He adds: 'With respect to every *mantra* – as in the case of Western
ceremonial – there must be *intent*, otherwise the words of a parrot
or of a gramophone would carry the full power.'

KRISHNA CONSCIOUSNESS

The Krishna Consciousness Movement, whose spiritual master is
A. C. Bhaktivedanta Swami Prabhupada, is based on studying the
Bhakti teachings of Lord Krishna in the *Bhagavad Gita* and on
chanting the *mantra*: HARE KRISHNA, HARE KRISHNA,
KRISHNA KRISHNA, HARE HARE, HARE RAMA, HARE
RAMA, RAMA RAMA, HARE HARE. Young people dancing

and chanting the preceding *mantra* have become a familiar sight in the major cities of the world.

Swami Prabhupada explains the purpose in chanting the *mantra* (159):

What is ego? I am pure soul, but with my intelligence and mind I am in contact with matter, and I have identified myself with matter. This is false ego. I am pure soul, but I am identifying falsely. For example, I am identifying with the land, thinking that I am an Indian, or that I am American. This is called *ahamkara*. *Ahamkara* means the point where the pure soul touches matter. That junction is called *ahamkara*. *Ahamkara* is still finer than intelligence.

Krishna says that these are the eight material elements: earth, water, fire, air, ether, mind, intelligence and false ego. False ego means false identification. Our nescient life has begun from this false identification – thinking that I am this matter, although I am seeing every day, at every moment, that I am not this matter. Soul is permanently existing, while matter is changing. This misconception, this illusion, is called *ahamkara* false ego. And your liberation means when you are out of this false ego. What is that status? *Aham brahmasmi.* I am *Brahman*, I am spirit. That is the beginning of liberation. . . .

Simply understanding that I am not matter, I am soul, is not perfection. The impersonalist, the void philosopher, simply thinks of the negative, that I am not this matter, I am not this body. This will not stay. You have to not only realize that you are not matter, but you have to engage yourself in the spiritual world. And that spiritual world means to be working in Krishna consciousness. That spiritual world, that functioning of our real life, is Krishna consciousness.

False ego I have already explained. It is neither matter nor spirit, but the junction – where the spirit soul comes into contact with matter and forgets himself. It is just as, in delirium, a man is diseased and his brain becomes puzzled, and gradually he forgets himself and becomes a madman. He is gradually forgetting. So there is the beginning of loss, and there is one point where he forgets. That beginning point is called *ahamkara*, or false ego.

Chanting the *mahamantra* – Hare Krishna, Hare Krishna, Krishna Krishna, Hare Hare, Hare Rama, Hare Rama, Rama Rama, Hare Hare – is the process not merely of putting an end to this false conception of the self, but it goes beyond that, to the point where the pure spirit soul engages in his eternal, blissful, all-knowing activities in the loving service of God. This is the height of conscious development, the ultimate goal of all living entities now evolving through the cycles and species of material nature.

Ahamkara is the 'I'-sense set up by the action of spirit on matter (*prakriti*). *Prakriti's* evolutes were discussed in the chapter entitled 'Yogic Philosophy.'

BHAKTI *SAMADHI*

Bhakti calls on the Raja Yoga techniques of concentration and contemplation – it cannot do otherwise if the devotional force is sincere and authentic. Its powerful content of love and unselfishness should also demand action and service to one's fellow men: that is, it should lead to working in harness with Karma Yoga. Concentration and contemplation can be sustained into *samadhi*. The *Gheranda Samhita* (90), one of the classic texts we consulted several times for *Yoga of Breathing*, describes Bhakti as one of the ways to Yoga's supreme goal of enlightenment– 'Let him contemplate within his heart his special Deity; let him be full of ecstasy by such contemplation; let him, with thrill, shed tears of happiness, and by so doing he will become entranced. This leads to *Samadhi* and *Manomani*.' *Manomani* is another word for *samadhi*.

Samadhi triggered by sustained emotional concentration in its initial stages will contain gross elements but, once established, can be purified and refined. The rapture of the Christian mystics often has this affective tone, for, like Bhakti, it is powered by personal devotion to God or to Christ. The ecstasy of St Teresa of Avila, which will be quoted in the chapter entitled 'Yoga of Sex: Tantrism', cannot be cited as a pure example of mystical illumination, for her experience clearly had a strong emotional, even erotic, content. The bliss of *samadhi* and its intuitive awareness are much finer, more lucid, and less supercharged.

D. T. Suzuji (169), who has done more than any other oriental to explain Zen Buddhism to the West, in one of his essays compares the affective tone of so much Christian mysticism with the impersonal tone of Eastern illumination – *samadhi* in Yoga, *satori* in Zen – and says that the emotional content is added by Christian doctrine and does not really belong to the universal experience.

Perhaps the most remarkable aspect of the Zen experience is that it has no personal note in it as is observable in Christian mystic experiences.

There is no reference whatever in Buddhist *satori* to such personal and frequently sexual feelings and relationships as are to be gleaned from these terms: flame of love, a wonderful love shed in the heart, embrace, the beloved, bride, bridegroom, spiritual matrimony, Father, God, the Son of God, God's child, etc. We may say that all these terms are interpretations based on a definite system of thought and really have nothing to do with the experience itself. At any rate, alike in India, China, and Japan, *satori* has remained thoroughly impersonal, or rather highly intellectual.

Bhakti, however, is the Yoga with the strongest affective tone, though it is true to say that Bhakti *samadhi* is not so emotional as the experiences related by some of the Christian mystics. But Christian mystics vary in temperament: Meister Eckhart is clearly intellectual (a Jnana Yogin), and St John of the Cross (St Teresa's compatriot) blends harmoniously two paths to illumination: love and understanding.

CHRISTIAN YOGAS

Bhakti and Christian worship have affinities: both direct devotion and adoration to divine figures. A little thought will show that Christianity, like Hinduism, has its Bhakti, Karma, and Jnana paths – those of devotion, social service, and intellection respectively. It has its Mantra Yoga in prayer, its Raja Yoga in meditation and contemplation. Only Hatha Yoga, with its physical exercises and breath controls, fails to find a correspondence. (The English emphasis on building moral fibre on the playing fields points in that direction, but is only faintly comparable.)

THE *GITA* ON BHAKTI YOGA

Bhakti Yogins have a special affection for the *Bhagavad Gita*, in particular those chapters which describe the Yoga of Devotion. Discourses 9 to 12 are mainly devotional – Discourse 12 is an account of Bhakti Yoga. Devotion to the Supreme is described in the following verses:

9, 18. I am the Goal, the Sustainer, the Lord, the Witness, the Abode, the Shelter and the Friend, the Origin, Dissolution and Stay; the Treasure-house, the Seed imperishable.

9, 22. Those men who, meditating on Me as non-separate, worship Me all around – to them who are ever devout, I secure gain and safety.

9, 26. When one offers to Me with devotion a leaf, a flower, a fruit, water – that I eat, offered with devotion by the pure-minded.

9, 27. Whatever thou doest, whatever thou eatest, whatever thou sacrificest, whatever thou givest, in whatever austerity thou engagest, do it as an offering to Me.

9, 28. Thus shalt thou be liberated from the bonds of actions which are productive of good and evil results; equipped in mind with the Yoga of renunciation, and liberated, thou shalt come to Me.

9, 34. Fix thy mind on Me, be devoted to Me, sacrifice to Me, bow down to Me. Thus steadied, with Me as thy Supreme Goal, thou shalt reach Myself, the Self.
'Steadied' in the above verse refers to keeping the pool of mind-stuff (*citta*) unruffled. 'The Self' refers to the Self of all beings. And Self equals Cosmic Self.

10, 20. I am the Self, O Gudakesa, seated in the heart of all beings; I am the beginning and the middle, as also the end, of all beings.
Sankaracharya, the most illustrious commentator on the *Gita*, considered the following verse to be 'the essence of the whole teaching . . . which conduces to Highest Bliss':

11, 55. He who does work for Me, who looks on Me as the Supreme, who is devoted to Me, who is free from attachment, who is without hatred for any being, he comes to Me, O Pandava.
Verses 13 to 20 of Discourse 12 are cherished by Bahkti Yogins:
12, 13-14. He who hates no single being, who is friendly and compassionate to all, who is free from attachment and egoism, to whom pain and pleasure are equal, who is enduring, ever content and balanced in mind, self-controlled, and possessed of firm conviction, whose thought and reason are directed to Me, he who is [thus] devoted to Me is dear to Me.

12, 15. He by whom the world is not afflicted and who is not afflicted by the world, who is free from joy, envy, fear and sorrow, he is dear to Me.

12, 16. He who is free from wants, who is pure, clever, unconcerned, untroubled, renouncing all undertakings, he who is [thus] devoted to Me is dear to Me.

12, 17. He who neither rejoices, nor hates, nor grieves, nor desires, renouncing good and evil, he who is full of devotion is dear to Me.

12, 18-19. He who is the same to foe and friend, and also in honour and dishonour; who is the same in cold and heat, in pleasure and pain; who is free from attachment; to whom censure and praise are equal; who is silent, content with anything, homeless, steady-minded, full of devotion; that man is dear to Me.

12, 20. They, verily, who follow this immortal Law described above, endued with faith, looking up to Me as the Supreme, and devoted, they are exceedingly dear to Me.

Sir Edwin Arnold's verse translation of the *Bhagavad Gita* presents the final lines of Discourse 12 less literally than the translation given above, but more poetically:

> Who fixed in faith on me
> Dotes upon none, scorns none; rejoices not,
> And grieves not, letting good or evil hap
> Light when it will, and when it will depart,
> That man I love! Who, unto friend and foe
> Keeping an equal heart, with equal mind
> Bears shame and glory; with an equal peace
> Takes heat and cold, pleasure and pain; abides
> Quit of desires, hears praise or calumny
> In passionless restraint, unmoved by each;
> Linked by no ties to earth, steadfast in Me,
> That Man I love!

XIII Yoga of Knowledge: Jnana

REASON AND BEYOND

Just as Karma Yoga is the way of action and Bhakti Yoga the way
of devotion, so Jnana Yoga is the way of knowledge. It does not
exclude assistance from other Yogas, but in itself stands out because
it makes use of conscious reasoning to penetrate the veils of ignorance
and illusion that prevent our seeing the light of that pure consciousness which Yogins consider the basis of life and its secret. But
intellectual understanding needs to be reinforced by the experience
of meditation in which thought is transcended because the meditator has gone to its source within.

Jnana Yoga uses the well-honed intellect to cut a way through
the tangle of mental impressions (*samskaras*) to find the truth that
dwells in the place the *upanishads* call 'the space within the heart'

The English poet Robert Browning wrote, in 'Paracelsus':

> Truth is within ourselves; it takes no rise
> From outward things, whate'er you may believe.
> There is an inmost centre in us all,
> Where truth abides in fullness; and around,
> Wall upon wall, the gross flesh hems it in,
> This perfect, clear perception – which is truth.
> A baffling and perverting carnal mesh
> Binds it, and makes all error: and, to *know*
> Rather consists in opening out a way
> Whence the imprisoned spendour may escape,
> Than in effecting entry for a light
> Supposed to be without.

The Jnana Yogin uses the penetrating power of thought to open
out a way to the 'inmost centre', but in the end thought is stilled,
falls silent, and is transcended. It is not a question of despising or

underestimating the powers of reason, but of taking them as far as they will go, which is to the taking-off point for transcendental consciousness, sometimes called bliss consciousness (*sat chit ananda*).

The greatest Yoga teachers look on Yoga as a science that does not contradict reason, though in the final stage it goes beyond it to the plane of Being. Swami Vivekananda taught that the lower and higher stages of consciousness belong to the same mind and that Yogic Enlightenment fulfils reason. This is how he put it (171):

> To get any reason out of the mass of incongruity we call human life, we have to transcend our reason, but we must do it scientifically, slowly, by regular practice, and we must cast off all superstition. We must take up the study of the super-conscious state just as any other science. On reason we must lay our foundation, we must follow reason as far as it leads; and when reason fails, reason itself will show us the way to the highest plane. When you hear a man say, 'I am inspired', and then talk irrationally, reject it. Why? Because these three states – instinct, reason and super-consciousness, or the unconscious, conscious, and super-conscious states – belong to one and the same mind. There are three minds in one man, but one state of it develops into the others. Instinct develops into reason, and reason into the transcendental consciousness; therefore not one of the states contradicts the others. Real inspiration never contradicts reason, but fulfils it. Just as you find the great prophets saying, 'I come not to destroy but to fulfil', so inspiration always comes to full reason, and is in harmony with it.

Vivekananda is repeating a teaching expressed in the sixth century BC in the *Bhagavad Gita*:

> 3, 42. They say that the senses are superior; superior to the sense is mind; superior to mind is reason; one who is even superior to reason is He.

The distinction made in Yoga between mind (*manas*), which is concerned with selection and rejection, assimilation and co-ordination, and reason or intellect (*buddhi*) is here brought out. The latter is higher than the former in the evolution towards Self-realization. Sankaracharya, the leading expounder of Jnana Yoga, comments on the above verse (164):

> The senses are five, the sense of hearing, etc. When compared with the physical body, which is gross, external, and limited, the senses are superior as they are comparatively more subtle and internal, and have a more extensive sphere of action. So say the wise. Superior to the senses is mind (*manas*, the impulsive nature) which is composed of

thoughts and desires, of errors and doubts (*sankalpa* and *vikalpa*). Superior to mind is reason (*buddhi*) characterized by determination (*nischaya*). So, He who is behind all things visible, inclusive of reason, the Dweller in the body, whom – it has been said – desire, seated in the senses and other quarters, bewilders by enveloping wisdom – He, the Self, the witness of reason, is superior to reason.

The concluding verse of Discourse 3 follows:

3, 43. Thus knowing Him who is superior to reason, subduing the self by the self, slay thou, O mighty-armed, the enemy in the form of desire, hard to conquer.

Lord Krishna is instructing the young warrior Arjuna. Understanding the Self, the *Atman* which is identical with the Absolute One or *Brahman*, is the heart of Jnana Yoga practice and experience.

REGRESSION OR EVOLUTIONARY ADVANCE?

The Western rationalist is wary of going beyond reason. He may also suspect that the superconscious state of mystical experience is a regression to primitive or fetal levels of existence. Sigmund Freud and other psycho-analysts have taken this view. Those Yogins who have attained Self-realization (*samadhi*) aver that the mystic experience is not a regression but an evolutionary advance based on an integration that is the highest possible development of human consciousness, in which the subject-object duality is reconciled in a new unity which is the essence of maturity.

Professor Eliade puts the case for the goal of Yogic meditation, Patanjali's eighth and final stage (120):

It would be a gross error to regard this supreme reintegration as a mere regression to primordial nondistinction. It can never be repeated too often that Yoga, like many other mysticisms, issues on the plane of paradox and not on a commonplace and easy extinction of consciousness. As we shall see, from time immemorial India has known the many and various trances and ecstasies obtained from intoxicants, narcotics, and all the other elementary means of emptying consciousness; but any degree of methodological conscience will show us that we have no right to put *samadhi* among these countless varieties of spiritual escape. Liberation is not assimilable with the 'deep sleep' of prenatal existence, even if the recovery of totality through undifferentiated enstasis seems to resemble the bliss of the human being's fetal preconsciousness. One essential fact must always be borne in mind: the yogin works on all levels of consciousness and of the subconscious, for the purpose of opening the way to transconsciousness (knowledge-possession of the Self, the *purusa*). He enters into 'deep sleep' and into the 'fourth state' (*turiya*, the cataleptic state) with the utmost lucidity; he does not sink into self-hypnosis. The importance that all authors ascribe to the yogic states of *super*consciousness shows us that the final reintegration takes place in *this* direction, and not in a trance, however profound. In other words: the recovery, through *samadhi*, of the initial nonduality introduces a new element in comparison with the primordial situation (that which existed before the twofold division of the real into object-subject). That element is *knowledge* of unity and bliss. There is a 'return to the beginning,' but with the difference that the man 'liberated in this life' recovers the original situation enriched by the dimensions of *freedom* and *transconsciousness*.

THE ONION GAME

Though the mystic experience is ineffable and can only be known by direct experience, nevertheless mystics sometimes feel drawn to attempt a negative description: if they cannot say what it is, they can at least say what it is not, the Hindu 'not this, not that' (*neti, neti*). And they continue the stripping process until nothing remains, or rather Nothing, for we speak now of what Buddhists call the Void, which is really a plenitude and the source of every manifest thing. Other names the experience goes by are Being, Self, Ultimate Reality, *Brahman*, *Atman*, Cosmic Consciousness, God, Godhead.

The *Tao Te Ching* says in its opening line: 'The Tao that can be expressed is not the eternal Tao.' And St John of the Cross speaks for all mystics when he says (134):

We receive this mystical knowledge of God [Being, Self, etc.] clothed in none of the kinds of images, in none of the sensible representations which our mind makes use of in other circumstances. Accordingly in this knowledge, since the senses and imagination are not employed, we get neither form nor impression, nor can we give any account or furnish any likeness, although the mysterious and sweet tasting wisdom comes here so directly to the innermost parts of the soul.

Father Augustin Baker (1575-1641), in one of his many treatises on the prayer of contemplation, states (105):

By reason of this habituation and absolute dominion of the Holy Spirit in the souls of the perfect (who have wholly neglected, forgotten, and lost themselves, to the end that God alone may live in them, whom they contemplate in the absolute obscurity of faith), hence it is that some mystic writers do call this perfect union the UNION OF NOTHING WITH NOTHING, that is, the union of the soul, which is nowhere corporally, that hath no images nor affections to creatures in her; yes, that hath lost the free disposal of her own faculties, acting by a portion of the spirit above all the faculties, and according to the actual touches of the Divine Spirit, and apprehending God with an exclusion of all conceptions and apprehensions; thus it is that the soul, being nowhere corporally or sensibly, is everywhere spiritually and immediately united to God, this infinite nothing.

A stripping away ('not this, not that') is basic to the meditative practice of the Jnana Yogin in answer to the key question: Who (or what) am I? Like so many onion skins, the 'not I' things are peeled away, until the last skin is discarded and only the fullness of Being remains. The goal of the Onion Game has then been reached. Any person can play, though the game suits the intellectual temperament, just as Bhakti Yoga suits the devotional temperament and Karma Yoga the active temperament.

Sufis are taught to pursue the 'Who am I?' inquiry in this meditation:

I am not the body.
I am not the senses.
I am not the mind.
I am not this.
I am not that.
What then am I? What is the Self?
It is in the body.
It is in everybody.
It is everywhere.
It is the All.
It is Self. I am It. Absolute oneness.

Sufism is the mystical wing of the Islamic religion. The Sufic final stage of *fana* or 'passing away' has close affinities with the Hindu *samadhi* and the Buddhist *nirvana*. Among the various mystical traditions, descriptions of stages of the 'way' parallel each other to a considerable extent, and the final stage is inevitably a transcending of the ego and a finding of the Self.

THE *CHANDOGYA UPANISHAD*

The oldest extant accounts of how to play the Onion Game are those of the *upanishads*, notably the *Chandogya Upanishad*, which is amongst the earliest. It is believed that the first *upanishads* were written about 800 BC. These metaphysical treatises, which instruct in Yoga, are mostly the records of schools of wisdom centred on forest sages – in a sense, school notes. A few of the sages' names are mentioned, but the majority remain anonymous.

The central teaching, expressed again and again using a variety of analogies, is the *raison d'être* of Yoga practice – the *Atman* (Self) within is one with *Brahman*, the subtle essence of all things. 'That thou art' (*tat atvam asi*).

In the *Chandogya Upanishad* Svetaketu, who is twenty-four years old and has studied for twelve years, has still to learn the fundamental message about Self and the All from his father (6, 12-13, translated by Max Muller):

'Fetch me from thence a fruit of the Nyagrodha tree.'

'Here is one, Sir,'

'Break it.'

'It is broken, Sir.'

'What do you see there?'

'These seeds, almost infinitesimal.'

'Break one of them.'

'It is broken, Sir.'

'What do you see there?'

'Not anything, Sir.'

The father said: 'My son, that subtile essence which you do not perceive there, of that very essence this great Nyagrodha tree exists.

'Believe it, my son. That which is the subtle essence, in it all that exists has its self. It is the True. It is the Self, and thou, O Svetaketu, art it.'

'Please, Sir, inform me still more,' said the son.

'Be it so, my child,' the father replied.

'Place this salt in water, and wait on me in the morning.'

The son did as he was commanded.

The father said to him: 'Bring me the salt, which you placed in the water last night.'

The son having looked for it, found it not, for, of course, it was melted.

The father said: 'Taste it from the surface of the water. How is it?'

The son replied: 'It is salt.'

'Taste it from the middle. How is it?'

The son replied: 'Is is salt.'

The father said: 'Throw it away and then wait on me.'

He did so; but salt exists for ever.

Then the father said: 'Here also, in this body, forsooth, you do not perceive the True (*sat*), my son; but there indeed it is.

'That which is the subtle essence, in it all that exists has its self. It is true. It is the Self, and thou, O Svetaketu, art it.'

In section 8 of the *Chandogya Upanishad* there is a long account of meditation in pursuit of the Self – 'I am not this, I am not that' The teacher is Prajapati, and his pupil is the god Indra. Here is Prajapati's concluding instruction, in the translation of Juan Mascaro (151):

It is true that the body is mortal, that it is under the power of death; but it is also the dwelling of *Atman*, the Spirit of immortal life. The body, the house of the Spirit, is under the power of pleasure and pain; and if a man is ruled by his body then this man can never be free. But when a man is in the joy of the Spirit, in the spirit which is ever free, then this man is free from all bondage, the bondage of pleasure and pain.

The wind has not a body, nor lightning, nor thunder, nor clouds; but when those rise into the higher spheres then they find their body of light. In the same way, when the soul is in silent quietness it arises and leaves the body, and reaching the Spirit Supreme finds there its body of light. It is the land of infinite liberty where, beyond its mortal body, the Spirit of man is free. There can he laugh and sing of his glory with ethereal women and friends. He enjoys ethereal chariots and forgets the cart of his body on earth. For as a beast is attached to a cart, so on earth the soul is attached to a body.

'Know that when the eye looks into space it is the Spirit of man that sees: the eye is only the organ of sight. When one says "I feel this perfume", it is the Spirit that feels: he uses the organ of smell. When one says 'I am speaking', it is the Spirit that speaks: the voice is the organ of speech. When one says 'I am hearing', it is the Spirit that hears: the ear is the organ of hearing. And when one says 'I think', it is the Spirit that thinks: the mind is the organ of thought. It is because of the light of the Spirit that the human mind can see, and can think, and enjoy this world.

'All the gods in the heaven of *Brahman* adore in contemplation their

Infinite Spirit Supreme. This is why they have all joy, and all the worlds and all desires. And the man who on this earth finds and knows *Atman*, his own Self, has all his holy desires and all the worlds and all joy.'

I AM

Patanjali named certain *klesas* (afflictions) that the Yogin needs to eliminate. They are metaphysical ignorance (*avidya*), not recognizing one's real nature, confusion as to the nature of Reality, identifying with the ego, the sense of I-am-ness (*asmita*), attractions and repulsions, the desire for life or death. The root *klesa* is *avidya*, the ignorance responsible for our bondage, the spirit's imprisonment in matter. Patanjali defines *asmita* as a mixing of pure consciousness (*purusha*) and cognition (*buddhi*). However, it is not the pure 'I am' that is the trouble, but wrong identification with its enmeshment in matter.

Thus a modern commentator on Patanjali's *Yoga Sutras* writes (89):

'I am' represents the pure awareness of self-existence and is therefore the expression ... of pure consciousness or the *purusha*. When the pure consciousness gets involved in matter and, owing to the power of *maya*, knowledge of its real nature is lost, the pure 'I am' changes into 'I am this', where 'this' may be the subtlest vehicle through which it is working, or the grossest vehicle, namely, the physical body. The two processes – namely, the loss of awareness of its real nature and the identification with the vehicles – are simultaneous.

Note Exodus 3: 14: 'And God said unto Moses, I AM THAT I AM: and he said, Thus shalt thou say unto the children of Israel, I AM hath sent me unto you.'

I AM experience is the *purusha* or *atman* of the Yogin. It is the Self beyond the ego, and the constant behind the changes of body, intellect, and feeling.

THE ELUSIVE *I*

Look within for your *I*. It is more elusive than the Scarlet Pimpernel. We seek it here, we seek it there – but each time it eludes your grasp by becoming the *I* of a moment ago in an infinite regression. This *I* is not the contents of consciousness, for they can become the objects of consciousness at any moment. Who then observes the contents of the mind? Observing the mind you see objects of consciousness but not consciousness itself. Introspective self-examination is always the study of things of the past, even when that past is just a moment ago. And if we identify the *I* with our thoughts, images, and emotions, then we make the disconcerting discovery that we are not a single *I* but a multiplicity of *I's* each, in P. D. Ouspensky's phrase, seeking to be caliph, for an hour, sometimes only for a minute.

Some of the great Western philosophers have been puzzled by their inability to locate or grasp the elusive *I*. 'I can never catch my *self*,' said David Hume, 'Whenever I try, I always stumble at some sense-impression or idea.' And William James said: 'The so-called "self" is only a stream of thought; the passing thought itself is the thinker.' Jean-Paul Sartre too, has played the Onion Game, coming up with a concept of man's radical 'freedom' that is an existentialist version of Yoga's *moksha*. Again, Sartre's concept that man as Being-for-itself – in contrast to Being-in-itself (such as rocks, trees, and clouds) – brings Nothingness into the world has affinities with Hindu and Buddhist ideas of the Void. Hazel Barnes (106), a lucid interpreter of Sartre's philosophy, here shows how the French philosopher answers the key question of Jnana Yoga: 'Who (or What) am I?'

If I probe inward to find out what I really am, the only demonstrable objective unity I can discover is inextricably bound up with my autobiography. Yet I feel that this accumulated essence is too inert to be that directing consciousness which projects itself towards the future. I sense confusedly that the subject consciousness cannot be identified without any given set of attitudes; yet I remain convinced that throughout my psychic experience there is some transcendent unity, something which is involved in every state of consciousness without being restricted to any one of them. The mystery is explained by Sartre's conclusion that each consciousness is particular but not personal. The personal ego is on the side of the psychic; that is, it belongs with all the psychological phenomena which we view objectively as the personality. But the personality is not a structure of consciousness in the sense that we might describe the makeup of an optical lens. It is that at which the lens is directed. Consciousness itself is not timid or courageous or avaricious or generous. These qualities exist *for* consciousness. It evokes them, brings them into the world, for others and for itself. . . .

The unity of my psychic life lies precisely in my accumulation of psychic experience. The 'I' and the 'Me' are respectively the active and passive ideal poles of all that I have experienced and will experience. Therefore, the feeling of frustration which comes over me when I try introspectively to find myself reflects exactly what I actually am. If I seek to find an 'I' endowed with personal qualities, I can find one objectively in my psychic history, but the 'I' is always in the past or, by imagination, in the future. The consciousness which continues to produce it is without personal qualities. Thus my dim comprehension that the active source of my awareness trascends any 'I' which even the most accurate self-analysis could evoke is exactly correct.

If consciousness stands aloof even from the personality, it is determined by nothing save itself. Here is the source of Sartre's radical freedom. My consciousness is not myself. . . .

Granted that this self-consciousness is impersonal, what *is* it? . . . Even if we are to say that the self-consciousness is not personal, it seems that it must be something or there could be no sense of self. Or if consciousness is process and not entity, of what is it a process? I am not sure that Sartre could – or would – claim that he could give a totally satisfactory answer to that basic question. This is partly because to do so would involve us in purely metaphysical speculations which seek to go behind reality.

At the crucial point Sartre draws back from metaphysics and the numinous, not acknowledging anything holy or worthy of worship in the pure consciousness uncovered by the stripping power of his intellect. Nor does he look at meditation as a technique for exploring consciousness and going 'behind reality'.

IN PURSUIT OF THE *I*

The climax of Dr Paul Brunton's *A Search in Secret India* (109) comes when he receives this instruction from a Maharishi:

'Pursue the enquiry "Who am I?" relentlessly. Analyse your entire personality. Try to find out where the I-thought begins. Go on with your meditations. Keep turning your attention within. One day the wheel of thought will slow down and an intuition will mysteriously arise. Follow that intuition, let your thinking stop, and it will eventually lead you to the goal.'

Dr Brunton gave an account of 'Who am I?' meditation in the *The Quest of the Overself* (110)published three years after *A Search in Secret India*.

An unorthodox account of playing the Onion Game is that given by Aubrey Menen in the concluding pages of his autobiography *The Space Within The Heart* (153). Mr Menen, the son of an Indian father and an Irish mother, tells how he isolated himself in a small room in the heart of the Thieves' Quarter of Rome and proceeded to examine his life, shedding layer after layer of his personality after holding each up to the light of his attention. Basing the stripping of his conditioned ego skins on the method taught in the *upanishads*, Mr Menen finally reached what that work calls 'the space within the heart'. It is here that he is most challenging and unorthodox:

'The philosophers of the *Upanishads*, after having led the reader into the very depths of his being, with shattering results to all his dearest beliefs, advise him to get up and go and enjoy himself like anybody else, with, they specify, horses, chariots, food and women. The verses in which this is said are as coarse as a hearty laugh and a slap on the back. How people manage to find God in such a book I cannot say, but I think it may be that they have a natural refinement which puts things decently straight.'

One may assume that Aubrey Menen would attribute Juan Mascaro's repeated use of the qualifying adjective 'ethereal' in the extract from the *Chandogya Upanishad* given earlier in this chapter, and his use of 'soul' rather than 'Self', to the 'natural refinement which puts things decently straight'.

Aubrey Menen returned to what he holds to be the unadulterated message of the *upanishads* in his book The New Mystics (152), published four years after his autobiography. He says that a 'gigantic fig-leaf' has been spread over the direct and simple teachings of the *upanishads*. He describes the Onion Game again, stressing the need for shedding the layers of personality put there by parents, teachers, and society. (A similar teaching of the necessity of not identifying the Self with our conditioned ideas, attitudes, and memories may be found in the books and recorded talks of Jiddu Krishnamurti).

'Disembodied laughter' is the nearest Mr Menen feels he can get to describing the feeling of being in 'the space within the heart'(153). 'Then a great tranquillity steals over you. It trickles like water through the cells of your mind, washing them clean. You think of nothing, nothing at all, but with a crystalline awareness, and it is the end of your search.'

Yogins call this centre of consciousness the Self or Atman. And to know the *Atman* is to know *Brahman*, which is the ground of all Being.

XIV Psychic Powers (Siddhis)

THE CORRECT ATTITUDE FOR YOGINS

Told that another Yogi master had walked across the waters of a broad and deep river, a famous Tibetan Yogi retorted: 'His feat wasn't worth the penny it would have cost him to take the ferry.' This attitude to occult powers is taken by the most respected Yoga masters, and by Patanjali in his *Yoga Sutras*, in which he lists the psychic attainments (*siddhis*) resulting from the Yoga of Meditation, but points out that they are obstacles in the way of attainment of Self-realization, Yoga's goal.

Possession of psychic powers, when made the primary aim of mastering the internal nature, leads to ego-inflation. Patanjali, and other authorities, therefore say that such awakened powers should be treated in a matter-of-fact manner, as extensions of the ordinary senses, and not allowed to become distractions from the goal of stilling the mind and uncovering the pure Self. Nor should telepathy, clairvoyance, or any such attainments be used for worldly ends. Patanjali says that *siddhis* can be produced by means other than meditation: by drugs, fasting, and incantations (*mantras*), for example. A few people are born with them.

A wide range of psychic powers is listed by Patanjali in Section 3 of the *Yoga Sutras*. These are variously interpreted, from a fundamentalist approach that believes in them literally to the viewpoint that every one of them should be taken symbolically. It should also be mentioned that Yoga meditation and respiratory control can induce the feelings that the body has shrunk to minute size, that it has become light as air, that it is floating, and so on.

PATANJALI'S LISTING OF PSYCHIC ATTAINMENTS

Patanjali listed various powers which arise when *samyama* – that is, concentration, contemplation, *samadhi* – is applied to certain things. It should be recalled that there is a qualitative change in *samyama* from the gross to the subtle.

3, 16. The knowledge of past and future, by *Samyama* on the three transformations.

The three transformations are 'property, character, and condition' (according to Dvivedi), or 'form, time, and state,' (according to Vivekananda).

3, 17. The word, its sense, and knowledge, are confused with one another on account of their being mutually mistaken for one another; hence by *Samyama* on the proper province of each [arises] the comprehension of [the meaning of] sounds uttered by any being.

3, 18. By mental presentation of the impressions, a knowledge of former class.

Vivekananda translates this as 'former life'.

3, 19. With reference to a sign, the knowledge of the mind of others.

3, 20. But not with its occupant, for that is not the subject.

'But not its contents', says Vivekananda.

3, 21. By *Samyama* on the form of the body, the power of comprehension being suspended, and the connection between light and eye being severed, there follows disappearance of the body.

3, 22. *Karma* is of two kinds: active and dormant. By *Samyama* on them [results] knowledge of cessation; as also by portents.

'Cessation' here means death.

3, 23. In sympathy, etc., strength.

By making *samyama* on sympathy, friendship, mercy, and so on, comes a strengthening of these qualities.

3, 24. In strength, that of the elephant, etc.

3, 25. The knowledge of the subtle, the obscure, and the remote, by contemplation of the inner light.

3, 26. By *Samyama* on the sun, the knowledge of space.

Vivekananda translates 'the knowledge of the world':

3, 27. In the moon, the knowledge of the starry regions.

3, 28. In the pole-star, knowledge of their motions.

That is, the motions of the stars.

3, 29. In the navel-circle, the knowledge of the arrangement of the body.

This refers to the subtle body and its energy centres (*chakras*), energy channels (*nadis*), and so on.

3, 30. In the pit of the throat, the cessation of hunger and thirst.

Compare this with the *Siva Samhita*: (171) 'Let the Yogi seat himself in the *Padmasana* [Lotus Posture] and fix his attention on the cavity of the throat, let him place his tongue at the base of the palate; by this he will extinguish hunger and thirst.'

3, 31. In the *Kurma-nadi*, steadiness.

Again compare this with the *Siva Samhita*: (171)'Below the cavity of the throat, there is a beautiful *Nadi* [vessel] called *Kurma*: when the Yogi fixes his attention on it, he acquires great concentration of the thinking principle [*citta*[.' Vivekananda translates this as 'fixity of body', not thought.

3, 32. In the light of the head, the sight of the *Siddhis*.

The *Siva Samhita* says (91): 'When the Yogi constantly thinks he has got a third eye – the eye of Siva – in the middle of his forehead, he then perceives a fire, brilliant like lightning. By contemplating on this light, all sins are destroyed, and even the most wicked person obtains the highest end. If the experienced Yogi thinks of this light day and night he sees *Siddhas* [adepts], and can certainly converse with them.'

3, 33. Or everything from the result of *Pratibha* [intuition].

3, 34. In the heart, knowledge of mind.

3, 35. Experience is the indistinctness of the mild conception of *Sattva* and *Purusha* which are absolutely apart; this enjoyment being for another, knowledge of *Purusha* arises from *Samyama* on himself.

3, 36. Thence is produced intuitional [cognition of] sound, touch, sight, taste, and smell.

It is at this point that Patanjali interpolates the admonition mentioned in the opening paragraph of this chapter:

3, 37. These are obstacles in the way of *Samadhi*, and are powers in moments of suspension.

The *Tattva-vaisaradi* of Vacaspati Misra (about 850 AD) comments (77): 'It is only he whose mind is active in going out that becomes proud of the possession of these as attainments. A beggar in life may think that the possession of a little wealth is the fullness of riches. The yogi, however, who is inclined to the attainment of trance [*samadhi*] must reject them whenever they come.'

3, 38. The mind enters another body, by relaxation of the cause of bondage, and by knowledge of the method of passing.

3, 39. By mastery over *Udana*, ascension, and non-contact with water, mud, thorns, and so on.

By gaining control over the energy current called *udana* within the subtle body a Yogi can cross rivers without paying a penny to the ferryman, walk with bare feet on thorns, and so on.

3, 40. Effulgence by mastery over *samana*.

Samana is a subtle energy current that operates between the pelvis and the navel.

3, 41. By *Samyama* on the relation between *akasa* and the sense of hearing, [arises] supernatural audition.

Akasa is space.

3, 42. By *Samyama* on the relation between the body and *akasas*, as also by being identified with light [things like] cotton, [there follows] passage through space.

Vyasa (fourth century AD) comments (77): 'Wherever there is the body, there is the *akasa*. The body becomes related to the *akasa*, because the latter gives room to the former. Having mastered the relation by the attainment of the state of thought transforming into light things such as cotton, etc., down to the atom, the yogi becomes light. Thence does he get the power of roaming through space and walking over water with his feet. He walks over a spider's web, and then walks over the rays of light. Then does he get the power of roaming through space at will.'

3, 43. The external, unthought-of transformation [of the mind] is the great incorporeal; hence the destruction of the covering of illumination.

3, 44. Mastery over the elements, by *Samyama* on the gross, the constant, the subtle, the all-pervading, and the fruition-bearing [in them].

Vivekananda comments (171): 'By making *Samyama* on the gross and fine forms of the elements, their essential traits, the inheritance of the *Gunas* in them and on their contributing to the experience of the soul, comes mastery of the elements.'

3, 45. Then the attainment of *anima* and others, as also of perfection of the body and the corresponding non-obstruction of its functions.

'*Anima* and others' refers to eight attainments, said also to result from mastery of *pranayama*. They are:

 i *Anima :* to become as small as an atom
 ii *Mahima :* to become very large
 iii *Laghima :* to become very light

iv *Garima* : to become very heavy
v *Prapti* : to be able to go anywhere
vi *Prakamya* : to have one's desires fulfilled.
vii *Vashitva* : to control all nature
viii *Ishitva* : to possess the power to create.

3, 46. Beauty gracefulness, strength, adamantine hardness, constitute perfection of the body.

3, 47. Mastery over the organs of sense by *Samyama* on the power of cognition, nature, egoism, all-pervasiveness, and fruition-giving capacity [of them].

3, 48. Thence fleetness [as of] mind, the being unobstructed by instruments, and complete mastery over the *pradhana*.

Pradhana is the first cause, the root of all – another name for *prakriti*.

3, 49. In him who is fixed upon the distinctive relation of *sattva* and *Purusha* [arise] mastery over all things and the knowledge of all.

3, 50. By non-attachment even thereto, follows *Kaivalya*, the seeds of bondage being destroyed.

Kaivalya is absolute independence and freedom. It is the subject-matter of Section 4 of Patanjali's *Yoga Sutras*.

3, 51. [There should be] entire destruction of pleasure and pride in the invitations by the powers [of various places], for there is possibility of a repetition of evil.

3, 52. Discriminative knowledge from *Samadhi* on moments. Their order.

3, 53. From it knowledge of similars, there being non-discrimination by class, characteristic, or position.

3, 54. The knowledge born of discrimination to *taraka*, relating to all objects, in every condition, and simultaneous.

Taraka is the highest knowledge possible to a Yogin.

3, 55. *Kaivalya* on the equality of purity between *Purusha* and *sattva*.

EXTRAORDINARY SENSE-PERCEPTIONS

In Section 1, *sutra* 35 Patanjali refers to 'forms of concentration that bring extraordinary sense-perceptions'. He adds that these encourage Yogins to persist with their meditation.

Swami Vivekananda commented on this (171):

This naturally comes with Dharana, concentration; the Yogis say, if the mind becomes concentrated on the tip of the nose, one begins to smell, after a few days, wonderful perfumes. If it becomes concentrated at the root of the tongue, one begins to hear sounds; if on the tip of the tongue, one begins to taste wonderful flavours; if on the middle of the tongue, one feels as if he were coming in contact with something. If one concentrates his mind on the palate he begins to see peculiar things. If a man whose mind is disturbed wants to take some of these practices of Yoga, yet doubts the truth of them, he will have his doubts set at rest when, after a little practice, these things come to him, and he will persevere.

XV   Yoga of Sex: Tantrism

YOGA AND SEXUAL ENERGY

A living Indian tradition, of ancient origin, aims at harnessing the great forces of sexual energy for the purpose of achieving higher consciousness. This tradition is divided into two contrasting ways of utilizing sexual power.

The first achieves its effects by concentrating and conserving sexual energy by chastity without repression. The celibacy a *guru* demands of his pupil (*chela*) is to conserve energy and to avoid distractions that could mar the single-mindedness and concentration required in Yogic disciplines. It has nothing to with a sense of guilt, shame, sin, or disgust in connection with sex. On the contrary, the sexual energies (even sexual fluid) are to be hoarded as though they were gold. And the reasons for celibacy are ascetic only in the original meaning of the word: *askesis* was the discipline voluntarily undergone by the Greek athlete in strict training.

The second approach sees in sexual union itself the means of expanding consciousness. Coitus becomes sacramental, an act of contemplation. It may be actual or imaginative; orgasm may or may not occur.

The married 'householder' Yogin (*grihastha*) is free to draw on both ways of harnessing sexual energy. He may choose chastity at times to focus the libido for spiritual ends, and at other times he will deepen sexual relations with his wife in the spirit of Tantrism, the second way, which makes coitus a sacrament representing the *unio mystica*.

WHAT IS TANTRISM?

Tantrism is unique among Yoga paths in its fundamental character and in tone. Its goal is that of all the Yogas, but the means is an exuberant 'yes-saying' to the experiences of living. It welcomes the dance of life, whether macabre or joyous, the play of universal energy which, as William Blake said, is eternal delight.

According to Tantric doctrine, human history is divided into four ages, representing a decline from the Golden Age to the Dark Age, which is our own. The *Tantras* (Tantric scriptures) are Siva's answer to the request of Shakti (the Divine Mother) for guidance for our pleasure-loving age (*Kali yuga*). One of the *Tantras* says: 'Eating and coitus are desired and natural to men, and their use is regulated for their benefit in the ordinance of Siva.' Another *Tantra* says: 'She [Shakti] does not exact from her weak and short-lived children of the *Kali yuga* long and trying *Brahmacharya* (celibacy) and austerity to show them the way to her Lotus Feet . . . The low and the high, all are equally taken care of, and for all the path has been made smooth and straighter.'

The word *tantra* derives from a root connected with the inter-dependence of warp and woof in weaving. The Tantrist does not withdraw from the world but faces, squarely and with heightened perception, its pain and pleasure, suffering and joy, destruction and construction, darkness and light – and, by meditation full of rich and subtle imagery, he transcends the polar opposites.

Tantrism is not, however a licence to 'do what you will' or to indulge in orgies of pleasure; though, inevitably, it has sometimes been taken as such, and the excesses of some sects have given it a bad name with orthodox Hindus and Buddhists. The person who makes Tantric ritual an excuse for licentiousness and who con-centrates on the physical pleasure instead of the mystical expansion of consciousness is held by Hindu and Buddhist alike to be a 'fool', for he is creating bad *karma* instead of liberating his spirit. Though sometimes a fool who persists in his folly becomes wise, as William Blake pointed out.

Tantrism requires a long preparatory training and careful initiation. Its character, and the dangers of abuse and misinter-pretation, led to its practices becoming closely-guarded secrets. One text puts it: 'Whereas the other scriptures are like a common woman, free to all, the Tantra is like a secret house-bride.'

Tantric texts can be read and interpreted at several levels: physiological, psychological, symbolical, occult, mystical, and so on. This gives them extraordinary depth. Occidental students of Tantrism in the nineteenth century missed the point and saw only raw sex, macabre rites, and a pursuit of magical and occult power; they failed to see the sophistication, subtlety, and spirituality that were there. Today the directness of the language at one level and the nature of the practices no longer shock, as they shocked Christian missionaries and scholars who sprang from a society guilt-ridden about sex.

Tantrism harnesses cosmic energy, which it sees in essence as sexual. Hundreds of years before the birth of Sigmund Freud, Hindu and Buddhist Tantrists were intensely aware of the power of the libido and had worked out ways of ritual and contemplation to channel this force for spiritual ends. Practice (*sadhana*) includes coitus as ritual and contemplation, the coming together of male and female bodies representing the coupling of god and goddess and the union of the great male (positive) and female (negative) polar forces in the cosmos – the energies which the Chinese named *yang* and *yin* respectively. Sexual intercourse thus enacts and represents the *unio mystica* that is the goal of all Yogas.

Tantrism takes its name from the *Tantras*, treatises which instruct in ritual and contemplation. Instructions that could be defined as being of an 'erotic' character make up only six to seven per cent of this literature – most of the passages concern the preparation of ingredients used in ritual, which *mantras* to repeat, the construction of *mandalas*, and so on. The erotic matters are also concerned with ritual and contemplation, including *maithuna* or sacramental coitus. *Saktisangama Tantra* means 'the *Tantra* about Shakti coition' and another text, *kamakalavilasa*, means 'erotic joy in love motion'.

Scholars disagree as to whether Buddhist Tantrism derived from Hindu Tantrism or the reverse. Other scholars say that both originated in a Yogic cult of ancient India, which on meeting with Hindu and Buddhist ideology became Tantric Hinduism and Tantric Buddhism respectively. Both became strong from about the fourth century AD. Tantric Hinduism is strongest in northern India, and Tantric Buddhism in Tibet and Nepal.

'Tantric' can be used as a general term applied to all Yogas using physiological techniques, including Hatha Yoga and Kundalini Yoga.

Tantric Yoga is an at times bizarre but always fascinating mixture of magic, occultism, body and mind mastery, esoteric knowledge, and mysticism of cosmic dimension. It has inspired much exuberant and excellent art and greatly influenced Indian aesthetics. Its insight that the physical union between man and woman in love and mindfulness represents a mystical way is valuable and can be reinterpreted for our age.

SEXUAL AND RELIGIOUS ECSTASY

Philip S. Rawson(162), an authority on Tantric art, has pointed out that 'quick and easy definitions' of Tantrism are impossible, because we are dealing with 'a special manifestation of Indian feeling, art and religion'. Another difficulty is that there is such a variety of belief and practice within Tantrism. 'However,' continues Mr Rawson, 'there is one thread which can guide us through the labyrinth; all the different manifestations of Tantra can be strung on it. This thread is the idea that Tantra is a cult of ecstasy, focused on a vision of cosmic sexuality. Life-styles, ritual, magic, myth, philosophy and a complex of signs and emotive symbols converge upon that vision.'

When Marghanita Laski, in compiling her study of ecstasy, questioned people who had experienced it in their lives, she found that art, nature, and sexual love were the three main triggers, scoring close together. Religion was the next most frequent trigger. In all ecstasies, whatever their cause, the ego sense is weakened and dissolves, and there is a sense of 'homecoming', of finding Reality. There may be physiological concomitants: Miss Laski's ecstatics experienced flashes of light, electrical tinglings in the spine, feelings of inner warmth, and the like (142). Similar sensations are reported by Tantric Yogins.

Sexual love offers the possibility of ecstasy. In this secular age great numbers of men and women make sex a substitute for religion and find in it a way of catching momentarily something of the non-duality, timelessness, and ego-obliteration experienced by the mystics. It is worth pausing to consider how the orgasm blots out both ego and time – two aims of esoteric psychologies. If men and women were granted the experience of orgasm only one or twice in their lives, one could well envisage a world religion being based on it.

Accounts of sexual and of religious ecstasy are unsatisfactory for the same reason: in either case an attempt is being made to describe the ineffable. In accounts of sexual ecstasy mere descriptions of behaviour are obviously inadequate, and the writer must take wing into language that could be applied just as aptly to an account of religious ecstasy. Conversely, descriptions of religious ecstasy often employ language of a sexual character. In particular this is so when religious adoration is operating, focused on a divine figure, as often in Bhakti Hinduism and Christian mysticism.

The ecstasy on the face of St Teresa of Avila (1515-82), as portrayed in white marble by Bernini, could be sexual rather than religious; and she described her visions and raptures in imagery and language so erotic as to embarrass the Church. She had a vision she said, in which an angel appeared carrying a long, golden spear with a fiery tip.

[He] plunged it into my deepest inward. When he drew it out, I thought my entrails would be drawn out too and when he left me I glowed in the hot fire of love for God. The pain was so strong that I screamed aloud, but simultaneously I felt such infinite sweetness that I wished the pain to last forever. It was the sweetest caressing of the soul by God.

Even so analytical and intellectual a mystic as St John of the Cross evokes the atmosphere of a lovers' tryst in one of his most beautiful poems:

> Upon an obscure night
> Fevered with Love's anxiety
> (O hapless, happy plight!)
> I went, none seeing me,
> Forth from my house, where all things quiet be.
>
> By night, secure from sight
> And by a secret stair, disguisedly,
> (O hapless, happy plight!)
> By night and privily
> Forth from my house, where all things quiet be.
>
> Blest night of wandering
> In secret, when by none might I be spied,
> Nor do I see anything;
> Without a light to guide
> Save that which in my heart burnt in my side.

That light did lead me on,
More surely than the shining of noontide
Where well I knew that One
Did for my coming bide;
Where He abode might none but He abide.

O night that didst lead thus,
O night more lovely than the dawn of light;
O night that broughtest us,
Lover to lover's sight,
Lover to loved, in marriage of delight!

Upon my flowery breast
Wholly for Him and Himself for none,
There did I give sweet rest
To my beloved one:
The fanning of the cedars breathed thereon.

                                        (trs. Arthur Symons)

The erotic element in Bhakti Hinduism is direct and unself-conscious. For millions of Indians the love story of Krishna and Rhada embodies Bhakti emotion. Bhakti *kirtans* or song-poems (like this by Vidyapati, translated by A. Coomaraswamy and A. Sen), can be erotic and at the same time exquisite:

She cries: Oh no, no, no! and tears are pouring from her eyes.
She lies outstretched upon the margin of the bed.
His close embrace has not unloosed her zone.
Even of handling her breast has been but little . . .
When Kanu lifts her to his lap, she bends her body back
Like a young snake, untamed by spells.

Vaisnava Sahajayists identify all men with Krishna and all women with Rhada.

GODS AND GODDESSES

It is significant that of the multiplicity of gods and goddesses of Hindusim the most popular has been Krishna. As an *avatar* or earthly incarnation of Vishnu, he pursued erotic adventures that have been a popular subject of Indian literature and art for many centuries.

He was brought up on a cattle farm, where the milkmaids, the wives of the cowherds, all fell in love with him. A popular story culminates in the *Rasa Mandala*, or round dance, in which Krishna dances with all the girls by moonlight, magically providing each cowgirl with a replica of himself, so that each believes she alone danced with him. They throw off their clothes and dance and sing and make love passionately for six months. Finally, they bathe in the Jumna River, and Krishna orders the girls to return to their homes. When they do so, no one is aware that they have not been there all the time.

With characteristic exaggeration, Hindu tradition says there are thirty-three *crores* (a *crore* is ten million) of gods and goddesses. But they are all manifestation of the One, the Absolute, *Brahman*. *Brahman* is not personified, but has a triune manifestation as Brahma the Creator, Vishnu the Preserver, and Siva the Destroyer. Each of these gods has a female helpmate, his *shakti* or earth-power. Hindu sculpture frequently depicts the gods and goddesses engaged in the dance of life or making love.

Indian temple sculpture fascinates and surprises tourists by its erotic exuberance. Piled in tier upon tier in rock recesses, the figures have a unique ripeness and voluptuousness of bodily curve, and their rhythms are those of the dance and sexual love. These male and female figures display all the erotic inventiveness and sportiveness we find in the classic Indian love-manuals, such as the *Kama Sutra* of Vatsayana and the *Ananga Ranga*, both now widely read in the West.

Siva, the Destroyer, also represents the universal force of generation, fertility, and fecundity, destroying only that new life may burgeon. Representations of his *lingam* or phallus are ubiquitous in Hindu temple art. Sometimes *lingam* and *yoni* (vagina) are depicted in union. B. Z. Goldberg (125), in his study of sex in religion, entitled *The Sacred Fire*, says: 'the symbol of the *limgan* is the father of the statue in religious worship'.

The legend behind *lingam* worship is this. Siva's mate had died, and he wandered about the land haggard and disconsolate. The sages who lived in the forest of Daruvanam, shocked to see the god in so piteous a state, saluted him with downcast eyes. But their wives were heartbroken on gazing upon the sad features of Siva and left their husbands to follow the god. Whereupon the sages angrily cursed the god with: 'May his *lingam* fall to the ground!' The curse must have worked, or perhaps Siva decided that, bereaved of his mate, he could dispense with his phallus – whatever way it was, Siva vanished and his *lingam* was found sticking in the ground.

B. Z. Goldberg continues the legend (125):

As the *lingam* fell, it penetrated the lower worlds. Its length increased and its top towered above the heavens. The earth quaked and all there was upon it. The *lingam* became fire and caused conflagration wherever it penetrated. Neither god nor man could find peace or security.

So both Vishnu and Brahma came down to investigate and to save the universe. Brahma ascended to the heavens to ascertain the upper limits of Siva's *lingam*, and Vishnu betook himself to the lower regions to discover its depth. Both returned with the news that the *lingam* was infinite: it was lower than the deep and higher than the heavens.

And the two great gods both paid homage to the *lingam* and advised man to do likewise. They further counselled man to propitiate Parvati, the goddess, that she might receive the *lingam* into her *yoni*.

This was done and the world was saved. Mankind was taught that the *lingam* is not to be cursed or ignored; that it is infinite in its influence for good or evil; and that rather than wishing it destroyed, they should worship it by offering it flowers and perfumes and by burning fires before it.

Whether it was the goddess Venus or the god Siva, whether it was the feminine principle or the masculine, the worship of the god or of the goddess came as a punishment for sex ignored. Love suppressed, offended, and imprisoned came to be rescued by the gods of religion. Siva's consort or *shakti* turns up variously as Parvati, Durga, Kali, Devi, and Uma. She is the Divine Mother. In Yoga's symbolism the union of Siva and *shakti* represents the mystic union of Self (*Atman*) and Over-Self (*Brahman*).

SACRAMENTAL COITUS

Bearing in mind the unselfconscious erotic element in Hinduism and its history of *lingam* worship and of temple prostitution in which sex was a sacred rite, it need occasion no surprise that schools of Yoga should have developed for which sexual union became a sacrament and a way to illumination.

Sacred prostitution flourished in India for many centuries and continued well into our own. Coupling took place between priest and temple prostitute (*Deva-dasi*) or female visitor, or between prostitute and male visitor. Most of the prostitutes also served as dancing girls and lived within the temple precincts; others lived outside and charged a fee which they passed on to the priests. By initiation the *Deva-dasi* was married to a god, whom she served by dancing and by prostitution. Indian temple harlotry continued into the twentieth century, persisting in some states of South India into the early thirties. Gandhi attacked the practice in 1927 (*Young India*, 6 October 1927, p. 335). The southern state of Travancore, which at the turn of the century had about four hundred *Deva-dasis*, abolished temple prostitution in 1930.

Tantric texts can be read at different levels according to the reader's esoteric knowledge, but statements that *maithuna* (ceremonial intercourse) represents only a symbolic technique and that no actual fleshly union takes place are not in accord with the evidence. While it is true that for some Tantric schools the coincidence of bodies refers to subtle or astral bodies, there can be no denying that within other sects coitus between man and woman in the flesh does occur, with or without orgasm, and that some Tantrists employ actual coitus in the early stages of training until their imaginative and meditative powers have developed enough 'muscle' to enable them to dispense with fleshly union.

Philip Rawson, in the *Catalogue for the Exhibition of Tantric Art Sponsored by the Arts Council of Great Britain* in the autumn of 1971; wrote (162):

Modern writers on Tantra tend to discuss its sexual rituals in an abstract way, as if they were purely imaginary or merely mechanical functions of Yoga. In fact, real intercourse with complete enjoyment can be treated as an icon of what it signifies. ... The true inner image behind sexual intercourse is a transcendent enjoyment in energetic love-play of the two-sexed divinity in Hinduism or Buddha-nature in Buddhism. The joy of actual sexual intercourse, undertaken in the same spirit as worship of an outer image, can help to awaken in the mind of the *Sadhaka* that permanent inner blissful image, of which human intercourse is another reflection.

Mr Rawson is saying, in effect, that coitus can be a contemplative act, a Yoga – which is what it is in Tantrism. This means that sexual coupling is to be approached with real reverence, the mood is to be built up for days or weeks, and that the union when it comes is not an attempt to extract maximum sensual excitement, but rather a contemplative joy, an *ekstasis*. To ensure this calm centre at the heart of the whirlpool, the couple stay immobile, locked in an embrace; orgasm may or may not be triggered. Such sexual control requires skill in Yogic posturing, breathing and meditation. Coital posture can contribute to stillness: the man sits in one of the traditional cross-legged meditative poses and then the woman sits down on the Yogin's lap with her legs around his waist. The couple then lock in an embrace and stay immobile in a spiritual communion that is given strength and support by their physical union, which is prolonged for many minutes, even several hours, and accompanied by a, contemplation that lifts the minds of Yogin and Yogini well above any concern with bodily sensation.

TANTRIC PRACTICE

Tantric meditation is a way of focusing the libido and harnessing its energies for transcendental ecstasy. Yogin and Yogini become god and goddess. The initiation of women for their roles is among the most closely guarded secrets of Tantrism. Those who favour actual rather than imaginative or symbolic intercourse are known as followers of the Left Hand Path. Nothing condemnatory is implied by 'left' – they take their name from the fact that the Yogini at the commencement of the ceremony sits to the left side of the Yogin.

Before one can harness power it is customary first of all to generate it. In Tantric Yoga practice (*sadhana*) the energy and heat is built up in the total organism and is not localized in genital erethism. Some 'left-hand' sects deliberately flout Brahmin and Buddhist convention and orthodoxy by eating forbidden foods and drinking alcohol. Their five sacraments, known as the five Ms, are eating fish (*matsya*), beef (*mamsa*), and parched grain (*mudra*); drinking alcoholic beverages (*madya*); and ceremonial coitus (*maithuna*). Aphrodisiacs and drugs (mainly *bhang* or *ganjam*, types of cannabis) may be taken. Doubtless a special excitement is engendered through partaking of food and drink normally forbidden.

Mantras – words imbued with sacred, magical, or psycho-physiological potency – are repeated, aloud or inwardly. Each Yogi is given a personal *mantra* on initiation into the cult. A *yantra* or mystic diagram is drawn on the ground.

Through meditation, Yogi and Yogini become god and goddess. They participate in ritual purification. Flowers are offered to the 'goddess", who is bathed and anointed with perfumed oils.

Coitus follows, an act of worship and contemplation. The male and female universal principles merge and unite, duality is over-come, the opposites are transcended.

Tantric practice (*sadhana*) is so profuse, complex and varied that it would be impossible to do it justice in the space available in this chapter. Nor does it readily come within our practical approach to Yoga. The ritual is long-drawn-out and makes wearisome reading for those outside the tradition.

SEMEN HOARDING

Sexual energy is at its most intense and explosive at orgasm, yet the Tantrists mostly avoid orgasm in ceremonial coition. One might expect to find in Tantrism a view of orgasm on lines similar to that expounded by Wilhelm Reich, the Austrian psycho-analyst and natural scientists, who saw the orgasm as the answer to man's main health and social problems. The Tantrists have two reasons for avoiding orgasm in *maithuna*.

The first reason is that the energy which normally goes into orgasm is in *maithuna* harnessed for meditative ends. The total effect of the contemplative embrace is one of spiritual communion, sexually sustained at what the sexologists call the plateau phase. Contemplation, which may go on for one or two hours, would be violently disrupted by the orgasm of either partner. And when *maithuna* takes place entirely within consciousness, attaining orgasm would clearly be difficult.

The second reason why the Tantrist may avoid orgasm is to be found in the strong belief that semen is the gross form of a con-centrated psychic power called *ojas*, and that by retaining semen (*bindu*) one builds up radiant energy (*tejas*) in the body. Thus one finds either chastity or coitus without ejaculation favoured in Yogic texts. Seminal fluid is precious, and to be hoarded. This concept is widespread in the East, though not supported in any way by medical science.

Magical power has been ascribed to semen from man's earliest history. In Indian folk-lore one finds the superstition that if you

cut the skin of one of India's wandering holy men the wound will
exude not blood but semen. The legends of the Naths depict woman
as a serpent or tigress who steals man's source of life power: his
semen. Similar stories are found in the folk tradition of many
cultures. There is a belief in Yoga schools that exceptional powers
(*siddhis*), such as telepathy and clairvoyance, result from transferring
semen or, more strictly speaking, *ojas* to the brain, the eyes, and
so on.

There is even a Yogic technique for reabsorbing the ejaculate,
which was described in the section on Yogic hygiene in *Yoga of
Breathing*. Nothing symbolic implied here, but an actual muscle
control whereby water can be drawn up the urethra and held for a
while in the gladder.

A story is told of the fifth Dalai Lama (who died about 1680)
which only makes sense if one knows about the Yogic technique of
reabsorbing the ejaculate. It appears that the fifth Dalai Lama had
a reputation as a womanizer. (He also wrote love songs still popular
with the Tibetans.) One day, standing on one of the upper terraces
of his palace, the Dalai Lama listened to criticisms of his way of life
from his advisers, to which he retorted: 'Yes, it is true that I have
women . . . but copulation for me is not the same thing as it is for
you.' He then stepped to the edge of the terrace and pissed over it.
The urine streamed downwards, from terrace to terrace, until it
reached the bottom of the palace. Then, to the great astonishment of
onlookers, it began to flow upwards, defying the law of gravity by
climbing terrace after terrace, and finally re-entering the Dalai
Lama's body at the point of its previous exit. He then turned to his
advisers and said: 'Unless you can do the same, you must realize
that my sexual relations are different from yours.'

The meaning behind the story lies in the spiritual power ascribed
to semen by the Tibetans and the technique whereby the ejaculate
can be reabsorbed. The Dalai Lama, it will be noted, was not
concerned with the sinfulness of sex or with the risk of making his
mistresses pregnant – but he was very much concerned with retaining his semen.

Taoists have used a more mechanical but simpler technique,
pressing on the perineum (between scrotum and anus) at the moment
of orgasm, and thereby diverting the seminal fluids into the bladder.

Medical knowledge indicates that reabsorbed or diverted semen
will pass into the bladder and not the testicles. Yogins reply that

even if this is so, the psychic force (*ojas*) will permeate the body.

A persistent superstition, found in many cultures, is that a drop of semen is equal to an ounce of blood. One recalls that less than a hundred years ago European and American doctors were terrifying boys by telling them of the dreadful perils to health and sanity caused by loss of 'vital fluids' through masturbation or 'wet dreams'. This warning is no longer heard. Belief that semen contains concentrated life force or that its loss is debilitating does not now accord with anything known to medical science, though we cannot dismiss it entirely on that account.

KAREZZA

The Tantric practice of prolonged intercourse without orgasm has been followed in many cultures and goes under a variety of names.

A comparable practice among the Bedouins called Udhrism or the cult of Beni Udhra was praised by some Arab poets and spread to Spain and parts of Europe. Men and women embraced either without penetration of the vagina, or with penetration, but without orgasm. The latter control was called *ismak* or 'retention'. The aims of the technique were spiritual bliss and illumination. The cult inspired some intensely erotic and mystical poetry.

In the West the technique has gone under various names, the best known of which are male continence, *coitus reservaturs*, and *karezza*. It has been practised by some mystical or semi-mystical cults. The best known example of male continence is the sect founded by John Humphrey Noyes (died 1886) at Oneida Creek, New York State, in the middle of the last century. At first Noyes advocated 'complex marriage', which meant that the sexes practised a form of free love, which he felt fulfilled biblical teaching. Sexual congress took place, without the male ejaculating. It was known at first as male continence, and later as *coitus reservatus*.

The more sophisiticated name *karezza* or *carezza* (a Persian word) was given to the withholding of orgasm by both partners by Alice Bunker Stockham in her book *Karezza*, published in 1896. Intercourse was sustained for from one to two hours, and the embrace repeatedly taken to the verge of climax. It was claimed for *karezza* that it led to rejuvenation, good health, a feeling of buoyancy and well-being, heightened perception of natural objects and, most important of all, the raising of levels of consciousness.

Karezza was vehemently attacked on moral grounds, and criticized for medical reasons. Prolonged tumescence, doctors said, could lead to inflammation of the genital organs, and psychological damage could result from the unreleased build-up of nervous force. Supporters of *karezza* replied that there were no reported cases of harm on either score: the moral criticisms they countered by saying that *karezza* 'spiritualized' sexual relations.

The sublimation of sexuality for purposes of spiritual illumination by sleeping chastely with virgins was castigated by St Paul in the First Epistle to the Corinthians. A more tolerant account is that by John Cowper Powys in his novel *Weymouth Sands;* in this the eccentric mystic Sylvanus Cobbold sleeps chastely with young girls.

YOGA AND SEXUAL FITNESS

Tantrists are familiar with the muscle contractions and locks, called *mudras* and *bandhas*, which we described in *Yoga of Breathing* as a means of enhancing sexual vigour. These controls, which belong to esoteric Yoga, strengthen and tone the sexual organs, muscles and glands.

It should be noted, too, that the postures (*asanas*) of Hatha Yoga aid sexual fitness in two ways. Firstly, they increase suppleness for what is after all an athletic or gymnastic performance of a kind. Secondly, they promote the health and tone of the spine, nervous system, glands, and vital organs. Blood is carried to the pelvis and feeds the spinal nerves. Such famous poses as the Cobra, Bow, Locust, Spinal Twist, Supine Thunderbolt, Shoulderstand, Spinal Rock, Fish, and Lotus are held by Yogins to enhance sexual health, and the muscle controls *Uddiyana* (Abdominal Retraction) and *Nauli* (Isolation of the Recti) are closely associated with sex fitness.

THE SPIRIT OF TANTRISM

For most readers it is the special spirit or feeling of Tantrism, rather than its complicated ritualistic practices, that will prove valuable. Tantric Yoga is a strange mixture of magical and occult belief and practice, often-macabre rites, bodily and mental mastery, and sexual and mystical wisdom. Disregarding the mumbo-jumbo, its insight that the physical union between partners in love and mindfulness represents a mystical way is valuable, and can be reinterpreted for our times and circumstances in ways productive of human happiness and self-actualization. It heightens our awareness and enjoyment of the present moment, not only in sex but in all of life's activities.

The follower of the Tantric way, says Alan Watts (172),

discovers that existence is basically a kind of dancing or music – an immensely complex energy pattern which needs no explanation other than itself – just as we do not ask what is the *meaning* of fugues by Bach or sonatas by Mozart. We do not dance to reach a certain point on the floor, but simply to dance. Energy itself, as William Blake said, is eternal delight – and all life is to be lived in the spirit of rapt absorption in an arabesque of rhythms.

The Tantrist worships the female principle, representing the negative, dark, and earthy aspects of the universe, and seeks union with this *shakti*. He accepts darkness with light, light with darkness, realizing that each is necessary to the Whole. Both are present and each leaps to the eye as figure or ground according to which viewpoint one adopts – like those double images that can be either two shaded faces in profile or a white chalice against a dark background. 'Some understanding of Tantra is therefore a marvellous and welcome corrective to certain excesses of Western civilization,' Alan Watts continues:

We over-accentuate the positive, think of the negative as 'bad', and thus live in a frantic terror of death and extinction which renders us incapable of 'playing' life with an air of noble and joyous detachment. Failing to understand the musical quality of nature, which fulfils itself in an eternal present, we live for a tomorrow which never comes – like an orchestra racing to attain the finale of a symphony. But through understanding the creative power of the female, of the negative, of empty space, and of death, we may at least become completely alive in the present.

XVI Press-button Yoga: Biofeedback

IS BIOFEEDBACK INSTRUMENTAL YOGA?

This chapter deals with Yoga with the aid of electrical equipment – instrumental or press-button Yoga, which is what biofeedback claims to be, and certainly in part is.

The part of biofeedback that corresponds with elements in Yoga is auto-control of the involuntary nervous system, that section responsible for such physiological functions as the heartbeat, blood pressure, and the different kinds of brain waves. This is the kind of body-mind control with which Indian fakirs and Yogins have on occasions surprised observing doctors and scientists. Now, with biofeedback instruments, these startling feats can be learned by most men and women. The mastery extends to producing those brain wave patterns observable in meditating Yogins and Zen monks.

The main feature of the learning process is that the working of functions in the human body hitherto thought involuntary can be translated into some sort of signal, by observing which we can train ourselves to regulate the internal body function. Of biofeedback, two American psychologists (137) have written that 'the ultimate possibilities of man's self-control are nothing less than the evolution of an entirely new culture where people can change their mental and physical states as easily as switching channels on a television set.'

Increasing the state of muscular relaxation, lowering the blood pressure, switching the brain's 'engine' into neutral gear and free-wheeling for a while – all these controls come within the capabilities of the majority of men and women training with biofeedback apparatus. The medical importance is obvious, and the personal importance for the layman is full of fascinating possibilities.

If Yoga is modification of the mind-stuff – Patanjali's classic definition – biofeedback is a kind of Yoga. But as yet there is no substantial evidence of meditators by machine having peak illuminative experiences that transform the personality permanently, which is what Yoga claims for the experience of *samadhi*. In regulating physiological processes hitherto thought inaccessible to direct conscious control, except as displayed occasionally by remarkable Yogins, biofeedback is, again, a kind of Yoga. As an aid to deep relaxation, biofeedback promotes one of Yoga's greatest benefits to harassed Western man.

The number of scientific papers (mostly American) on biofeedback is already considerable. Valuable and startling gains in auto-control are objectively recorded.

BIOFEEDBACK EXPLAINED

Biofeedback instruments may be intricate, but the principle of feedback is simple enough and in practice known to everyone. Like Molière's M Jourdain, who discovered to his great surprise that he had been speaking prose all his talking life, we find on examination that each of us depends on feedback for learning efficiency in every-day living. The term itself belongs to the early days of radio, but its operation in the human organism belongs to the total history of man.

Say you visit a funfair and decide to try your luck at dislodging coconuts by throwing balls at them. Your first throw misses a coconut by several inches to the right hand side. You now make a mind-body adjustment for the next throw, but you over-compensate so that the ball misses its target by a few inches to the left hand side. The third throw now has a more hopeful chance of success, for past performance – the first two throws – has been imprinted and the information has been processed for the third throw. That is the way efficient motor performance is acquired. As babies we learned to use our hands by watching them, and by trial and error, and we learned to speak on the basis of listening to our first attempts and improving upon them. So we know what feedback means – we have been using it all of our lives.

Biofeedback (the Greek word *bios* means 'life') is a special kind of feedback that is concerned with such life processes as the beating of the heart, the pressure and circulation of the blood, and the energy waves of the brain. Through biofeedback training we develop control over inner physiological functions in the same way as, by feedback learning, we have developed manual and other human skills which we use to survive in a complex and hazardous environment. Every animal owes its performance and survival to feedback.

The reason why biofeedback training is an exciting new advance is that modern technology offers us the opportunity to become aware of inner functioning by translating it into an outward signal – visual (a flashing light, a moving needle, oscillating pens on a graph) or aural (a sustained tone, 'bleeps' or clicks, amplified breathing or heartbeats). The translated signals open up new territories of self-regulation. We tune into physiological processes we had thought involuntary and beyond conscious direction. The senses of sight and hearing which all our lives we have been accustomed to use to guide our movements, are now employed for monitoring the functioning of our inner organs. We raise or lower the pitch of a tone or take note of what subtleties of sensation accompany a 'bleep', and in doing so are able to regulate normally involuntary physiological mechanisms. We learn, as one American psychologist put it, 'to play our internal organs'. Yogins sometimes achieve this tuning in without the aid of electrical instruments; but few of us can develop such sensitivity of awareness that, without assistance, we can listen to the circulation of the blood and to other internal bodily activities normally outside the reach of conscious attention. Biofeedback equipment provides that assistance.

THE TWO NERVOUS SYSTEMS

The two nervous systems are the voluntary and the involuntary systems. The voluntary system gives us control over the nerves responsible for movements of the skeletal muscles, that is, for deliberate body movements. The involuntary or autonomic nervous system controls the functions of the heart, glands, and digestion, and controls temperature adjustment – physiological processes that normally can be allowed to get on with their vital work without interference, interruption, or direction from consciousness. Yet when something goes wrong with these processes it can clearly be of value if the person concerned is able to regulate his inner functioning to the benefit of his health and efficiency.

In *Yoga of Breathing* we described the Yogic technique of *tumo*, by which heat can be engendered in any part of the body – say a foot or a hand — by directing consciousness to that place. Biofeedback equipment brings *tumo*, which the Yogi takes months, even years, to master, within the reach of the majority of users in a matter of hours.

Professor Neal E. Miller (117), of Rockefeller University, New York, taught rats whose voluntary nervous systems had been paralysed by curare to gain mastery over their involuntary nervous systems. One of his rats learned to blush one ear at a time. Yet Professor Miller had great difficulty in finding people to work with him on experiments based on what seemed too far-fetched a possibility.

BIOFEEDBACK THERAPY

The areas of medical treatment in which biofeedback has been found helpful are cases of migraine and tension headaches, high blood pressure, heart trouble, insomnia, muscular tics, and anxiety.

At a number of hospitals and medical schools in America patients have been taught to monitor and regulate their heartbeats, an ability retained outside the laboratory. The importance of such a skill in cases of heart disease and irregularity is obvious.

Biofeedback training opens up many possibilities of auto-healing. However, attempts at self-cure should not be taken beyond relaxation to tampering with the functioning of vital organs and processes without prior medical consultation. This is an area in which to 'go it alone' could be highly dangerous.

REDUCING ANXIETY

Dr Paul Grim (127) has achieved rapid results in reducing anxiety by using respiration biofeedback. The subjects were ninety-five nursing students. A psychological test prior to relaxation was used to determine their general level of anxiety. The students then were taught to let go from tension by listening to their amplified breathing while lying limp on the bed. Following the period of training in relaxation, the psychological test measuring anxiety was taken again by each subject. The result? A significant reduction of the level of anxiety. Listening to the amplified breathing led to respiration becoming smoother and more rhythmic – exactly what happens in Yogic *pranayama* (breath control), which also induces relaxation. Amplifying the sound of breathing could be an aid to making rapid progress in some aspects of *pranayama*. A similar monitoring effect can be obtained in two ways without electrical apparatus – by covering the ears with the hands, and by lying back in the bath so that the water covers the ears but the nose is held out of the water. Awareness of emptying and filling the lungs with air is popular as a meditative practice in Buddhism and in some schools of Yoga.

Other biofeedback methods aim at relaxing the forehead muscles, which are intimately linked with anxiety. Electrodes pick up any movement of the fontalis muscle, and this is fed into an EMG (electromyograph) machine. The signal is a tone which rises when the muscle contracts and falls when it relaxes. This and related equipment is available to the general public as well as to clinicians. One can learn to recognize subtle rises in tension that normally escape awareness, and to let go from them.

But the biofeedback method of dissolving anxiety and inducing mental calm which most interests us here is that which produces alpha electrical activity in the brain. This is the activity found in meditating Yogins.

BRAIN WAVES

Hans Berger, a German scientist, discovered the presence of brain waves shortly after the First World War. In July 1924 he attached two electrodes from a galvanometer to the scalp of a seventeen-year-old mental patient and found that the brain emits a form of electrical energy. During the following five years Berger established the existence of two distinct brain wave patterns, which he named 'alpha' and 'beta'. He saw that beta registered during concentrated mental work, whereas alpha was associated with a relaxed passive state. Berger was dismissed in 1938 by the Nazis from his position at the University of Jena, and committed suicide three years later.

The modern EEG machine (electroencephalograph) records brain wave patterns by means of a row of oscillating inked pens 'writing' on a continuously winding roll of graph paper.

Beta brain wave, with a frequency of over 14 cycles per second, is the commonest pattern in active minds. It is produced in mental work, such as adding up figures or solving a crossword puzzle. Beta rhythms are marked by much electrical static.

Alpha activity has a frequency of 8-13 cycles per second, with associated feelings of passivity. Not everyone finds the sensation pleasant, but most people do. The mind in the alpha state is neither active nor drowsy, but in neutral. When the brain rhythms of meditating Yogins were tested with EEG equipment, alpha patterns were recorded. For reasons not yet understood, a few people produce alpha patterns almost all the time, and some others cannot produce them at all.

Since Berger's time two more electrical brain patterns have been found, and named 'delta' and 'theta'.

Theta waves have a frequency of 4-7 cycles per second. This is a rhythm characteristic of the period just before the onset of sleep. Delta waves, with a frequency of $\frac{1}{2}$-6 cycles per second, are rarely found except in sleep.

An intriguing feature of brain wave activity is that at any moment one pattern may be observable in one part of the brain, while a different pattern is observable in another part of the brain. It is usually alpha and beta that are thus simultaneously engaged, and they may suddenly reverse locations. Alpha rhythm is recorded at its intensest at the back of the head, though the wave usually sweeps from the front to the back of the cortex.

CONTROLLING BRAIN RHYTHMS

The discovery of self-regulation of brain waves is accredited to Dr Joe Kamiya (136), who was researching sleep at the University of Chicago in 1958. 'I became fascinated by the alpha rhythm that came and went in the waking EEGs and wondered if, through laboratory experiments with this easily traced rhythm, a subject could be taught awareness of an internal state,' he was to recall. A subject was placed in a darkened room and Dr Kamiya observed the brain wave rhythms on an EEG machine. At various intervals a bell was rung. The subject had to say whether alpha rhythm was present or not. 'The first day, he was right only about 50 per cent of the time, no better than chance. The second day he was right 65 per cent of the time; the third day, 85 per cent. By the fourth day, he guessed right on every trial – 400 times in a row.' Dr Kamiya had an additional surprise with further subjects. 'They were able to control their minds to the extent to entering and sustaining either [alpha or beta] state upon our command.'

From this initial experiment Dr Kamiya went on to using bio-feedback for speedier learning of brain wave identification. In his procedure, each time a subject produced alpha waves an auditory signal, a tone, was sustained, cutting off when the brain changed from alpha activity. This kind of training procedure has been followed since, and it normally takes only a few hours to master the technique and produce alpha waves at will. Dr Kamiya observed: 'I generally tend to have more positive liking for the individual who subsequently turns out to learn alpha control more readily.' Other investigators have trained subjects to produce beta, theta, and delta to order.

Some people experience a strange apprehension on changing from beta to alpha activity. They are usually people who like to be 'on the go' all the time, who find it positively uncomfortable to relax and just let the brain 'tick over' for a while. But most people find that alpha rhythm soothes the nervous system. Why listening to or seeing a signal representing brain wave activity should give us power to control consciousness remains a mystery.

Tremors of the eyelids cause bursts of alpha activity in the brain. Two other findings are of interest to the student of Yoga: alpha waves may be produced by holding the breath (as in pranayama), and by looking steadily at some object (as in *trataka*).

BIOFEEDBACK AND MEDITATION

When the brain wave patterns of meditating Yogins have been recorded, alpha rhythms have invariably been observed. Zen monks also showed alpha activity, but some went into the theta wave state. Two Japanese researchers, Akira Kasamatsu and Tomio Hirai (1966), of Tokyo University, studied the brain wave patterns of Zen meditators, and discerned four distinct stages in their meditation.

  i The appearance of alpha, even though the meditator's eyes were open

  ii An increase in alpha amplitude

  iii A decrease of alpha frequency

iv The appearance of a 'rhythmical theta train'. The fourth state is that preceding the onset of sleep – those pre-sleep minutes which are often productive of ideas for writers, composers, artists, and other creative people.

Green, Green, and Walters (1970) found (126) that some of their most relaxed subjects produced theta waves accompanied by dreamlike imagery, and in some cases by the emergence of the deeply-buried contents of the unconscious.

Another study (Anand, 1961) found that the people who normally produce a well-defined alpha pattern are those with the greatest enthusiasm for taking up meditation, and that they show marked ability in the practice.

Researcher Dr Johann Stoyva says that the 'blank mind' state of Zen and Yoga may, with biofeedback procedure, be reached in 'months or even weeks'. Dr Kamiya (the man who discovered that electrical brain patterns could be changed by conscious control), thinks that alpha rhythms are but one factor in meditation, but that the missing factors can be discovered. 'I do think . . . it will be possible to find the unique neurophysiological signature of meditation by checking out other channels – besides alpha. Once we have the complete physiological pattern that characterises meditation, there's no reason why we can't train people, with feedback, to mimic it in a relatively short space of time,' he says.

But would 'the complete physiological pattern' of meditation be identical with the experience of meditation as found in Yoga or Zen? There are many people who doubt it. They also doubt whether *samadhi* or *satori* could ever be duplicated by putting chemicals into the bloodstream or by inducing neurophysiological responses with electrical instruments. The real test will be whether these 'reproduction' peak illuminative experiences of Yoga and Zen will transform the personality totally and lastingly. A few subjects in biofeedback investigation have reported that alpha activity produced states of consciousness superior to those produced by drugs, with the additional advantages of self-control throughout the experiment and no hangovers subsequently.

Mystical illumination is a rare enough experience within the traditional oriental psychologies, and it may be argued that acquiring some of the practical benefits of meditation rapidly by biofeedback makes it of value. Further: this is a push-button age, and many people who feel at home in it will be encouraged to start meditating through the appeal of biofeedback. Dr Eleanor Criswell, director of the Humanistic Psychology Institute, says: 'It has been said that Americans need gadgets in order to be able to do things, so if this is America's gadget way of giving itself permission to meditate, then it's worth it.'

BRINGING TOGETHER THE TWO PSYCHOLOGIES

The scientific method of testing, observing, recording, and presenting the recorded data in papers for scientific journals has been made applicable to psychology by limiting study to observable behaviour. As a result, psychologists split into two camps: behaviourists following investigations by the respected scientific method, and others willing to study and speculate about states of consciousness. Biofeedback studies and controls states of consciousness in a scientific manner, and so helps to draw together the two schools of approach to psychological study and experiment.

BIOFEEDBACK INSTRUMENTS

We conclude this section on biofeedback by indicating the kinds of equipment that are available for home use. Compact, battery-operated instruments are produced for the general public. The following are sold in America and Britain:

i.   The EEG machine for regulating brain waves. Electrodes on the scalp pick up and amplify signals from the brain, in particular those with the frequency range known as alpha, each peak of which produces a 'beep' from the instrument's loudspeaker. The user learns when he is producing alpha waves. The concomitant mental state is one of neutral-gear coasting, distinct from concentration, drowsiness, or trance. Alpha is a feature – though not the whole story – of oriental-style meditation.

For reasons not fully understood, some people cannot produce alpha waves and others do so almost all the time. The manufacturers make a part refund to such customers.

ii   The EMG (electromyographic) machine, used to gain mastery over physiological processes normally involuntary. Trade name

'Myophone'. It has medical uses, but should not become a substitute for a doctor's care.

iii   The GSR (galvanic skin response) machine, which operates by producing a continuous tone. This rises if the user becomes tense or excited in any way. The pitch of the tone drops as relaxation increases. The electrodes are placed on the user's fingertips, and measure the electrical resistance of the skin, which lowers when tension or excitement causes changes in the sweat glands. Conversely relaxation raises skin resistance.

Galvanic skin response provides a rapid method of training a person to recognize both tension and relaxation in the body – the the latter a 'letting go' from the former. Skill in relaxation benefits health, conserves energy, and increases efficiency in work, creativity, and play.

XVII   The Future of Yoga

EAST AND WEST – A NEW SYNTHESIS

Interest in Yoga and other Eastern esoteric psychologies has never been so great in the Western world as now – not only among the general public seeking mental energy, peace of mind, and Self-realization, but also among psychologists, psychiatrists, neurologists, and other specialists. This interest marks a slackening, at least among some sections of Western society, of what has been the predominant orientation of occidental civilization for many centuries. The direction of Western civilization has been towards outward achievement, dissecting, classifying, building, producing – and also, indisputably, towards killing, destroying, self-aggrandizement, greed for material possessions and a ruthless competitiveness.

The history of Western Man has been one of conquering nature. He has sought for the meaning of life outside of human consciousness. In contrast, the Eastern truth-seeker has looked within himself. He has sought to learn the secret of nature (the Tao) not by dissecting or conquering it but by recognizing that he is part of the Whole, the One of the mystics.

There is now widespread acknowledgment in both East and West that these contrasting directions of development have been lopsided and harmful.

Eastern religions and philosophies have been criticized, notably by Albert Schweitzer, as life-negating. The measure of truth in this criticism was then accepted by Swami Vivekananda, Rabindranath Tagore, Mahatma Ghandi, and other Indian reformers, and is now widely accepted. Yoga meditation *can* be escapist and world-renouncing; but it is not so in its modern presentation.

Just as the life-negating, passive, and other-worldly side of Eastern thought is being recognized and countered, so, too, occidentals are increasingly aware of the need to counterbalance Western self-aggrandizement, materialism, and compulsive busyness. Among the young there is a spiritual quest that is universalist in outlook and transcends the worn-out dogmas, doctrinal rigidities, and shibboleths of the traditional institutionalized religions. One aspect of the Western counterbalancing is the growing interest in Eastern methods of relaxation and meditation. Meditation is a degree subject at some American universities. Meditation centres are a feature of many European and American cities. Meditation is taught to air pilots, to hospital patients, to business executives, to factory workers, and to schoolchildren to reduce stress and to improve psychophysical efficiency.

There are many signs of a new synthesis of Eastern and Western attitudes, ideas, and techniques of self-development. In terms of recent scientific research into the workings of the brain, this represents a harmonizing of the functioning of the right and left hemispheres, and in psychological terms the production of spiritual ambiverts instead of introverts and extraverts.

SCIENCE LOOKS AT YOGA

'There is a new conception of man's capacities forming within the scientific community,' says Dr James Fadiman of Stanford University. 'During the twentieth century academic science has radically underestimated man – his sensitivity to subtle sources of energy, his capacity for love, understanding and transcendence, his self-control.'

The new approach is marked by less rigidity in drawing specialist boundaries and a zestful exploration of fields of inquiry hitherto labelled 'fringe science'. Biofeedback is one of the new developments and there are many others.

The new intellectual adventurousness is revealed by some of the contents of college and university curricula and the text-books that go with them. A book of readings called *The Nature of Human Consciousness* (157) includes papers drawn from scientific, medical, psychiatric, and psychological journals on, to mention a few titles, 'Bimodal Consciousness', 'Deautomatization and the Mystic Experience', 'The Physiology of Meditation', and Electroencephalographic Study on the Zen Meditation (Zazen),' and 'Implications of Physiological Feedback Training'. There are also extracts from books on Yoga, Zen, Sufism, and the *I Ching*.

Laboratory tests have been carried out on meditating Yogins in India, Zen monks in Japan, and Transcendental Meditators in America. Consciousness is being studied from new angles and in new ways, and Yoga is being subjected to scientific examination. Most leading Yoga Masters welcome the new studies. Yoga will benefit from losing any superstitious accretions. Out of the scientific investigation should come a clearer understanding of what is valuable in Yogic techniques. It should lead to old methods being streamlined and freshened up and to new methods being introduced.

THE EVOLUTION OF HUMAN CONSCIOUSNESS

An East-West synthesis harbours much that is valuable for the psychological development and future history of mankind.

In his introduction to his translation of the *Brahma Sutra*, S. Radhakrishnan, a great Indian philosopher and a President of India, wrote (161):

Man's quest for perfection consists in organizing the things of body, mind and soul into a whole. The activities of the human spirit are interrelated, the artistic and the ethical, the religious and the rational. Man is a miniature of the universe in which he lives. Man, as he is, is a transitional being, an unfinished experiment. When he is awakened, he is at peace with himself, he thinks and acts in a new way. For this awakening, man has to take another step in his evolution.

In any step upward on the evolutionary ladder, the Yoga of Meditation is likely to have a major role to play.

English Posture Index

ENGLISH POSTURE INDEX

530

ENGLISH POSTURE INDEX

Sanskrit Posture Index

Glossary of Sanskrit Terms

Abhyasa Yoga – Yoga of Steady Effort
Acharya – religious teacher
Advaita Vedanta – branch of the Vedanta philosophy whose central tenet is non-duality
Aham Brahma asmi – I am Brahman
Ahamkara – the 'I'-sense
Ahimsa – non-violence
Ajna chakra – brow centre
Anahata chakra – heart centre
Anga – limb; Patanjali lists eight *angas* of Yoga
Antaranga – the three internal practices of meditation
Apara – lower
Aparigraha – non-possessiveness
Asamprajnata samadhi – unconscious *samadhi*
Asanas – bodily postures
Ashram – Yoga centre or school
Asmita – the sense of I-am-ness
Asramas – stages of life for the Hindu
Asteya – non-stealing
Atman – the Self
Atman Yoga – Yoga of Self
AUM – see OM
Avatar – earthly incarnation of a divinity
Avidya – metaphysical ignorance
Bandha – muscular lock; binding
Bhakti Yoga – Yoga of Devotion
Bija – seed
Bindu – point; semen; seed
Brahmacharya – continence
Brahman – the Absolute; the One; Ultimate Reality; Universal Spirit
Brahmins – the highest, priestly caste
Buddhi – intellect; widsom
Buddhi Yoga – Yoga of Wisdom
Chakra – an energy centre in the subtle body; literally, a vortex
Chela – a pupil
Cit – pure consciousness

Citta – mind-stuff

Crore – ten million

Darshama – viewpoint or vision

Deva-dasi – temple prostitute

Dharana – concentration; holding the attention steadily on an object

Dharma – way of life; civilization; national consciousness

Dhyana – contemplation; the free-flowing continuation of *dharana*

Dhyana Yoga – Yoga of Meditation

Drashta or *drashtri* – the Seer, Witness, or Looker

Ekagra – one-pointed; concentrated

Ekamevadvitiyam – one without a second

Gunas – the three inherent qualities of Nature

Guru – teacher

Hatha Yoga – Yoga of Bodily Control

Ida – left nerve channel of the subtle body

Isvara or *Ishvara* – Supreme Being; God

Japa – repetition of a *mantra*

Jivatma or *Jivatman* – the individual soul

Jnana Yoga – Yoga of Self-knowledge

Jyotir or *tajo dhyana* – luminous contemplation

Kaivalya – absolute independence and freedom

Kali yuga – our pleasure-loving age

Karma – action; the law of cosmic cause and effect

Karma Yoga – Yoga of Action

Klesas – afflictions; suffering

Kshatriyas– the caste of princes, aristocrats and warriors

Kundalini – serpent power; latent energy at the base of the spine

Lingam – phallus

Mahat – cosmic consciousness

Maithuna – sacramental coitus, representing the *unio mystica*

Manas – mind

Mandala – circle; the most important oriental symbol for unity and wholeness

Manipura chakra – solar plexus centre

Mantra – a sound-symbol; incantation

Maya – illusion; the illusory world

Mimansa – one of the six schools of Indian philosophy

Moksha or *mukti* – liberation; spiritual freedom

Mudra – a muscular contraction

Mukti – see *moksha*

Muladhara chakra – root centre

Nada – internal sound

Nadi – a channel of the subtle body

Naishkaramya karma – actionless action

Nauli – isolation of the recti muscles in the central abdomen

Nirbija samadhi – *samadhi* without seed

Nirodhah – restraint

Nirvicara – a grade of *samprajnata samadhi*

Nirvitarka – a grade of *samprajnata samadhi*

Niyamas – observances
Nyaya – one of the six schools of Indian philosophy
Ojas – concentrated psychic power
OM (AUM) – sacred syllable representing the Absolute; the chief *mantra*
Pada – part of a book
Padmasana – Lotus Posture
Para – higher
Pingala – right nerve channel of the subtle body
Prakriti – eternal Nature; basic substance; the Uncaused Cause
Prana – cosmic energy; life force; breath of life
Pranava – OM, representing the Absolute
Pranayama – breath control
Pratyahara – sense withdrawal; turning the attention inwards
Purusha – soul; pure consciousness
Raja Yoga – Yoga of Mental Mastery
Rajas – one of the three *gunas*; activity; energy; the kinetic principle
Sabija samadhi – *samadhi* with seed
Sadhaka – a seeker or aspirant
Sadhana – practice
Sahasrara chakra – crown of the head centre
Samadhi – the highest stage of Yoga meditation; Self-realization; Absorption
Samkhya – one of the six schools of Indian philosophy
Samkhya Yoga – Yoga of Science; literally, number
Samprajnata samadhi – conscious *samadhi*
Samskaras – mental impressions
Samyama – the final three stages of meditation taken together: *dharana*,
    dhyana and *samadhi*
Sannyasa Yoga – Yoga of Renunciation
Sannyasi – one who has renounced the world
Santosha – contentment
Sat chit ananda – bliss consciousness; literally, being-consciousness-bliss
Sattva – the finest of the three *gunas*; purity; intelligence; orderliness; illumin
    ation
Satya – truthfulness
Saucha – purity
Savicara – a grade of *samprajnata samadhi*
Savitarka – a grade of *samprajnata samadhi*
Shakti – female creative power; earth power; goddess
Siddhasana – Perfect Posture or Adept's Posture
Siddhi – psychic attainment or power
Sthiti – state
Sthula dhyana – gross contemplation, with form
Sudras – the caste of servants and labourers
Sukhasana – Easy Posture
Sukshma sharira – the subtle or astral body
Suksma dhyana – subtle contemplation
Sushumna – central channel carrying *kundalini* energy
Sutra – thread; highly condensed, aphoristic method of literary expression

Svadhyaya – study

Swadhisthana chakra – pelvic centre

Tajo dhyana – see *jyotir dhyana*

Tamas – one of the three *gunas*; inertia; mass; resistance; stability; solidity; durability

Tanmatras – the five potentials of matter: light, sound, smell, taste, and touch

Tantras – treatises of the Tantric schools

Tantric Yoga – Yoga practice based on physiological disciplines

Tapas – austerity

Tat tvam asi – 'That thou art'

Tattwas – the categories or thatnesses, of which there are twenty-four

Tejas – radiant energy

Trataka – gazing steadily at an object; one of the six purifying processes of Hatha Yoga

Uddiyana – retraction of the abdomen

Vairagya – non-attachment; literally, uncolouredness

Vaisesika – one of the six schools of Indian philosophy

Vaisyas – the caste of merchants, farmers, and professional people

Vedanta – one of the six schools of Indian philosophy; literally, the end of the *vedas*

Vibhuti – divine power

Vijnana Yoga – Yoga of Comprehension

Vishudda Chakra – throat centre

Vritti – literally, whirlpool; agitation in the mind-stuff

Yamas – abstinences

Yantra – a form or design symbol

Yoga – Union; mystical Absorption; *Atman* and *Brahman* known as One; literally, to yoke, to join; one of the six schools of Indian philosophy

Yoni – vagina

Bibliography

Works on Hatha Yoga
1. Acharya, Pundit, *Breath Is Life*, Prana Press, New York, 1939.
2. Aiyengar, Srinivasa, (tr.), *Hatha Yoga Pradipika*, Tkaram Tastya, Bombay, 1933.
3. Alain, *Yoga for Perfect Health*, Thorsons, 1957.
4. Atkinson, W., *Hatha Yoga*, Yogi Publishing Society, Chicago, 1904.
   Avalon, Arthur, *see* Woodroffe, Sir John.
5. Bahm, Archie J., *Yoga for Business Executives*, Stanley Paul, 1967.
6. Behanan, Kovoor Y., *Yoga: A Scientific Evaluation*, Macmillan, New York, 1937; Dover, New York, 1959.
7. Bernard, Theos, *Hatha Yoga*, Columbia University Press, New York, 1944; Rider, London, 1950.
8. Bragdon, Claude, *Yoga for You*, Alfred A. Knopf, New York, 1943.
9. Brahmachari, Dhirendra, *Yogasana Vijnana*, Asia Publishing House, 1970.
10. Brena, S. F., *Yoga and Medicine*, Julian Press, New York, 1972.
11. Briggs, G. W., *Gorakhnath and the Kanphata Yogis*, Oxford University Press, 1938.
12. Carr, Rachel, *Yoga for All Ages*, Simon and Schuster, New York, 1972.
13. Chrishop, E. D., *Keep Young Through Yoga*, Health For All, 1956.
14. Danielou, Alain, *Yoga: The Method of Reintegration*, University Books, New York, 1949; Johnson Publications, London, 1949.
15. Day, Harvey, *Study and Practice of Yoga*, Thorsons, 1953.
16. Day, Harvey, *Practical Yoga for the Business Man*, Pelham Books, 1970; Drake Publishers, New York, 1970.
17. Day, Harvey, *Yoga Illustrated Dictionary*, Kaye and Ward, 1971.
18. De, Sushil Kumar, 'The Bhakti-Rasa-Sastra of Bengal Vaishnavism', *Indian Historical Quarterly* (Calcutta), viii,4(1932)
19. Dechanet, J. M., O. S. B., *Yoga in Ten Lessons*, Harper, New York, 1965; Burns and Oates, London, 1965.
   Devi, Indra, *see* Strakaty, Eugenie.
20. Dey, P., *Yogic System of Exercise*, Luzac, 1934.
21. Dukes, Sir Paul, *The Yoga of Health, Youth, and Joy*, Cassell, 1960.
22. Dvivedi, Manilal Nabhubhai (tr.), *The Yoga Sutras of Patanjali*, Madras, 1890.
23. Garde, R. V., *Principles and Practice of Yoga Therapy*, Taraporevala, Bombay, 1972.
24. Garrison, O. V., *Tantra: The Yoga of Sex*, Julian Press, New York, 1965.
   Gheranda Samhita, *see* Vasu, Sris Chandra.

25. Goswami, S. S., *Hatha Yoga*, Fowler, 1963.
26. Gould, J., *Yoga for Health and Beauty*, Thorsons, 1969.
27. Gunaji, N. V., *Scientific and Efficient Breathing*, N. V. Gunaji, Bombay, 1948.
28. Gupta, Yogi, *Yoga and Long Life*, Dodd Mead, Toronto, 1958; Y. Gupta, New York, 1965.
    Guyot, Felix, *see* Kerneiz, C.
    Hatha Yoga Pradipika, *see* Sinh, Pancham.
29. Hewitt, James, *Teach Yourself Yoga*, The English Universities Press, 1960; retitled *A Practical Guide to Yoga*, Funk and Wagnalls, New York, 1968.
30. Hewitt, James, *Yoga and You*, Anthony Gibbs, 1966; Tandem, 1967; Pyramid, New York, 1967.
31. Hittleman, R. L., *Be Young with Yoga*, Prentice-Hall, Englewood Cliffs, N.J., 1962; A. Thomas, Preston, 1963.
32. Hittleman, R. L., *Yoga for Physical Fitness*, Prentice-Hall, Englewood Cliffs, N.J.; A. Thomas, Preston, 1967.
33. Hittleman, R. L., *The Yoga Way to Figure and Facial Beauty*, Hawthorn Books, New York, 1969.
34. Hutchinson, Ronald, *Yoga: A Way of Life*, Hamlyn, 1975.
35. Iyengar, B. K. S., *Light on Yoga*, Allen and Unwin, 1966; Schocken Books, New York, Rev. Ed., 1977.
36. Johns, June, with Mehr. S. Fardoonjhi, *Practical Yoga*, David and Charles, Newton Abbot, 1975.
37. Kerneiz, C. (Guyot, Felix), *Yoga: The Science of Health*, Dutton, New York, 1937; Rider, London, 1937.
38. Kiss, M., *Yoga for Young People*, Bobbs-Merrill, New York, 1971.
39. Krishnananda, R., *Mystery of Breath*, Para-vidya Centre, New York, 1940.
40. Kumar, N., *Aerobics and Yoga*, Whitmore, Philadelphia, 1973.
41. Krishna, Gopi, *Higher Consciousness*, Julian Press, New York, 1975.
42. Krishna, Gopi, *The Biological Basis of Religion and Genius*, New York Press, New York, 1971.
43. Krishna, Gopi, *The Secret of Yoga*, Harper, New York, 1972; Turnstone, London, 1973.
44. Kuvalayananda, Swami, *Yoga Mimansa Journals*, Lonavla, Bombay, 1924.
45. Kuvalayananda, Swami, *Pranayama*, Lonavla, Bombay, 1931.
46. Kuvalayananda, Swami, *Srimat Asanas*, Lonavla, Bombay, 1931.
47. Kuvalayananda, Swami, *Popular Yoga Asanas*, Prentice-Hall, Englewood Cliffs, N.J., 1972.
48. Lee-Richardson, J., *Manual of Yoga*, Foulsham, 1956.
49. Lee-Richardson, J., *Yoga Made Easy*, Prentice-Hall, Englewood Cliffs, N.J., 1961.
50. Liebers, A., *Relax with Yoga*, Oak Tree Press, 1960.
51. Louis-Frederick, *Yoga Asanas*, Thorsons, 1959.
52. Lysebeth, Andre van, *Yoga Self-Taught*, Harper, New York, 1972; Allen and Unwin, London, 1972.

53. Marwaha, B. S., *Health and Efficiency through Yoga Asanas*, Army Educational Publications, New Delhi, 1965.
54. Mia, T., *Get in Touch with Yourself through Yoga*, Prentice-Hall, Englewood Cliffs, N.J., 1972; Luscombe, London, 1975.
55. Mumford, J., *Psychosomatic Yoga*, Thorsons, 1962.
56. Murphet, H., *Yoga for Busy People*, Old Bourne Press, London, 1964; Soccer Associates, New Rochelle, N.Y., 1965.
57. Mazumar, S., *Yogic Exercises*, Longmans, 1954.
58. Narayananda, Swami, *Secrets of Prana, Pranayama, and Yoga-asanas*, N. K. Prasad, Rishikesh, 1959.
59. Oki, M., *Practical Yoga*, Japan Publications, Tokyo and New York, 1971.
60. Oman, J. C., *The Mystics, Ascetics, and Saints of India*, Unwin, London, 1899.
61. Phelan, N. C. and Volin, M., *Yoga For Women*, Harper, New York, 1963; Pelham, London, 1963.
62. Phelan, N. C. and Volin, M., *Yoga For Beauty*, London, 1965.
63. Phelan, N. C. and Volin, M., *Yoga Breathing*, Pelham, 1966.
64. Phelan, N. C. and Volin, M., *Sex and Yoga*, Harper, New York, 1967; Pelham, London, 1967.
65. Phelan, N. C. and Volin, M., *Growing Up with Yoga*, Harper, New York, 1969; Pelham, London, 1969.
66. Pratinidhi, S. B. P., *The Ten-Point Way to Health*, Dent, 1938.
67. Rawls, E. S., *A Handbook of Yoga for Modern Living*, Parker, West Nyack, N.Y., 1966.
68. Rawls, E. S. and Diskin, E., *Yoga for Beauty and Health*, Horwitz, Sydney, 1969.
69. Rele, V. G., *The Mysterious Kundalini*, Taraporevala, Bombay, 1927.
70. Rele, V. G., *Yogic Asanas*, Taraporevala, Bombay, 1939.
71. Rieker, Hans-Ulrich (tr.), *The Yoga of Light: Hatha Yoga Pradipika, India's Classical Handbook*, Allen and Unwin, 1972.
72. Roy, A. T., *Nervous System of the Ancient Hindu*, Hazaribagh, 1930.
73. Ruchpaul, E., *Hatha Yoga*, Funk and Wagnalls, New York, 1970.
74. Saraswati, S., *Hatha Yoga*, Yoga Vedanta Forest University, Rishikesh, 1939.
75. Saraswati, S., *Yogic Home Exercises*, Taraporevala, Bombay, 1939; Kegan Paul, London, 1939.
76. Satchidananda, Swami, *Integral Hatha Yoga*, Holt, Rinehart, and Winston, New York, 1970.
77. Sinh, Pancham, (tr.), *Hatha Yoga Pradipika*, Lalit Mohan Basu, The Panini Office, Allahabad, 1915.
78. Sivananda, Swami, *Yoga Asanas*, Madras, 1934.
79. Sivananda, Swami, *Yogic Home Exercises*, Taraporevala, Bombay, 1944.
80. Sivananda, Swami, *Kundalini Yoga*, Divine Light Society, Rishikesh.
81. Sivananda, Swami and Vishnudevananda, Swami, *Practical Guide for Students of Yoga*, Divine Light Society, Hong Kong.
    Siva Samhita, *see* Vidyarnava, R. B. S. C.

82. Spring, C. and Goss, M. G., *Yoga for Today*, Holt, Rinehart and Winston, New York, 1959; A. Thomas, Preston, 1959.
83. Stearn, Jess, *Yoga, Youth, and Reincarnation*, Neville Spearman, 1966.
84. Strakaty, Eugenie (Indra Devi), *Forever Young, Forever Healthy*, Prentice-Hall, Englewood Cliffs, N.J., 1953; A. Thomas, Preston, 1955.
85. Strakaty, Eugenie, *Yoga for Americans*, Prentice-Hall, Englewood Cliffs, N.J., 1959; retitled *Yoga For You*, A. Thomas, Preston, 1960.
86. Strakaty, Eugenie, *Renew Your Life Through Yoga*, Prentice-Hall, Englewood Cliffs, N.J., 1963; Allen and Unwin, London, 1963.
87. Sundaram, S., *Yogic Physical Culture*, Bandalore, 1931.
88. Sunita, Y., *Pranayama Yoga*, West Midlands Press, Walsall, 1966.
89. Taimini, I. K., *The Science of Yoga*, The Theosophical Publishing House, Wheaton, Illinois, 1967.
90. Vasu, Sris Chandra, (tr.), *Gheranda Samhita*, Adyar, Madras, 1933.
91. Vidyarnava, Rai Bahadur Srisa Chandra, (tr.), *Siva Samhita*, Sudhindra Nath Basu, The Panini Office, Allahabad, 1923.
92. Vishnudevananda, Swami, *The Complete Illustrated Book of Yoga*, Julian Press, New York, 1960; Souvenir Press, London, 1961.
93. Vithaldas, Yogi, *The Yoga System of Health*, Faber, 1939; Greenberg, New York, 1950.
94. Wood, Ernest, *Yoga*, Penguin Books, 1959.
95. Woodroffe, Sir John (Arthur Avalon), *The Serpent Power*, Ganesh, Madras, 1918.
96. Woodroffe, Sir John, *Shakti and Shakta*, Ganesh, Madras, 1929.
97. Yesudian, S. R. and Haich, E., *Yoga and Health*, Allen and Unwin, 1966.
98. Yogendra, Shri, *Physical Education*, The Yoga Institute, Bombay, 1928.
99. Yogendra, Shri, *Yoga: Personal Hygiene*, The Yoga Institute, Bombay, 1943.
100. Yogendra, Sita Devi, *Yoga For Women*, The Yoga Institute, Bombay, 1943.
101. Young, F. R., *Yoga For Men Only*, Parker, West Nyack, N.Y., 1969.
102. Zorn, William, *Body Harmony: The Easy Yoga Exercise Way*, Hawthorn, New York, 1971; retitled *The Easy Yoga Exercise Book*, Pelham, London, 1971.

General Works
103. Ashe, Geoffrey, *The Art of Writing Made Simple*, W. H. Allen, 1972.
104. *Asiatic Monthly Journal*, Madras, 1829. Included in H. H. Wilson, *A Sketch of the Religious Sects of the Hindus*, London, 1862; Calcutta, 1958.
105. Baker, Father Augustin, *Holy Wisdom, or Directions for the Prayer of Contemplation*, Burns, Oates & Washbourne, 1876.
106. Barnes, Hazel E., *Sartre*, J. B. Lippincott Co., New York, 1973; Quartet Books, London, 1974.

107. Baudouin, Charles, *Suggestion and Auto-suggestion,* Dodd, Mead & Co., New York, 1922, Allen & Unwin, 1949.
108. Bouquet, A. C., (ed.), *Sacred Books of the World,* Penguin Books, 1954.
109. Brunton, Paul, *A Search in Secret India,* Rider & Co., 1934.
110. Brunton, Paul, *The Quest of the Overself,* Rider & Co., 1937.
111. Cannon, Alexander, *The Invisible Influence,* Rider, 1933; Acquarian Press, 1969.
112. Cooper, Kenneth H., M.D., *Aerobics,* Evans, New York, 1968.
113. David-Neel, Alexandra, *With Mystics and Magicians in Tibet,* John Lane, 1931.
114. Deikman, Arthur J., 'Implications of Experimentally Induced Contemplative Meditation', *Journal of Nervous and Mental Disease,* 142, No. 2, 101–16.
115. Deikman, Arthur J., 'Meditation and the Mystic Experience', *Psychiatry,* 29 (1966), 324–38. Included in Robert E. Ornstein (ed.), *The Nature of Human Consciousness,* W. H. Freeman & Co., San Francisco, 1973.
116. Deussen, P., *Outlines of Indian Philosophy,* Carl Curtus, Berlin, 1907.
117. Di Cara, L., and N. Miller, 'Instrumental Learning.of Vasomotor Responses by Rats: learning to respond differentially in the ears', *Science,* 159 (1968), 1485–6.
118. Ebdon, Martin (ed.), *Maharishi, The Guru: An International Symposium,* New American Library, New York, 1968.
119. Eliade, Mircea, *Images and Symbols,* Paris, 1952; Harvill Press, 1961.
120. Eliade, Mircea, *Yoga: Immortality and Freedom,* Routledge & Kegan Paul, 1958.
121. Evans-Wentzl W. Y. (ed)., *The Tibetan Book of the Dead,* Oxford University Press, 1927.
122. Freuchen, Peter, *The Book of the Eskimos,* Fawcett World Library, New York, 1959.
123. Furlong, Monica, *Contemplating Now,* Hodder & Stoughton, 1971.
124. Garbe, Richard von, *Philosophy of Ancient India,* The Open Court Publishing Co., Chicago, 1897.
125. Goldberg, B. Z., *The Sacred Fire: The Story of Sex in Religion,* Grove Press, New York, 1958.
126. Green, E., A. Green and E. Walters, 'Voluntary Control of Internal States', *Psychological and Physiological Journal of Transpersonal Psychology* 2, No. I (1970), 1–26.
127. Grim, Paul, 'Anxiety changes produced by self-induced muscular tension and by relaxation with respiration feedback', *Behavior Therapy,* 12 (1971), 11–17.
128. Happold, F. C., *Mysticism: A Study and An Anthology,* Penguin Books, 1963.
129. Hewitt, James, *Techiques of Sex Fitness,* Universal, New York, 1969.
130. Honigberger, John Martin, *35 Years in the East,* London, 1852.
131. Jaffe, Aniela, in *Man and His Symbols,* by C. G. Jung, Aldus Books, 1964.

132. James, William, *On Vital Reserves,* Henry Holt & Co., New York, 1911.

133. James, William, *Varieties of Religious Experience,* Longmans, Green & Co., New York and London, 1902.

134. John of the Cross, St., *The Complete Works of St. John of the Cross,* Newman Press, 1953.

135. Kafka, Franz, *The Diaries of Franz Kafka* (1914–23), Martin Secker & Warburg, 1949; Schocken Books, New York, 1949.

136. Kamiya, Joe, 'Conscious control of brain waves', *Psychology Today* 1, (1968), 57–60.

137. Karlins, Marvin and Lewis M. Andrews, *Biofeedback: Turning on the Power of Your Mind,* Garnstone Press, 1973.

138. Kimura, S., Ashiba, M., and Matsushima, I., 'Influence of the Air Lacking in Light Ions and the Effect of its Artificial Ionization Upon Human Beings in Occupied Rooms', *Japanese Journal of Medical Science,* 7 (1939).

139. Koestler, Arthur, *The Lotus and the Robot,* Hutchinson, 1966.

140. Kotaka, S. and Krueger, A. P., 'Studies on Air Ionized-Induced Growth Increase in Higher Plants', *Advancing Frontiers of Plant Sciences,* 20 (1967).

141. Kreuger, A. P., 'Preliminary Consideration of the Biological Significance of Air Ions', *Scientia,* 104 (Sept-Oct 1969). Included in Robert E. Ornstein (ed.), The Nature of Human Consciousness, Freeman, San Francisco, 1973.

142. Laski, Marghanita, *Ecstasy, A Study of Some Secular and Religious Experiences,* Cresset Press, 1961.

143. Le Vay, David, *Teach Yourself Human Anatomy and Physiology,* The English Universities Press, 1972.

144. Linssen, Robert, *Zen: The Art of Life,* Pyramid Communications, New York, 1972.

145. Luk, Charles (Lu k'uan Yu), *The Secrets of Chinese Meditation,* Rider & Co.. 1964.

146. Mahesh Yogi, Maharishi, *On the Bhagavad Gita,* SRM Publications, 1967; Penguin Books, 1969.

147. Mahesh Yogi, Maharishi, *The Science of Being and the Art of Living,* SRM Publications, 1963.

148. Mann, W. Edward, *Orgone, Reich and Eros,* Simon & Schuster, New York, 1973.

149. Maraini, Fosco, *Secret Tibet,* Bari, Italy, 1951; Hutchinson, 1952.

150. Maspero, Henri, 'Les Procedes de "nourrir le principe vital" dans la religion Taoiiste ancienne', *Journal Asiatique,* Paris, ccxxvii (1937). Included in Mircea Eliade, *Yoga: Immortality and Freedom,* Routledge and Kegan Paul, 1958.

151. Mascaro, Juan (tr.), *The Upanishads,* Penguin Books, 1965.

152. Menen, Aubrey, *The New Mystics,* Thames & Hudson, 1974.

153. Menen, Aubrey, *The Space Within the Heart,* Hamish Hamilton, 1970.

154. Miller, Benjamin F. and Goode, Ruth, *Man and His Body,* Gollancz, 1961.
155. Muller, Max (tr.), *The Upanishads: The Sacred Books of the East,* vol. 1, 1879 and vol. xv, 1884, Clarendon Press, Oxford.
156. Naranjo, Claudio, and Robert E. Ornstein, *On the Psychology of Meditation,* The Viking Press, New York, 1971.
157. Ornstein, Robert E. (ed.), *The Nature of Human Consciousness: A Book of Readings,* W. H. Freeman & Co., San Francisco, 1973.
158. Ornstein, Robert E., *The Psychology of Consciousness,* Freeman, San Francisco, 1972.
159. Prabhupada, Swami A. C. Bhaktivedanta, *Our Real Life: The Krishna Consciousness Movement,* N.D.
160. Radhakrishnan, S., *The Hindu View of Life,* Allen & Unwin, 1927.
161. Radhakrishnan, S., (tr.), *The Brahma Sutra,* Allen & Unwin, 1960.
162. Rawson, Philip S., *Catalogue of the Exhibition of Tantric Art Sponsored by the Arts Council of Great Britain,* 1971.
163. Reich, Wilhelm, *The Discovery of the Orgone,* Noonday Press, New York, 1942.
164. Sastri, A. Mahadeva (tr.) *The Bhagavad Gita,* with commentary of Sri Sankaracharya, Mysore, second edition, 1901.
165. Sen, K. M., *Hinduism,* Penguin Books, 1961.
166. Shah, Idries, *The Sufis,* Doubleday & Company, New York, 1964.
167. Spiegelberg, Frederick, *Spirtual Practices of India,* Citadel Press, New York, 1962.
168. *Strand Magazine,* vol. xiii, pages 176–180 (1897).
169. Suzuki, D. T., *Essays in Zen Buddhism,* Luzac & Co., 1927; Rider & Co., 1949.
170. Tchijevsky, A. L., Transactions of the Central Laboratory Science Research Ionification, The Commune Publication House, Veronej, 1933.
171. Vivekananda, Swami, *Raja Yoga: The Yoga of Conquering Internal Nature,* Advaita Ashrama, Calcutta, 1901.
172. Watts, Alan, *Cloud Hidden, Whereabouts Unknown: A Mountain Journal,* Cape, 1974.
173. Werner, H. *Comparative Psychology of Mental Development,* International Universities Press, 1957.
174. Wood, Ernest, *The Occult Training of the Hindus,* Ganesh, Madras, 1931.
175. Yasutani Roshi, quoted by Philip Kapleau in *The Three Pillars of Zen,* Beacon Press, Boston, 1967.